Henke's
Med-Math

First Canadian Edition

Brenda Predham, RN, BScN, MAEd (c)
Nursing Instructor
Keyano College
Fort McMurray, Alberta

Susan Buchholz, RN, MSN
Associate Professor
Georgia Perimeter College
Clarkston, Georgia

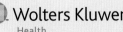 Wolters Kluwer | Lippincott Williams & Wilkins
Health

Philadelphia • Baltimore • New York • London
Buenos Aires • Hong Kong • Sydney • Tokyo

Acquisitions Editor: Hilarie Surrena
Managing Editor: Michelle Clarke
Product Manager: Betsy Gentzler
Editorial Assistant: Victoria White
Design Coordinator: Holly Reid McLaughlin
Cover Designer: Caitlin Anderson
Art Director, Illustration: Brett MacNaughton
Manufacturing Coordinator: Karin Duffield
Production Services: Spearhead Global, Inc.

9 8 7 6 5 4 3 2 1

Printed in China

Library of Congress Cataloging-in-Publication Data

Predham, Brenda.
  Henke's med-math / Brenda Predham, Susan Buchholz. — 1st Canadian ed.
     p. ; cm.
  Includes index.
  ISBN-13: 978-0-7817-9986-7
  ISBN-10: 0-7817-9986-4
  1. Pharmaceutical arithmetic. I. Buchholz, Susan, RN. II. Henke, Grace. III. Title. IV. Title: Med-math.
  [DNLM: 1. Pharmaceutical Preparations—administration & dosage—Nurses' Instruction.
2. Pharmaceutical Preparations—administration & dosage—Programmed Instruction. 3. Drug Dosage Calculations—Nurses' Instruction. 4. Drug Dosage Calculations—Programmed Instruction.   QV 18.2 P923h 2010]
  RS57.H46 2010
  615'.1401513—dc22

                                2009028785

Care has been taken to confirm the accuracy of the information presented and to describe generally accepted practices. However, the authors, editors, and publisher are not responsible for errors or omissions or for any consequences from application of the information in this book and make no warranty, expressed or implied, with respect to the currency, completeness, or accuracy of the contents of the publication. Application of this information in a particular situation remains the professional responsibility of the practitioner; the clinical treatments described and recommended may not be considered absolute and universal recommendations.

The authors, editors, and publisher have exerted every effort to ensure that drug selection and dosage set forth in this text are in accordance with the current recommendations and practice at the time of publication. However, in view of ongoing research, changes in government regulations, and the constant flow of information relating to drug therapy and drug reactions, the reader is urged to check the package insert for each drug for any change in indications and dosage and for added warnings and precautions. This is particularly important when the recommended agent is a new or infrequently employed drug.

Some drugs and medical devices presented in this publication have U.S. Food and Drug Administration (FDA) clearance for limited use in restricted research settings. It is the responsibility of the healthcare provider to ascertain the FDA status of each drug or device planned for use in his or her clinical practice.

LWW.COM

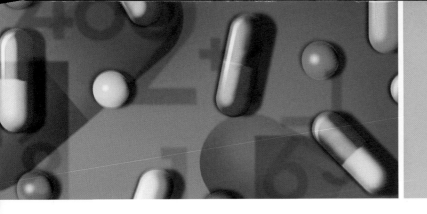

Reviewers

Katherine R. Saulnier, BSCN, RN, CCNP
Clinical Associate
St. Francis Xavier University
Antigonish, NA

Julie Duff Cloutier, MSc, RN
Assistant Professor
Laurentian University
Sudbury, ON

Kim Love, BSN, RN
Professor
Malaspina University-College
Nanaimo, BC

Sharon Aka, MSN, BSc Phys Ed & N, RN, CK
Professor
Humber Institute of Technology & Advanced Learning
Toronto, ON

Jane Mighton, MSN, BSN, RN
Nursing Instructor
Langara College
Vancouver, BC

Sarah Malo, MN, BN, RN
Instructor
Red Deer College
Red Deer, AB

Carly Hall, BSN, RN
Instructor
Camosun College
Victoria, BC

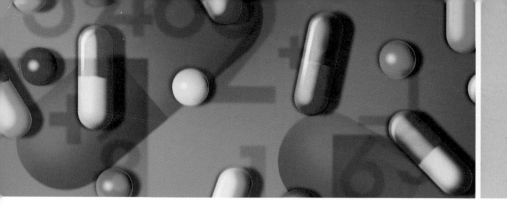

The examples and practice opportunities in this text will help you learn the steps in dosage calculation to begin the process of safe medication administration. Learning to give the right amount of the right drug to the right patient at the right time by the right route is as convoluted as it sounds; however, with practice, nursing students can safely and competently fulfill this task.

This *First Canadian Edition* of *Henke's Med-Math* has been fully adapted to reflect Canadian standards in measurement and drug language. As with previous editions of Henke's text, the Canadian edition is designed to meet the needs of students in every type of nursing program. Previous editions of Sister Henke's text have been widely used by other healthcare professionals who administer medications and are recommended to practicing nurses in need of review or nurses who wish to return to practice. Students in introductory courses should complete all the chapters. Practicing nurses may wish to do the proficiency tests at the end of each dosage chapter to target areas of weakness for content review.

Text Organization

The first five chapters of this workbook lay the foundation for further study in Chapters 6 through 13.

Chapter 1 concentrates on the arithmetic needed to calculate doses.

Chapter 2 identifies the language used in prescriptions and explains how to interpret it.

Chapter 3 explains the metric dosage measurement system and teaches students how to convert units of measurement when the order differs from the available stock medication.

Chapter 4 clarifies information printed on Canadian drug labels and types of drug packaging.

Chapter 5 defines the forms in which drugs are prepared and the equipment used in administration.

Chapters 6 to 10 concentrate on calculating doses through the application of simple rules for
- Oral solids and liquid problems
- Injections from liquids and powders
- Intravenous medications and pediatric doses

Chapter 11 explains the dimensional analysis method of drug calculations.

Chapters 12 and 13 present information and techniques for safe administration, including standard precautions, basic drug knowledge, and legal and ethical considerations. Also included is information on systems of administration and drug administration by a variety of different routes.

Numerous examples, self tests, and proficiency tests enable students to achieve mastery of the material.

Content Highlights

- Canadian content and metric measurements
- Information that reflects Canadian Food and Drugs Act and Health Canada standards
- Institute for Safe Medication Practices Canada recommended "Do Not Use" list of abbreviations
- Dosage problems that simulate actual clinical experience
- Simple to complex organization of the text
- Colourful drug labels and tables representing Canadian content
- Easy-to-learn formulas and a step-by-step approach in solving problems
- Examples showing three methods of calculation (formula, ratio, proportion)
- Chapter on the dimensional analysis method, as well as answers that demonstrate this method
- Rule and Example style of presentation that highlights important rules of thumb, followed by their application to clarify student learning
- Intravenous calculations for basic, advanced, and special types of intravenous administration
- Principles of drug administration that reflect current nursing practice

Key Features

- **Self Tests** interspersed throughout the chapters offer opportunities to review and apply content as you read; answers are given at the end of each chapter.
- **Proficiency Tests** at the end of each chapter help you test your understanding and show four methods of calculations (formula, ratio, proportion, and dimensional analysis), with an easy-to-locate answer key in Appendix A.
- **Critical Thinking: Test Your Clinical Savvy** feature presents clinical situations and poses "what if" questions.
- **Putting It Together** presents case studies for application of dosage calculations and critical thinking questions; suggested answers are provided in Appendix B.
- **Glossary** at the end of the text provides definitions for important terms and abbreviations.
- **Quick-Reference Card** in the back of the book lists common conversions and formulas.

Teaching/Learning Package
Resources for Instructors

Tools to assist you with teaching your course are available upon adoption of this text on the Point
at http://thePoint.lww.com/Predham1e and on the Instructor's Resource CD-ROM:

- The **Test Generator** lets you put together tests from a bank containing hundreds of questions that correspond with each book chapter to help you in assessing your students' understanding of the material.
- **PowerPoint Presentations** for each chapter provide an easy way for you to integrate the textbook with your students' classroom experience, either via slide shows or handouts. Multiple-choice and

true/false questions are integrated into the presentations to promote class participation and allow you to use i-clicker technology.

- An **Image Bank** lets you use the photographs and illustrations from this textbook in your PowerPoint slides or as you see fit in your course.

Resources for Students

Interactive resources are available to help students review material. Students can access these resources on the free CD-ROM bound in this book or online at the **Point** at http://thePoint.lww.com/Predham1e using the codes printed in the front of this book.

- **Watch & Learn** video clips review important concepts and skills related to medication administration.

- **Dosage Calculators** and **Dosage Calculation Quizzes** provide additional opportunities to practice essential calculation skills.

Brenda Predham, RN, BScN, MAEd (c)
Susan Buchholz, RN, MSN

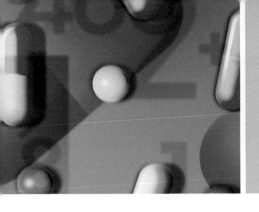

Dedication and Acknowledgments

I dedicate this book to my daughter Elizabeth; I love you.

I would like to thank the following people for helping make this book possible:

Sister Grace Henke, the original author

Sue Buchholz, author of previous American editions of *Henke's Med-Math*

Hilarie Surrena, Senior Acquisitions Editor, Wolters Kluwer Health | Lippincott Williams & Wilkins

Michelle Clarke, Managing Editor, Wolters Kluwer Health | Lippincott Williams & Wilkins

Corey Wolfe, Senior Account Manager, Wolters Kluwer Health | Lippincott Williams & Wilkins, who first approached me with the idea

Barb Johnston for sharing her "love" of math that made this whole thing possible

Colleagues and nursing students at both Keyano College in Fort McMurray, Alberta, and the University of Calgary in Calgary, Alberta

Pharmaceutical companies that provided labels

Christine Koczmara, Institute for Safe Medication Practices Canada

Carol Vorster, pharmacist, Northern Lights Regional Health Centre, Fort McMurray, Alberta

Lorraine, pharmacist, Canada Safeway, Calgary

Leisa and Bonnie for always being supportive

And Graham, for loving me

Brenda Predham

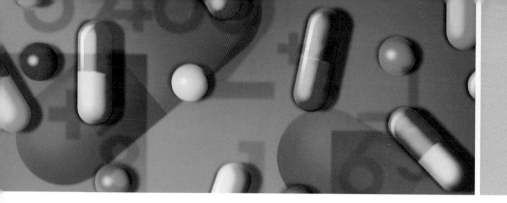

Contents

CHAPTER

8

Calculation of Basic IV Drip Rates   197

CHAPTER 12

Information Basic to Administering Drugs 341

CHAPTER 13

Administration Procedures   364

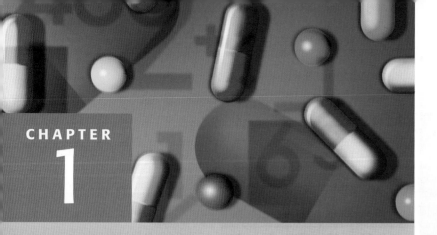

CHAPTER

1

Arithmetic Needed for Dosage

When a medication order differs from the fixed amount at which a drug is supplied, you must calculate the dose needed. Calculation requires knowledge of the systems of dosage measurements (see Chapter 3) and the ability to solve arithmetic. This chapter covers the common arithmetic functions needed for the safe administration of drugs.

Beginning students invariably express anxiety that they will miscalculate a dose and cause harm. Although *everyone* is capable of error, no one has to *cause* an error. The surest way to prevent a mistake is to exercise care in performing basic arithmetic operations.

For students who believe their arithmetic skills are already satisfactory, this chapter contains self tests and a proficiency exam. Once you pass the proficiency exam, you can move on to other chapters in the book.

Students with math anxiety and those with deficiencies in performing arithmetic will want to work through this chapter page by page. Examples demonstrate how to perform calculations; the self tests provide practice and drill. FINE POINTS boxes explain details about the calculation. After you've mastered the content, take the proficiency exam to verify your readiness to move on.

Since calculators are readily available, why go through all the arithmetic? For one thing, using a calculator can actually complicate the process, because you must know what numbers and functions to enter. In clinical situations, you may encounter some problems that require a calculator's help, but it's good to know how to make calculations on your own. Solving the arithmetic problems yourself helps you think logically about the amount ordered and the relative dose needed. And when you can mentally calculate dosage, you increase your speed and efficiency in preparing medications. None of the arithmetic problems in this chapter requires a calculator.

1	2	3	4	5	6	⑦	8	9	10	11	12
2	4	6	8	10	12	14	16	18	20	22	24
3	6	9	12	15	18	㉑	24	27	30	33	36
4	8	12	16	20	24	28	32	36	40	44	48
5	10	15	20	25	30	35	40	45	50	55	60
6	12	18	24	30	36	42	48	54	60	66	72
7	14	㉑	28	35	42	49	56	63	㊀70	77	84
⑧	16	24	32	40	48	㊚56	64	72	80	88	96
9	18	27	36	45	54	63	72	81	90	99	108
10	20	30	40	50	60	70	80	90	100	110	120
11	22	33	44	55	66	77	88	99	110	121	132
12	24	36	48	60	72	84	96	108	120	132	144

FIGURE 1-1

The multiplication table. The numbers going down the left side (from 1 to 12) are the row numbers. The numbers going across the top (from 1 to 12) are the column numbers. To multiply any two numbers from 1 to 12, find the column for one number, find the row for the other number, and read across the row until you intersect the column.

Multiplying Whole Numbers

If you need a review, first study the multiplication table (Fig. 1-1) for the numbers 1 through 12. Then do the problem, aiming for 100% accuracy without referring to the table.

Example   Multiply 8 by 7 (8×7).

1. Find row 8.

2. Find column 7.

3. Read across row 8 until you intersect column 7. The answer is 56.

SELF TEST 1   **Multiplication**

After studying the multiplication table, write the answers to these problems. Answers are given at the end of the chapter; aim for 100%.

1. $2 \times 6 =$ _____

2. $9 \times 7 =$ _____

3. $4 \times 8 =$ _____

4. $5 \times 9 =$ _____

5. $12 \times 9 =$ _____

6. $8 \times 3 =$ _____

7. $11 \times 10 =$ _____

8. $2 \times 7 =$ _____

9. $8 \times 6 =$ _____

10. $8 \times 9 =$ _____

11. $3 \times 5 =$ _____

12. $6 \times 7 =$ _____

13. $4 \times 6 =$ _____

14. $9 \times 6 =$ _____

15. $8 \times 8 =$ _____

16. $7 \times 8 =$ _____

17. $2 \times 9 =$ _____

18. $8 \times 11 =$ _____

19. $4 \times 9 =$ _____

20. $3 \times 8 =$ _____

21. $12 \times 11 =$ _____

22. $9 \times 5 =$ _____

23. $9 \times 9 =$ _____

24. $7 \times 5 =$ _____

1	2	3	4	5	6	7	8	⑨	10	11	12
2	4	6	8	10	12	14	16	18	20	22	24
3	6	9	12	15	18	21	24	27	30	33	36
4	8	12	16	20	24	28	32	36	40	44	48
5	10	15	20	25	30	35	40	45	50	55	60
6	12	18	24	30	36	42	48	54	60	66	72
7	14	21	28	35	42	49	56	63	70	77	84
8	16	24	32	40	48	56	64	72	80	88	96
9	18	27	36	45	54	63	72	81	90	99	108
10	20	30	40	50	60	70	80	90	100	110	120
11	22	33	44	55	66	77	88	99	110	121	132
⑫	24	36	48	60	72	84	96	(108)	120	132	144

FIGURE 1-2

Division table. The numbers going down the left side (from 1 to 12) are the row numbers. The numbers going across the top (from 1 to 12) are the column numbers. To divide, find the divisor (the number performing the division) in the row. Read across the row to the dividend (the number to be divided). The number at the top of that column is the answer.

Dividing Whole Numbers

The division table is helpful when you're dividing large numbers by smaller ones. Study the table (Fig. 1-2) for the division of numbers 2 through 12. Again, aim for 100% accuracy without referring to the table.

Example Divide 108 by 12 (108 ÷ 12).

1. Find 12 (the smaller number) in the left row.
2. Read across that row until you find 108 (the larger number).
3. The number at the top of that column is the answer: 9.

Remember, because 9 × 12 = 108, then 108 ÷ 12 = 9 (see Fig. 1-2).

SELF TEST 2 Division

After studying the division of larger numbers by smaller numbers, write the answers to the following problems. Answers are given at the end of the chapter.

1. 63 ÷ 7 = _____
2. 24 ÷ 6 = _____
3. 36 ÷ 12 = _____
4. 42 ÷ 6 = _____
5. 35 ÷ 5 = _____
6. 96 ÷ 12 = _____
7. 12 ÷ 3 = _____
8. 27 ÷ 9 = _____
9. 49 ÷ 7 = _____
10. 18 ÷ 3 = _____
11. 72 ÷ 8 = _____
12. 48 ÷ 8 = _____
13. 28 ÷ 7 = _____
14. 21 ÷ 7 = _____
15. 24 ÷ 8 = _____
16. 84 ÷ 12 = _____
17. 81 ÷ 9 = _____
18. 32 ÷ 8 = _____
19. 36 ÷ 6 = _____
20. 18 ÷ 9 = _____
21. 21 ÷ 3 = _____
22. 48 ÷ 4 = _____
23. 144 ÷ 12 = _____
24. 56 ÷ 8 = _____

Fractions

A *fraction* is a portion of a whole number. The top number in a fraction is called the *numerator* and the bottom number is called the *denominator*. The line between the numerator and the denominator is a division sign. Therefore, you can read the fraction $\frac{1}{4}$ as "one divided by four."

Example	$\frac{1}{4}$	$\rightarrow$ numerator
		$\rightarrow$ denominator

Types of Fractions

In a *proper* fraction, the numerator is smaller than the denominator.

Example	$\frac{2}{5}$ (Read as "two fifths.")

In an *improper* fraction, the numerator is larger than the denominator.

Example	$\frac{5}{2}$ (Read as "five halves.")

A *mixed number* has a whole number plus a fraction.

Example	$1\frac{2}{3}$ (Read as "one and two thirds.")

In a *complex* fraction, both the numerator and the denominator are already fractions.

Example	$\frac{\frac{1}{2}}{\frac{1}{4}}$ (Read as "one half divided by one fourth.")

RULE   **REDUCING FRACTIONS**

Find the largest number that can be divided evenly into the numerator *and* the denominator. ■

Example

EXAMPLE 1

Reduce $\frac{4}{12}$

$$\frac{\overset{1}{4}}{\underset{3}{12}} = \frac{1}{3}$$

EXAMPLE 2

Reduce $\frac{7}{49}$

$$\frac{\overset{1}{7}}{\underset{7}{49}} = \frac{1}{7}$$

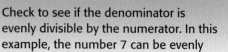

FINE POINTS ○

Check to see if the denominator is evenly divisible by the numerator. In this example, the number 7 can be evenly divided into 49.

Sometimes fractions are more difficult to reduce because the answer is not obvious.

Example

EXAMPLE 1

Reduce $\frac{56}{96}$

$$\frac{56}{96} = \frac{\overset{1}{\cancel{8}} \times 7}{\underset{1}{\cancel{8}} \times 12} = \frac{7}{12}$$

FINE POINTS

Use the multiplication table (see Fig. 1-1) to change the numbers to their multiples.

EXAMPLE 2

Reduce $\frac{54}{99}$

$$\frac{54}{99} = \frac{\overset{1}{\cancel{9}} \times 6}{\underset{1}{\cancel{9}} \times 11} = \frac{6}{11}$$

When you need to reduce a very large fraction, it may be difficult to determine the largest number that will divide evenly into both the numerator and the denominator. You may have to reduce the fraction several times.

Example

EXAMPLE 1

Reduce $\frac{189}{216}$

Try to divide both by 3 $\dfrac{\overset{63}{\cancel{189}}}{\underset{72}{\cancel{216}}} = \dfrac{63}{72}$

FINE POINTS

Prime numbers cannot be reduced any further. Examples are 2, 3, 5, 7, and 11.
When reducing, if the last number is even or a 0, try 2.
If the last number is a 0 or 5, try 5.
If the last number is odd, try 3, 7, or 11.

Then use multiples $\dfrac{63}{72} = \dfrac{\overset{1}{\cancel{9}} \times 7}{\underset{1}{\cancel{9}} \times 8} = \dfrac{7}{8}$

EXAMPLE 2

Reduce $\frac{27}{135}$

Try to divide both by 3 $\dfrac{\overset{\overset{1}{\cancel{9}}}{\cancel{27}}}{\underset{\underset{5}{\cancel{45}}}{\cancel{135}}} = \dfrac{\overset{1}{\cancel{9}}}{\underset{5}{\cancel{45}}} = \dfrac{1}{5}$

SELF TEST 3 | **Reducing Fractions**

Reduce these fractions to their lowest terms. Answers are given at the end of the chapter.

1. $\frac{16}{24}$

2. $\frac{36}{216}$

3. $\frac{18}{96}$

4. $\frac{70}{490}$

5. $\frac{18}{81}$

6. $\frac{8}{48}$

7. $\frac{12}{30}$

8. $\frac{68}{136}$

9. $\frac{55}{121}$

10. $\frac{15}{60}$

Adding Fractions

If you need to add two fractions that have the *same* denominator, first add the two numerators; write that sum over the denominator and, if necessary, reduce again.

$$\frac{1}{5} + \frac{3}{5} = \frac{4}{5}$$

If two fractions have *different* denominators, first, make the denominators the same by finding the lowest common denominator (in this example, 15) and convert each fraction. Then, add the two new numerators together. If necessary, reduce again.

$$\frac{3}{5} + \frac{2}{3} =$$

$$\frac{3(\times 3)}{5(\times 3)} = \frac{9}{15}$$

$$\frac{2(\times 5)}{3(\times 5)} = \frac{10}{15}$$

$$\frac{9}{15} + \frac{10}{15} = \frac{19}{15}$$

Subtracting Fractions

To subtract two fractions that have the *same* denominator, first subtract their numerators and then write the difference over the denominator. Reduce if necessary.

$$\frac{27}{32} - \frac{18}{32} = \frac{9}{32}$$

If the two fractions have *different* denominators, first convert each fraction using the lowest common denominator (just as you did in the adding example, above). Then subtract the numerators, and reduce again if necessary.

$$\frac{7}{8} - \frac{2}{3} =$$

$$\frac{7(\times 3)}{8(\times 3)} = \frac{21}{24}$$

$$\frac{2(\times 8)}{3(\times 8)} = \frac{16}{24}$$

$$\frac{21}{24} - \frac{16}{24} = \frac{5}{24}$$

SELF TEST 4 Adding and Subtracting Fractions

Add and subtract these fractions. Answers are given at the end of the chapter.

1. $\frac{3}{7} + \frac{2}{7} =$

2. $\frac{3}{5} + \frac{1}{5} =$

3. $\frac{2}{4} + \frac{1}{4} =$

4. $\frac{2}{3} + \frac{1}{6} =$

5. $\frac{1}{2} + \frac{1}{3} =$

6. $\frac{15}{16} - \frac{5}{16} =$

7. $\frac{3}{7} - \frac{2}{7} =$

8. $\frac{3}{5} - \frac{2}{15} =$

9. $\frac{11}{15} - \frac{7}{10} =$

10. $\frac{8}{9} - \frac{5}{12} =$

Multiplying Fractions

There are two ways to multiply fractions. Use whichever method is more comfortable for you.

First Way

Multiply the numerators across. Multiply denominators across. Reduce the answer to its lowest terms.

Example $\frac{2}{7} \times \frac{3}{4} = \frac{2 \times 3}{7 \times 4} = \frac{6}{28}$

$$\frac{6}{28} = \frac{3 \times \overset{1}{\cancel{2}}}{14 \times \underset{1}{\cancel{2}}} = \frac{3}{14}$$

Second Way (When You Are Multiplying Several Fractions)

First, reduce each fraction by dividing its numerator evenly into its denominator. Multiply the remaining numerators across. Multiply the remaining denominators across. Check to see if further reductions are possible. In example 1, because of several fractions, you can use any numerator to divide into any of the denominators.

Example *EXAMPLE 1*

$$\frac{3}{14} \times \frac{7}{10} \times \frac{5}{12} = \frac{\overset{1}{\cancel{3}}}{\underset{2}{\cancel{14}}} \times \frac{\overset{1}{\cancel{7}}}{\underset{2}{\cancel{10}}} \times \frac{\overset{1}{\cancel{5}}}{\underset{4}{\cancel{12}}} = \frac{1}{16}$$

> **FINE POINTS**
>
> $14 \div 7 = 2$ The denominators are
> $10 \div 5 = 2$ being divided by the
>   numerators to reduce.
> $12 \div 3 = 4$

If you're multiplying mixed numbers, you first need to change each of them into an improper fraction. The process: For each fraction, multiply the whole number by the denominator; then add that total to the numerator.

EXAMPLE 2

$$1\frac{1}{2} \times \frac{4}{6} = \frac{\overset{1}{\cancel{3}}}{\underset{1}{\cancel{2}}} \times \frac{\overset{2}{\cancel{4}}}{\underset{2}{\cancel{6}}} = \frac{2}{2} = 1$$

EXAMPLE 3

$$\frac{4}{5} \times 6\frac{2}{3} = \frac{4}{5} \times \frac{\overset{4}{\cancel{20}}}{3} = \frac{16}{3}$$

SELF TEST 5 **Multiplying Fractions**

Multiply these fractions. Answers are given at the end of the chapter.

1. $\frac{1}{6} \times \frac{4}{5} \times \frac{5}{2} =$

2. $\frac{4}{15} \times \frac{3}{2} =$

3. $1\frac{1}{2} \times 4\frac{2}{3} =$

4. $\frac{1}{5} \times \frac{15}{45} =$

5. $3\frac{3}{4} \times 10\frac{2}{3} =$

6. $\frac{7}{20} \times \frac{2}{14} =$

7. $\frac{9}{2} \times \frac{3}{2} =$

8. $6\frac{1}{4} \times 7\frac{1}{9} \times \frac{9}{5} =$

Dividing Fractions

To divide two fractions, first invert the fraction that is after the division sign, then change the division sign to a multiplication sign.

Example   *EXAMPLE 1*

$$\frac{1}{50} \div \frac{1}{150} = \frac{1}{\cancel{50}} \times \frac{\cancel{150}^{3}}{1} = 3$$

EXAMPLE 2

$$\frac{\frac{1}{4}}{\frac{3}{8}} = \frac{1}{4} \div \frac{3}{8} = \frac{1}{\cancel{4}} \times \frac{\cancel{8}^{2}}{3} = \frac{2}{3}$$

EXAMPLE 3

$$\frac{1\frac{1}{5}}{\frac{2}{3}} = \frac{6}{5} \div \frac{2}{3} = \frac{\cancel{6}^{3}}{5} \times \frac{3}{\cancel{2}_{1}} = \frac{9}{5}$$

FINE POINTS ● ○ ● ●

Complex fractions such as

$$\frac{\frac{1}{4}}{\frac{3}{8}}$$ are read as $\frac{1}{4} \div \frac{3}{8}$

The vertical arrangement acts just like a division sign.

SELF TEST 6   **Dividing Fractions**

Divide these fractions. Answers are given at the end of the chapter.

1. $\frac{1}{50} \div \frac{1}{150} =$

2. $\frac{1}{8} \div \frac{1}{4} =$

3. $2\frac{2}{3} \div \frac{1}{2} =$

4. $75 \div 12\frac{1}{2} =$

5. $\frac{7}{25} \div \frac{7}{75} =$

6. $\frac{1}{2} \div \frac{1}{4} =$

7. $\frac{3}{4} \div \frac{8}{3} =$

8. $\frac{1}{60} \div \frac{7}{10} =$

Changing Fractions to Decimals

To change a fraction into a decimal, begin by dividing the numerator by the denominator. Remember that the line between the numerator and the denominator is a division sign; so $\frac{1}{4}$ can be read as $1 \div 4$.

In a division problem, each number has a name. The number that's being divided (your fraction's numerator) is the *dividend;* the one that does the dividing (your fraction's denominator) is the *divisor*; and the answer is the *quotient*.

$$
\begin{array}{r}
40. \leftarrow \text{quotient} \\
\text{divisor} \rightarrow 16\overline{)640.} \leftarrow \text{dividend} \\
\underline{64} \\
0
\end{array}
$$

1. Look at the fraction $\frac{1}{4}$

$\frac{1}{4}$ $\leftarrow$ numerator = dividend
$\phantom{\frac{1}{4}}$ $\leftarrow$ denominator = divisor

2. Write

$$4\overline{)1}$$

3. Some people find it easier to simply extend the fraction's straight line to the right, and then strike out the numerator and place that same number down into the "box."

$$\frac{1}{4} = \frac{\cancel{1}}{4\overline{)1}}$$

4. Once you've set up the structure for your division problem, place a decimal point immediately after the dividend. Put another decimal point on the quotient line (above), lining up that point exactly with the decimal point below.

   By placing your decimal points carefully, you can avoid serious dosage errors.

$$\frac{\cancel{1}}{4}\overline{}\ \text{.} \leftarrow \text{quotient}$$
$$4\overline{)1.}\ \leftarrow \text{dividend}$$

5. Complete the division.

$$\frac{\cancel{1}}{4}\underset{4\overline{)1.00}}{\overset{.25}{}} = 0.25$$
$$\begin{array}{r} \underline{8} \\ 20 \\ \underline{20} \\ 0 \end{array}$$

FINE POINTS ● ○ ● ●

If the answer does not have a whole number, place a zero before the decimal point. .25 is incorrect; 0.25 is correct.

   The number of places to carry out the decimal will vary depending on the drug and equipment used. For these exercises, carry answers to the thousandths place (three decimal places).

Example

EXAMPLE 1

$$\frac{5}{16} = \frac{\cancel{5}}{16\overline{)5.000}}\overset{0.312}{} = 0.312$$
$$\begin{array}{r} \underline{4\,8} \\ 20 \\ \underline{16} \\ 40 \\ \underline{32} \\ 8 \end{array}$$

EXAMPLE 2

$$\frac{640}{8} = \frac{\cancel{640}}{8}\overline{)640.}\overset{80.}{} = 80$$

FINE POINTS ● ○ ● ●

In the answer, note the space between 8 and the decimal point. When such a space occurs, fill it with a zero to complete your answer.

EXAMPLE 3

$$\frac{1}{75} = \frac{\cancel{1}}{75\overline{)1.000}}\overset{0.013}{} = 0.013$$
$$\begin{array}{r} \underline{75} \\ 250 \\ \underline{225} \\ 25 \end{array}$$

SELF TEST 7 **Converting Fractions to Decimals**

Divide these fractions to produce decimals. Answers are given at the end of the chapter. Carry the decimal point to three decimal places if necessary.

1. $\frac{1}{6}$ 4. $\frac{9}{40}$

2. $\frac{6}{8}$ 5. $\frac{1}{8}$

3. $\frac{4}{5}$ 6. $\frac{1}{7}$

Decimals

Medication orders are written in the metric system, which uses decimals.

Reading Decimals and Converting Decimals to Fractions

Start by counting how many places come after the decimal point. One space after the decimal point is the *tenths* place. Two spaces is the *hundredths* place. Three places is the *thousandths* place; and so on. When you read the decimal aloud, it sounds like you're reading a fraction:

0.1 is read as "one tenth" $\left(\frac{1}{10}\right)$.

0.01 is read as "one hundredth" $\left(\frac{1}{100}\right)$

0.001 is read as "one thousandth" $\left(\frac{1}{1000}\right)$.

Always read the number by its name first, and then count off the decimal places. If a whole number precedes the decimal, read it just as you normally would.

Since decimals are parts of a whole number, you can write them as fractions:

Example
0.56 = "fifty-six hundredths" $\left(\frac{56}{100}\right)$

0.2 = "two-tenths" $\left(\frac{2}{10}\right)$

0.194 = "one hundred ninety-four thousandths" $\left(\frac{194}{1000}\right)$

0.31 = "thirty-one hundredths" $\left(\frac{31}{100}\right)$

1.6 = "one and six-tenths" $\left(1\frac{6}{10}\right)$

17.354 = "seventeen and three hundred fifty-four thousandths" $\left(17\frac{354}{1000}\right)$.

SELF TEST 8   Reading Decimals

Write these decimals in longhand and as fractions. Answers are given at the end of the chapter.

1. 0.25 _____

2. 0.004 _____

3. 1.7 _____

4. 0.5 _____

5. 0.334 _____

6. 136.75 _____

7. 0.1 _____

8. 0.150 _____

Addition and Subtraction of Decimals

To add decimals, stack them vertically, making sure that all the decimal points line up exactly. Starting at the far right of the stack, add each vertical column of numbers. In your answer, be sure your decimal point lines up exactly with the points above it.

EXAMPLE 1

$$\begin{array}{r} 0.8 \\ +\,0.6 \\ \hline 1.4 \end{array}$$

EXAMPLE 2

$$\begin{array}{r} 10.30 \\ +\ \ 3.28 \\ \hline 13.58 \end{array}$$

To subtract decimals, stack your two decimals as you did for addition, lining up the decimal points as before. Starting at the far right of the stack, subtract the numbers; and again, make sure that the decimal point in your answer aligns with those above it.

EXAMPLE 1

$$13-12.54 = \begin{array}{r} \overset{2\ \ 9}{13.00} \\ -\,12.54 \\ \hline 0.46 \end{array}$$

EXAMPLE 2

$$14.56-0.47 = \begin{array}{r} \overset{4\ 16}{14.56} \\ -\,0.47 \\ \hline 14.09 \end{array}$$

Add and subtract these decimals. Answers are given at the end of the chapter.

1. $0.9 + 0.5 =$ **6.** $98.6 - 66.5 =$

2. $5 + 2.999 =$ **7.** $0.45 - 0.38 =$

3. $10.56 + 357.5 =$ **8.** $1.724 - 0.684 =$

4. $2 + 3.05 + 0.06 =$ **9.** $7.066 - 0.2 =$

5. $15 + 0.19 + 21 =$ **10.** $78.56 - 5.77 =$

Multiplying Decimals

Line up the numbers on the right. Do not align the decimal points. Starting on the right, multiply each digit in the top number by each digit in the bottom number, just as you would with whole numbers. Add the products. Place the decimal point in the answer by starting at the right and moving the point the same number of places equal to the sum of the decimal places in both numbers multiplied, count the number of places that you totalled earlier. If you end up with any blank spaces, fill each one with a zero.

Example   *EXAMPLE 1*

$$2.6 \times 0.03 = \quad 2.6 \text{ (1 decimal place)}$$
$$\underline{\times 0.03} \text{ (2 decimal places)}$$
$$0.078 \text{ (3 decimal places from the right)}$$

EXAMPLE 2

$$200 \times 0.03 = \quad 200 \text{ (no decimal place)}$$
$$\underline{0.03} \text{ (2 decimal places)}$$
$$6.00 \text{ (2 decimal places from the right)}$$
$$\text{or}$$
$$6$$

Dividing Decimals

A reminder: The number being divided is called the *dividend;* the number doing the dividing is called the *divisor;* and the answer is called the *quotient.*

$$\text{divisor} \rightarrow 16 \overline{)5.000} \rightarrow \text{dividend}$$
$$0.312 \rightarrow \text{quotient}$$

Note: As soon as you write your dividend, place a decimal point immediately after it. Then place another decimal point directly above it, on the quotient line.

Example $\frac{13}{16}$ $16\overline{)13.}$

$$\begin{array}{r} 0.812 \\ 16\overline{)13.000} \\ \underline{12\ 8} \\ 20 \\ \underline{16} \\ 40 \\ \underline{32} \\ 8 \end{array}$$

Clearing the Divisor of Decimal Points

Before dividing one decimal by another, clear the divisor of decimal points. To do this, move the decimal point to the far right. Move the decimal point in the dividend *the same number of places* and, directly above it, insert another decimal point in the quotient.

Example

EXAMPLE 1

$$0.2\overline{)0.004} = 0.\underset{\smile}{2}\,\overline{)0.0\underset{\smile}{0}4}$$

Hence, $2\overline{)00.04}$ with quotient 0.02

EXAMPLE 2

$4.3\overline{)5.427}$ becomes

$$\begin{array}{r} 1.262 \\ 43.\overline{)54.270} \\ 43 \\ \hline 11\,2 \\ 8\,6 \\ \hline 2\,67 \\ 2\,58 \\ \hline 90 \\ 86 \\ \hline 4 \end{array}$$

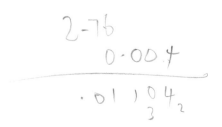

> **FINE POINTS**
>
> When you're dividing, the answer may not come out even. The dosage calculation problems give directions on how many places to carry out your answer. In Example 2, the answer is carried out to three decimal places.

SELF TEST 10   Multiplication and Division of Decimals

Do these problems in division of decimals. The answers are given at the end of this chapter. If necessary, carry the answer to three places.

1. $3.14 \times 0.02 =$

2. $100 \times 0.4 =$

3. $2.76 \times 0.004 =$

4. $7.8\overline{)140}$

5. $6\overline{)140}$

6. $0.025\overline{)10}$

Rounding Off Decimals

How do you determine the number of places to carry out division? The answer depends on the way the drug is dispensed and the equipment needed to administer the drug. Some tablets can be broken into halves or fourths. Some liquids are prepared in units of measurement: tenths, hundredths, or thousandths. Some syringes are marked to the nearest tenth, hundredth, or thousandth place. Intravenous rates are usually rounded to the nearest whole number. As you become familiar with dosage, you'll learn how far to round off your answers. To practice, first review the general rule for rounding off decimals.

RULE	**ROUNDING OFF DECIMALS**
	To round off a decimal, you simply drop the final number. Exception: If the final number is 5 or higher, drop it and then increase the adjacent number by 1.

Example

0.864 becomes 0.86

1.55 becomes 1.6

0.33 becomes 0.3

4.562 becomes 4.56

2.38 becomes 2.4

To obtain an answer that's rounded off to the nearest tenth, look at the number in the hundredth place and follow the above rule for rounding off.

Example

0.12 becomes 0.1

0.667 becomes 0.7

1.46 becomes 1.5

If you want an answer that's rounded off to the nearest hundredth, look at the number in the thousandth place and follow the above rule for rounding off.

Example

0.664 becomes 0.66

0.148 becomes 0.15

2.375 becomes 2.38

And if you want an answer that's rounded off to the nearest thousandth, look at the number in the ten-thousandths place and follow the same rules.

Example

1.3758 becomes 1.376

0.0024 becomes 0.002

4.5555 becomes 4.556

SELF TEST 11 Rounding Decimals

Round off these decimals as indicated. Answers are given at the end of the chapter.

Nearest Tenth	Nearest Hundredth	Nearest Thousandth
1. 0.25 = _____	**6.** 1.268 = _____	**11.** 1.3254 = _____
2. 1.84 = _____	**7.** 0.750 = _____	**12.** 0.0025 = _____
3. 3.27 = _____	**8.** 0.677 = _____	**13.** 0.4520 = _____
4. 0.05 = _____	**9.** 4.539 = _____	**14.** 0.7259 = _____
5. 0.63 = _____	**10.** 1.222 = _____	**15.** 0.3482 = _____

Comparing the Value of Decimals

Understanding which decimal is larger or smaller can help you solve dosage problems. Example: "Will I need more than one tablet or less than one tablet?"

RULE   **DETERMINING THE VALUE OF DECIMALS**

The decimal with the higher number in the tenth place has the greater value.

Example   Compare 0.25 with 0.5.

Since 5 is higher than 2, the greater of these two decimals is 0.5.

SELF TEST 12 Value of Decimals

In each pair, underline the decimal with the greater value. Answers are given at the end of the chapter.

1. 0.125 and 0.25

2. 0.04 and 0.1

3. 0.5 and 0.125

4. 0.1 and 0.2

5. 0.825 and 0.44

6. 0.9 and 0.5

7. 0.25 and 0.4

8. 0.7 and 0.350

Percents

Percent means "parts per hundred." Percent is a fraction, containing a variable numerator and a denominator that's always 100. You can write a percent as a fraction, a ratio, or a decimal. (To write a ratio, use two numbers separated by a colon. Example: 1:100. Read this ratio as "one is to a hundred.")

Percent written as a fraction: $5\% = \frac{5}{100}$

Percent written as a ratio: $5\% = 5:100$

Percent written as a decimal: $5\% = 0.05$

Whole numbers, fractions, and decimals may all be written as percents.

Example   Whole number: 4% (four percent)

Decimal: 0.2% (two-tenths percent)

Fraction: $\frac{1}{4}$% (one-fourth percent)

Percents That Are Whole Numbers

Example   *EXAMPLE 1*

Change to a fraction.

$$4\% = \frac{4}{100} = \frac{1}{25}$$

EXAMPLE 2

Change to a decimal.

$$4\% = \frac{4}{100} \quad 100\overline{)4.00}^{.04} = 0.04$$

Percents That Are Decimals

These may be changed in three ways:

1. By moving the decimal point two places to the left

$$0.2\% = 00.2 = 0.002$$

2. By keeping the decimal, placing the number over 100, and then dividing

$$0.2\% = \frac{0.2}{100} \quad 100\overline{)0.200}^{0.002} = 0.002$$

3. By turning it into a complex fraction. If you're using this method, remember to invert the number after the division sign and then multiply. A whole number always has a denominator of 1.

$$0.2\% = \frac{\frac{2}{10}}{100} =$$

$$\frac{2}{10} \div \frac{100}{1} =$$

$$\frac{2}{10} \times \frac{1}{100} = \frac{2}{1000}$$

$$\frac{\overset{1}{\cancel{2}}}{\underset{500}{\cancel{1000}}} = \frac{1}{500}$$

Percents That Are Fractions

Example   *EXAMPLE 1*

$$\tfrac{1}{4}\% = \frac{\tfrac{1}{4}}{100} = \tfrac{1}{4} \div \tfrac{100}{1} = \tfrac{1}{4} \times \tfrac{1}{100} = \tfrac{1}{400}$$

EXAMPLE 2

$$\tfrac{1}{2}\% = \frac{\tfrac{1}{2}}{100} = \tfrac{1}{2} \div \tfrac{100}{1} = \tfrac{1}{2} \times \tfrac{1}{100} = \tfrac{1}{200}$$

ALTERNATIVE WAY. Because $\tfrac{1}{2} = 0.5$, $\tfrac{1}{2}\%$ could also be written as 0.5%. If you follow the rule of clearing a percent by moving the decimal point two places to the left, you get $00.5\% = 0.005$. Note that 0.005 is $\tfrac{5}{1000} = \tfrac{1}{200}$. You could also write $\tfrac{0.5}{100}$.

SELF TEST 13   **Conversion of Percents**

*Change these percents to both a **fraction** and a **decimal**. Answers are given at the end of the chapter.*

1. 10%	¹/₁₀	·1	**7.** 20%	·20
2. 0.9%		·009	**8.** 0.4%	¹/₂₅₀
3. ⅕%	¹/₅₀₀	·005	**9.** ¹⁄₁₀ %	·001
4. 0.01%	1/10000	·0001	**10.** 2½%	
5. ⅔%	¹/₁₅₀	·0066	**11.** 33%	
6. 0.45%	45/1000	·00045	**12.** 50%	

Fractions, ratios, and decimals also can be converted to percents. Again, remember that percent means "parts of a hundred."

Fractions Converted to Percents

If the denominator is 100, simply write the numerator as a percent:

$$\tfrac{5}{100} = 5\%$$

If the denominator is not 100, you must convert the fraction, using 100 as the common denominator:

$$\tfrac{3}{5} = \tfrac{60}{100} = 60\%$$

Ratios Converted to Percents

If the second number in the ratio is 100, simply write the first number as a percent:

$$1:100 = 1\%$$

If the second number in the ratio is not 100, you must convert the ratio, using 100 as the common number:

$$4:5 = 80:100 = 80\%$$

Decimals Converted to Percents

Move the decimal point two places to the right, and then write the percent sign:

$$0.1 = 0.\underline{10} = 10\%$$

$$0.05 = 0.\underline{05} = 5\%$$

SELF TEST 14   **Fractions, Ratios, and Decimals**

Change these percents to a fraction, a ratio, and a decimal. Answers are given at the end of the chapter. Do not reduce.

	Fraction	**Ratio**	**Decimal**
1. 32% =	16/50	32:100	.32
2. 8.5% =	8·5		
3. 125% =	1.129x	1.25:1	1.25
4. 64% =			
5. 11.25%			

Now change these fractions, ratios and decimals to a percent.

6. $\frac{7}{10}$ = 70%

7. 2:5 = 40%

8. 0.08 = 8%

9. 0.56 = 56%

10. 3 = 300%

◖◗ Fractions, Ratio, and Proportion

Fractions show how the part (numerator) relates to the whole (denominator). *Ratio* indicates the relationship between two numbers. In this book, ratios are written as two numbers separated by a colon (1:10). Read this ratio as "one is to ten." *Proportion* indicates a relationship between two ratios or two fractions.

Example $\frac{2}{8} = \frac{10}{40}$ (Read the proportion like this: *"two is to eight as ten is to forty."*)

5:30 :: 6:36 (Read as *"five is to thirty as six is to thirty-six."*)

Proportions written with two ratios and the double colon can also be written as fractions. 5:30 :: 6:36 becomes

$$\frac{5}{30} = \frac{6}{36}$$

Solving Proportions With an Unknown

When one of the numbers in a proportion is unknown, the letter x substitutes for that missing number. By following three steps you can determine the value of x in a proportion.

Step 1.   Cross-multiply.

Step 2.   Clear x.

Step 3.   Reduce.

Here's how the three steps work.

Proportions Expressed as Two Fractions

Suppose you want to solve this proportion:

$$\frac{1}{0.125} = \frac{x}{0.25}$$

Step 1.   Cross-multiply the numerators and denominators.

$$\frac{1}{0.125} \diagdown\!\!\!\!\diagup \frac{x}{0.25}$$

$$0.125x = 0.25$$

Step 2.   Clear x by dividing both sides of the equation with the number that precedes x.

$$x = \frac{0.25}{0.125}$$

Step 3.   Reduce the number.

$$0.125\overline{)0.250.}\;\;^{2.}$$

$$x = 2$$

| **Example** | $\dfrac{45}{180} = \dfrac{3}{x}$ |

$$45x = 540$$

$$x = \frac{540}{45}$$

$$x = 12$$

Proportions Expressed as Two Ratios

Suppose you start with this proportion:

$$4 : 3.2 :: 7 : x$$

Step 1.   Cross-multiply the two outside numbers (called *extremes*) and the two inside numbers (called *means*).

$$4 : 3.2 :: 7 : x$$

$$4x = 22.4$$

Step 2.   Clear x by dividing both sides of the equation with the number that precedes x.

$$x = \frac{22.4}{4}$$

Step 3.   Reduce the number.

$$4\overline{)22.4} = 5.6$$

$$x = 5.6$$

Example   11 : 121 :: 3 : x

11x = 363

$$11\overline{)363.} = 33.$$
$$\underline{33}$$
$$33$$
$$\underline{33}$$

x = 33

SELF TEST 15   Solving Proportions

Solve these proportions. Answers are given at the end of the chapter.

1. $\frac{120}{4.2} = \frac{16}{x}$

2. 750 : 250 :: x : 5

3. $\frac{14}{140} = \frac{22}{x}$

4. 2 : 5 :: x : 10

5. $\frac{81}{3} = \frac{x}{15}$

6. 0.125 : 0.5 :: x : 10

Ratio and Proportion in Dosage

When the amount of drug ordered by a physician or healthcare provider differs from the supply, you can solve the dosage problem with proportion, using either two ratios or two fractions.

Example   Order: 0.5 mg of a drug

Supply: A liquid labelled 0.125 mg per 4 mL

You know that the liquid comes as 0.125 mg in 4 mL. And you know that the amount you want is 0.5 mg. You don't know, however, what amount of liquid is needed to equal 0.5 mg. So, you need one more piece of information: the unknown, or x.

You can set up and solve this arithmetic operation as a proportion, using either two fractions or two ratios separated by colons. Notice that both methods eventually become the same calculation.

Two Fractions   *Two Ratios Using Colons*

$$\frac{0.5}{0.125} \times \frac{x}{4}$$

$$0.125x = 2$$

$$\downarrow$$

$$0.5 : 0.125 :: x : 4$$

$$0.125x = 2$$

$$\frac{0.125x}{0.125} = \frac{2}{0.125}$$

$$\downarrow$$

$$\downarrow$$

$$\frac{0.125x}{0.125} = \frac{2.0}{0.125}$$

$$\downarrow$$

$$x = \frac{2}{0.125}$$

$$x = \frac{2}{0.125}$$

$$\downarrow$$

$$\downarrow$$

$$x = \frac{2}{0.125} \quad 0.125\overline{\smash{\big)}2.000.} \quad \begin{array}{r} 16. \\ \hline 1\ 25 \\ 750 \\ 750 \\ \hline \end{array}$$

$$x = \frac{2}{0.125} \quad 0.125\overline{\smash{\big)}2.000.} \quad \begin{array}{r} 16. \\ \hline 1\ 25 \\ 750 \\ 750 \\ \hline \end{array}$$

$$x = 16$$

So far, you've learned two ways to solve dosage calculation problems: the *ratio method* (i.e., the proportion of two ratios) and the *proportion method* (i.e., the proportion of two fractions). Chapter 6 introduces the simpler *formula method,* which is derived from ratio and proportion. And Chapter 11 explains another less complicated way: the *dimensional analysis method.* Throughout the book, proficiency test problems illustrate solutions reached by all four methods of calculation.

Name: _____

These arithmetic operations are needed to calculate doses. See Appendix A for answers. Your instructor can provide other practice tests if necessary.

A. Multiply

    a) $\begin{array}{r} 647 \\ \times\, 38 \\ \hline \end{array}$ **b)** $\frac{8}{9} \times \frac{12}{32}$ **c)** $\begin{array}{r} 0.56 \\ \times\, 0.17 \\ \hline \end{array}$

B. Divide. If necessary, report to two decimal places.

    a) $82\overline{)793}$ **b)** $5\frac{1}{4} \div \frac{7}{4}$ **c)** $0.015\overline{)0.3}$

C. Add and reduce

    a) $\frac{7}{15} + \frac{8}{15}$ **b)** $\frac{3}{8} + \frac{2}{5}$ **c)** $0.825 + 0.1$

D. Subtract and reduce

    a) $\frac{11}{15} - \frac{7}{10}$ **b)** $\frac{8}{15} - \frac{4}{15}$ **c)** $1.56 - 0.2$

E. Change to a decimal. If necessary, report to two decimal places.

    a) $\frac{1}{18}$ **b)** $\frac{3}{8}$

F. Change to a fraction and reduce to lowest terms.

    a) 0.35   **b)** 0.08

G. In each set, which number has the greater value?

    a) _____ 0.4 and 0.162

    b) _____ 0.76 and 0.8

    c) _____ 0.5 and 0.83

    d) _____ 0.3 and 0.25

H. Reduce these fractions to their lowest terms as decimals. Report to two decimal places.

    a) $\frac{20}{12}$ **b)** $\frac{7}{84}$ **c)** $\frac{6}{13}$

I. Round off these decimals as indicated.

    a) nearest tenth   5.349 _____

    b) nearest hundredth   0.6284 _____

    c) nearest thousandth   0.9244 _____

J. Change these percents to a fraction, ratio and decimal.

    a) $\frac{1}{3}\%$ **b)** 0.8%

K. Change these fractions, ratios and decimals to a percent.

    a) $\frac{7}{100}$ **b)** $1:10$ **c)** 0.008

L. Solve these proportions.

    a) $\frac{32}{128} = \frac{4}{x}$

    b) $8:72::5:x$

    c) $\frac{0.4}{0.12} = \frac{x}{8}$ (nearest whole number)

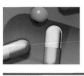

Answers to Self Tests

Self Test 1 Multiplication

1. 12	**5.** 108	**9.** 48	**13.** 24	**17.** 18	**21.** 132
2. 63	**6.** 24	**10.** 72	**14.** 54	**18.** 88	**22.** 45
3. 32	**7.** 110	**11.** 15	**15.** 64	**19.** 36	**23.** 81
4. 45	**8.** 14	**12.** 42	**16.** 56	**20.** 24	**24.** 35

Self Test 2 Division

1. 9	**5.** 7	**9.** 7	**13.** 4	**17.** 9	**21.** 7
2. 4	**6.** 8	**10.** 6	**14.** 3	**18.** 4	**22.** 12
3. 3	**7.** 4	**11.** 9	**15.** 3	**19.** 6	**23.** 12
4. 7	**8.** 3	**12.** 6	**16.** 7	**20.** 2	**24.** 7

Self Test 3 Reducing Fractions

1. $\frac{16}{24} = \frac{4}{6} = \frac{2}{3}$ (Divide by 4, then 2.)

Alternatively: $\frac{16}{24} = \frac{2}{3}$ (Divide by 8.)

2. $\frac{36}{216} = \frac{6}{36} = \frac{1}{6}$ (Divide by 6, then 6.)

3. $\frac{18}{96} = \frac{9}{48} = \frac{3}{16}$ (Divide by 2, then 3.)

4. $\frac{70}{490} = \frac{7}{49} = \frac{1}{7}$ (Divide by 10, then 7.)

5. $\frac{18}{81} = \frac{2}{9}$ (Divide by 9.)

6. $\frac{8}{48} = \frac{1}{6}$ (Divide by 8.)

7. $\frac{12}{30} = \frac{6}{15} = \frac{2}{5}$ (Divide by 2, then 3.)

Alternatively: $\frac{12}{30} = \frac{2}{5}$ (Divide by 6.)

8. $\frac{68}{136} = \frac{34}{68} = \frac{1}{2}$ (Divide by 2, then 34.)

9. $\frac{55}{121} = \frac{5}{11}$ (Divide by 11.)

10. $\frac{15}{60} = \frac{1}{4}$ (Divide by 15.)

Alternatively: $\frac{15}{60} = \frac{3}{12} = \frac{1}{4}$ (Divide by 5, then 3.)

Self Test 4 Adding and Subtracting Fractions

1. $\frac{5}{7}$

2. $\frac{4}{5}$

3. $\frac{3}{4}$

4. $\frac{(2 \times 2)}{\underset{6}{3}} + \frac{1}{6} = \frac{4}{6} + \frac{1}{6} = \frac{5}{6}$

5. $\frac{1}{2} + \frac{1}{3} = \frac{3}{6} + \frac{2}{6} = \frac{5}{6}$

6. $\frac{10}{16}$ or $\frac{5}{8}$

7. $\frac{1}{7}$

8. $\frac{(3 \times 3)}{\underset{15}{5}} - \frac{2}{15} = \frac{9}{15} - \frac{2}{15} = \frac{7}{15}$

9. $\frac{11}{15} - \frac{7}{10} = \frac{22}{30} - \frac{21}{30} = \frac{1}{30}$

10. $\frac{8}{9} - \frac{5}{12} = \frac{32}{36} - \frac{15}{36} = \frac{17}{36}$

Self Test 5 Multiplying Fractions (Two Ways to Solve)

First Way

1. $\frac{1}{6} \times \frac{4}{5} \times \frac{5}{2} = \frac{20}{60} = \frac{1}{3}$

2. $\frac{4}{15} \times \frac{3}{2} = \frac{\overset{2}{12}}{\underset{5}{30}} = \frac{2}{5}$

   (Divide by 6.)

3. $1\frac{1}{2} \times 4\frac{2}{3} = \frac{3}{2} \times \frac{14}{3} = \frac{\overset{7}{42}}{\underset{1}{6}} = 7$

   (Divide by 6.)

4. $\frac{1}{5} \times \frac{15}{45} = \frac{\overset{3}{15}}{\underset{45}{225}} = \frac{3}{45} = \frac{1}{15}$

   (Divide by 5.)

5. $3\frac{3}{4} \times 10\frac{2}{3} = \frac{15}{4} \times \frac{32}{3}$

   (Too confusing! Use the second way.)

6. $\frac{7}{20} \times \frac{2}{14}$

   (Too difficult. Use the second way.)

7. $\frac{9}{2} \times \frac{3}{2} = \frac{27}{4}$

   (Cannot reduce.)

8. $6\frac{1}{4} \times 7\frac{1}{9} \times \frac{9}{5} = \frac{25}{4} \times \frac{64}{9} \times \frac{9}{5}$

   (Too difficult. Use the second way.)

Second Way

1. $\frac{1}{\underset{3}{6}} \times \frac{\overset{1}{4}}{5} \times \frac{\overset{1}{5}}{\underset{1}{2}} = \frac{\overset{1}{2}}{\underset{3}{6}} = \frac{1}{3}$

2. $\frac{\overset{2}{4}}{\underset{5}{15}} \times \frac{\overset{1}{3}}{2} = \frac{2}{5}$

3. $1\frac{1}{2} \times 4\frac{2}{3} = \frac{3}{\underset{1}{2}} \times \frac{\overset{7}{14}}{\underset{1}{3}} = 7$

4. $\frac{1}{5} \times \frac{\overset{1}{15}}{\underset{3}{45}} = \frac{1}{15}$

5. $\frac{\overset{5}{15}}{\underset{1}{4}} \times \frac{\overset{8}{32}}{\underset{1}{3}} = 40$

6. $\frac{\overset{1}{7}}{\underset{10}{20}} \times \frac{\overset{1}{2}}{\underset{2}{14}} = \frac{1}{20}$

8. $\frac{\overset{5}{25}}{\underset{1}{4}} \times \frac{\overset{16}{64}}{\underset{1}{9}} \times \frac{\overset{1}{9}}{\underset{1}{5}} = 80$

Self Test 6 Dividing Fractions

1. $\frac{1}{75} \div \frac{1}{150} = \frac{1}{\underset{1}{75}} \times \frac{\overset{2}{150}}{1} = 2$

2. $\frac{1}{8} \div \frac{1}{4} = \frac{1}{\underset{2}{8}} \times \frac{\overset{1}{4}}{1} = \frac{1}{2}$

3. $2\frac{2}{3} \div \frac{1}{2} = \frac{8}{3} \times \frac{2}{1} = \frac{16}{3}$

4. $75 \div 12\frac{1}{2} = 75 \div \frac{25}{2} = \frac{\overset{3}{75}}{1} \times \frac{2}{\underset{1}{25}} = 6$

5. $\frac{7}{25} \div \frac{7}{75} = \frac{\overset{1}{7}}{\underset{1}{25}} \times \frac{\overset{3}{75}}{\underset{1}{7}} = 3$

6. $\frac{1}{2} \div \frac{1}{4} = \frac{1}{\underset{1}{2}} \times \frac{\overset{2}{4}}{1} = 2$

7. $\frac{3}{4} \div \frac{8}{3} = \frac{3}{4} \times \frac{3}{8} = \frac{9}{32}$

8. $\frac{1}{60} \div \frac{7}{10} = \frac{1}{\underset{6}{60}} \times \frac{\overset{1}{10}}{7} = \frac{1}{42}$

Self Test 7 Converting Fractions to Decimals

1.
$$\frac{1}{6}\overline{\big)1.000} \quad \frac{.166}{} = 0.166$$
$$\underline{6}$$
$$40$$
$$\underline{36}$$
$$40$$
$$\underline{36}$$
$$4$$

3.
$$\frac{4}{5}\overline{\big)4.0} \quad \frac{.8}{} = 0.8$$
$$\underline{4\,0}$$
$$0$$

5.
$$\frac{1}{8}\overline{\big)1.000} \quad \frac{.125}{} = 0.125$$
$$\underline{8}$$
$$20$$
$$\underline{16}$$
$$40$$
$$\underline{40}$$
$$0$$

2.
$$\frac{\overset{3}{\cancel{6}}}{\underset{4}{\cancel{8}}} = \frac{3}{4}\overline{\big)3.00} \quad \frac{.75}{} = 0.75$$
$$\underline{2\,8}$$
$$20$$
$$\underline{20}$$
$$0$$

4.
$$\frac{9}{40}\overline{\big)9.000} \quad \frac{.225}{} = 0.225$$
$$\underline{8\,0}$$
$$1\,00$$
$$\underline{80}$$
$$200$$
$$\underline{200}$$
$$0$$

6.
$$\frac{1}{7}\overline{\big)1.000} \quad \frac{.145}{} = 0.142$$
$$\underline{7}$$
$$30$$
$$\underline{28}$$
$$20$$
$$\underline{14}$$
$$6$$

Self Test 8 Reading Decimals

1. Twenty-five hundredths $\left(\frac{25}{100}\right)$

2. Four thousandths $\left(\frac{4}{1000}\right)$

3. One and seven tenths $\left(1\frac{7}{10}\right)$

4. Five tenths $\left(\frac{5}{10}\right)$

5. Three hundred thirty-four thousandths $\left(\frac{334}{1000}\right)$

6. One hundred thirty-six and seventy-five hundredths $\left(136\frac{75}{100}\right)$

7. One tenth $\left(\frac{1}{10}\right)$

8. One hundred fifty thousandths $\left(\frac{150}{1000}\right)$. The zero at the end of 0.150 is not necessary. The number could be read as fifteen hundredths $\left(\frac{15}{100}\right)$.

Self Test 9 Addition and Subtraction of Decimals

1.
$$\begin{array}{r} 0.9 \\ + 0.5 \\ \hline 1.4 \end{array}$$

2.
$$\begin{array}{r} 5.000 \\ + 2.999 \\ \hline 7.999 \end{array}$$

3.
$$\begin{array}{r} 10.56 \\ + 357.50 \\ \hline 368.06 \end{array}$$

4.
$$\begin{array}{r} 2.00 \\ 3.05 \\ + 0.06 \\ \hline 5.11 \end{array}$$

5.
$$\begin{array}{r} 15.00 \\ 0.19 \\ + 21.00 \\ \hline 36.19 \end{array}$$

6.
$$\begin{array}{r} 98.6 \\ - 66.5 \\ \hline 32.1 \end{array}$$

7.
$$\begin{array}{r} 0.\overset{3}{\cancel{4}}5 \\ - 0.38 \\ \hline 0.07 \end{array}$$

8.
$$\begin{array}{r} 1.\overset{6}{\cancel{7}}24 \\ - 0.684 \\ \hline 1.040 \end{array} \text{ or } 1.04$$

9.
$$\begin{array}{r} \overset{6}{\cancel{7}}.066 \\ - 0.200 \\ \hline 6.866 \end{array}$$

10.
$$\begin{array}{r} 7\overset{7}{\cancel{8}}.\overset{4}{\cancel{5}}6 \\ - \quad 5.77 \\ \hline 72.79 \end{array}$$

Self Test 10 Multiplication and Division of Decimals

1.
$$\begin{array}{r} 3.14 \\ \times\,0.02 \\ \hline 0.0628 \end{array}$$

2.
$$\begin{array}{r} 100 \\ \times\,0.4 \\ \hline 40.0 \end{array} \text{ or } 40$$

3.
$$\begin{array}{r} 2.76 \\ \times\,0.004 \\ \hline 0.01104 \end{array}$$

4. $7.8\overline{\smash{)}140.0}$ Now it is $78\overline{\smash{)}1400.000}$

$$\begin{array}{r} 17.948 \\ \underline{78} \\ 620 \\ \underline{546} \\ 74\,0 \\ \underline{70\,2} \\ 3\,80 \\ \underline{3\,12} \\ 680 \\ \underline{624} \\ 56 \end{array}$$

5. $6\overline{\smash{)}140.000}$

$$\begin{array}{r} 23.333 \\ \underline{12} \\ 20 \\ \underline{18} \\ 20 \\ \underline{18} \\ 20 \\ \underline{18} \\ 20 \\ \underline{18} \\ 2 \end{array}$$

6. $0.025\overline{\smash{)}10.000}$ Now it is $25\overline{\smash{)}10000.}$ → 400.

Note that because there are two places between the 4 and the decimal, you had to add two zeros.

Self Test 11 Rounding Decimals

Nearest Tenth	*Nearest Hundredth*	*Nearest Thousandth*
1. 0.3	**6.** 1.27	**11.** 1.325
2. 1.8	**7.** 0.75	**12.** 0.003
3. 3.3	**8.** 0.68	**13.** 0.452
4. 0.1	**9.** 4.54	**14.** 0.726
5. 0.6	**10.** 1.22	**15.** 0.348

Self Test 12 Value of Decimals

1. 0.25	**4.** 0.2	**7.** 0.4
2. 0.1	**5.** 0.825	**8.** 0.7
3. 0.5	**6.** 0.9	

Self Test 13 Conversion of Percents

1. Fraction $10\% = \dfrac{\frac{1}{10}}{\frac{100}{10}} = \frac{1}{10}$

   Decimal $10\% = \dfrac{10}{100}\,\overline{\smash{)}10.0}\;.1 = 0.1$

   Quick-rule decimal $10.\% = 0.1$

2. Fraction $\quad 0.9\% = \frac{\frac{9}{10}}{100} = \frac{9}{10} \div 100 = \frac{9}{10} \times \frac{1}{100} = \frac{9}{1000}$

Decimal $\quad 0.9\% = \frac{0.9}{100} \begin{array}{r} .009 \\ 100\overline{)0.900} \end{array} = 0.009$

Quick-rule decimal $\quad \underset{\smile}{00}.9\% = 0.009$

3. Fraction $\quad \frac{1}{5}\% = \frac{\frac{1}{5}}{100} = \frac{1}{5} \div 100 = \frac{1}{5} \times \frac{1}{100} = \frac{1}{500}$

Decimal $\quad \frac{1}{5}\% = \frac{1}{5} \div 100 = \frac{1}{500} \begin{array}{r} .002 \\ 500\overline{)1.000} \end{array} = 0.002$

Quick-rule decimal $\quad \frac{1}{5}\% = \frac{1}{5} \begin{array}{r} .2 \\ 5\overline{)1.0} \end{array} = 0.2\%$

$\underset{\smile}{00}.2 = 0.002$

4. Fraction $\quad 0.01\% = \frac{\frac{1}{100}}{100} = \frac{1}{100} \div \frac{100}{1} = \frac{1}{100} \times \frac{1}{100} = \frac{1}{10000}$

Decimal $\quad 0.1\% = \frac{0.01}{100} \begin{array}{r} 0.0001 \\ 100\overline{).0100} \end{array} = 0.0001$

Quick-rule decimal $\quad \underset{\smile}{00}.01 = 0.0001$

5. Fraction $\quad \frac{2}{3}\% = \frac{\frac{2}{3}}{100} = \frac{2}{3} \div \frac{100}{1} = \frac{2}{3} \times \frac{1}{100} = \frac{2}{300} = \frac{1}{150}$

Decimal $\quad \frac{2}{3}\% = \frac{2}{3} \div \frac{100}{1} = \frac{2}{3} \times \frac{1}{100} = \frac{2}{300} \begin{array}{r} .0066 \\ 300\overline{)2.000} \end{array} = 0.0066$

Quick-rule decimal $\quad \frac{2}{3}\% = \frac{2}{3} \begin{array}{r} .66 \\ 3\overline{)2.00} \end{array} = 0.66\% = \underset{\smile}{00}.66 = 0.0066$

6. Fraction $\quad 0.45\% = \frac{\frac{45}{100}}{100} = \frac{45}{100} \div \frac{100}{1} = \frac{45}{100} \times \frac{1}{100} = \frac{45}{10000} = \frac{9}{2000}$

Decimal $\quad 0.45\% = \frac{.45}{100} \begin{array}{r} .0045 \\ \overline{)0.4500} \end{array} = 0.0045$

Quick-rule decimal $\quad \underset{\smile}{00}.45\% = 0.0045$

7. Fraction $\quad \frac{\frac{1}{20}}{\underset{5}{100}} = \frac{1}{5}$

Decimal $\quad 20\% = \frac{20}{100} \begin{array}{r} 0.2 \\ \overline{)20.0} \end{array}$

Quick-rule decimal $\quad \underset{\smile}{20}.\% = 0.2$

8. Fraction $0.4\% = \dfrac{\frac{4}{10}}{100} = \dfrac{4}{10} \div \dfrac{100}{1} = \dfrac{\overset{1}{\cancel{4}}}{10} \times \dfrac{1}{\underset{25}{\cancel{100}}} = \dfrac{1}{250}$

Decimal $0.4\% = \dfrac{0.4}{100} \overset{0.004}{\overline{)0.400}} = 0.004$

Quick-rule decimal $\underset{\smile}{00}.4\% = 0.004$

9. Fraction $\dfrac{1}{10}\% = \dfrac{\frac{1}{10}}{100} = \dfrac{1}{10} \div \dfrac{100}{1} = \dfrac{1}{10} \times \dfrac{1}{100} = \dfrac{1}{1000}$

Decimal $\dfrac{1}{10}\% = \dfrac{1}{10} \div \dfrac{100}{1} = \dfrac{1}{10} \times \dfrac{1}{100} = \dfrac{1}{1000} \overset{0.001}{\overline{)1.000}} = 0.001$

Quick-rule decimal $\dfrac{1}{10}\% = \dfrac{1}{10} \overset{0.1}{\overline{)1.0}} = 0.1\% = \underset{\smile}{00}.1 = 0.001$

10. Fraction $2\tfrac{1}{2}\% = 2.5\% = \dfrac{\frac{25}{10}}{100} = \dfrac{25}{10} \div \dfrac{100}{1} = \dfrac{25}{10} \times \dfrac{1}{100} = \dfrac{25}{1000} = \dfrac{1}{40}$

Decimal $2.5\% = \dfrac{2.5}{100} \overset{0.025}{\overline{)2.50}} = 0.025$

Quick-rule decimal $\underset{\smile}{000}.2.5\% = 0.025$

11. Fraction $33\% = \dfrac{33}{100}$

Decimal $33\% = \dfrac{33}{100} \overset{.33}{\overline{)33.00}} = 0.33$

Quick-rule decimal $\underset{\smile}{33}.\% = 0.33$

12. Fraction $50\% = \dfrac{50}{100} = \dfrac{1}{2}$

Decimal $50\% = \dfrac{50}{100} \overset{.5}{\overline{)50.0}} = 0.5$

Quick-rule decimal $\underset{\smile}{50}.\% = 0.5$

Self Test 14 Fractions, Ratios and Decimals

	Fraction	*Ratio*	*Decimal*
1. 32% =	$\dfrac{32}{100}$	32:100	$\underset{\smile}{32}\% = 0.32$
2. 8.5% =	$\dfrac{8.5}{100}$ or $\dfrac{85}{1000}$	8.5:100	$\underset{\smile}{08}.5\% = 0.085$
3. 125% =	$\dfrac{125}{100}$	125:100	$\underset{\smile}{125}\% = 1.25$

4. $64\% =$ $\dfrac{64}{100}$ $64:100$ $64\% = 0.64$

5. $11.25\% =$ $\dfrac{11.25}{100}$ or $\dfrac{1125}{10000}$ $11.25:100$ $11.25\% = 0.1125$

6. $\dfrac{7}{10} = \dfrac{70}{100} = 70\%$

7. $2:5 = 40:100 = 40\%$

8. $0.08 = 8\%$

9. $0.56 = 56\%$

10. $3.00 = 300\%$

Self Test 15 Solving Proportions

1. $\dfrac{120}{4.2} = \dfrac{16}{x}$
$120x = 67.2$
$x = 0.56$

$$120\overline{)67.20}^{\,0.56}$$
$$\underline{60\ 0}$$
$$7\ 20$$
$$\underline{7\ 20}$$

2. $750 : 250 :: x : 5$
$250x = 750 \times 5$
$x = 15$

$$\dfrac{\overset{3}{750} \times 5}{\underset{1}{250}} = 15$$

3. $\dfrac{14}{140} = \dfrac{22}{x}$
$14x = 22 \times 140$
$x = 220$

$$\dfrac{22 \times \overset{10}{140}}{\underset{1}{14}} = 220$$

4. $2:5::x:10$
$5x = 20$
$x = 4$

5. $\dfrac{81}{3} = \dfrac{x}{15}$
$3x = 81 \times 15$
$x = 405$

$$\dfrac{81 \times \overset{5}{15}}{\underset{1}{3}} = 405$$

6. $0.125 : 0.5 :: x : 10$

$0.5x = 0.125 \times 10 = \dfrac{\overset{1}{0.125}}{\underset{4}{0.500}} \times 10 = \dfrac{10}{4}\overline{)10.0}^{\,2.5}$

$x = 2.5$

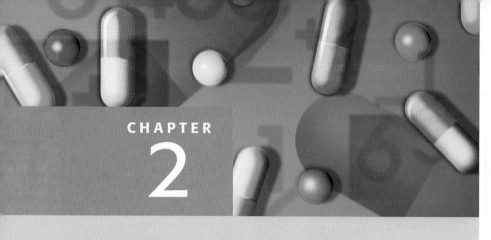

Interpreting the Language of Prescriptions

When you're calculating drug dosages, it's important to understand medical abbreviations. Misunderstanding them can lead to medication errors. If you're unsure about what a medical abbreviation stands for, if the handwriting is illegible, or if you have any question about the medication order, *do not prepare the dose.* Clarify the order or abbreviation with the healthcare provider who prescribed the medication.

Below are three sample medication orders. They may look confusing now, but after you've worked your way through this chapter, they'll make perfect sense:

- Morphine sulfate 15 mg sub Q stat and 10 mg q4h prn

- Chloromycetin 0.01% Ophth Oint left eye bid

- Ampicillin 1 g IVPB q6h

In 2004, the Joint Commission on Accreditation of Healthcare Organizations (JCAHO) issued a list of "Do Not Use" abbreviations: the ones that were often misread and thus led to medication errors. In 2006, the Institute for Safe Medication Practices Canada (ISMP Canada) proposed the abbreviations, symbols, and dose designations contained in Table 2-1 be eliminated from use by Canadian healthcare providers. Additionally, each institution or Health Region may also have its own "Do Not Use" list. As a nurse, you need to make careful note of abbreviations that are prohibited or dangerous.

TABLE 2-1 Do Not Use: Dangerous Abbreviations, Symbols, and Dose Designations

The abbreviations, symbols, and dose designations found in this table have been reported as being frequently misinterpreted and involved in harmful medication errors. They should NEVER be used when communicating medication information.

Abbreviation	Intended Meaning	Problem	Correction
U	unit	Mistaken for "0" (zero),"4" (four), or cc.	Use "unit."
IU	international unit	Mistaken for "IV" (intravenous) or "10" (ten).	Use "unit."
Abbreviations for drug names		Misinterpreted because of similar abbreviations for multiple drugs; e.g., MS, MSO_4 (morphine sulphate), $MgSO_4$ (magnesium sulphate) may be confused for one another.	Do not abbreviate drug names.
QD QOD	Everyday Every other day	QD and QOD have been mistaken for each other, or as "qid." The Q has also been misinterpreted as "2" (two).	Use "daily" and "every other day."
OD	Every day	Mistaken for "right eye" (OD = oculus dexter)	Use "daily."
OS, OD, OU	Left eye, right eye, both eyes	May be confused with one another.	Use "left eye", "right eye", or "both eyes."
D/C	Discharge	Interpreted as "discontinue whatever medications follow" (typically discharge medications).	Use "discharge."
cc	cubic centimetre	Mistaken for "u" (units).	Use "mL" or "millilitre."
μg	microgram	Mistaken for "mg" (milligram) resulting in 1000-fold overdose.	Use "mcg."

Symbol	Intended Meaning	Potential Problem	Correction
@	at	Mistaken for "2" (two) or "5" (five).	Use "at".
>	Greater than	Mistaken for "7" (seven) or the letter "L."	Use "greater than"/ "more than" or
<	Less than	Confused with each other.	"less than"/"lower than".

Dose Designation	Intended Meaning	Potential Problem	Correction
Trailing zero	X.0 mg	Decimal point is overlooked resulting in 10-fold dose error.	Never use a zero by itself after a decimal point. Use "x mg".
Lack of leading zero	.X mg	Decimal point is overlooked resulting in 10-fold dose error.	Always use a zero before a decimal point. Use "0.x mg".

Adapted from ISMP's List of *Error-Prone Abbreviations, Symbols,* and *Dose Designations 2006*

Report actual and potential medication errors to ISMP Canada via the web at https://www.ismp-canada.org/err_report.htm or by calling 1-866-54-ISMPC. ISMP Canada guarantees confidentiality of information received and respects the reporter's wishes as to the level of detail included in publications.

⬤▭ Time of Administration of Drugs

The abbreviations for the times of drug administration, which come from Latin words, appear in the following table. Memorize the abbreviations, their meanings, and the sample times that indicate how the abbreviations are interpreted. However, follow your institutional policy for administration times.

Time Abbreviation	Meaning	Explanation	Do Not Use
ac	Before meals	Latin, *ante cibum*	
		Sample Time 7:30 AM, 11:30 AM, 4:30 PM	
pc	After meals	Latin, *post cibum*	
		Sample Time 10 AM, 2 PM, 6 PM	
daily	Every day, daily	Latin, *quaque die*	qd
		Sample Time 10 AM	
bid	Twice a day	Latin, *bis in die*	
		Sample Time 10 AM, 6 PM	
tid	Three times a day	Latin, *ter in die*	
		Sample Time 10 AM, 2 PM, 6 PM	
qid	Four times a day	Latin, *quater in die*	
		Sample Time 10 AM, 2 PM, 6 PM, 10 PM	
qh	Every hour	Latin, *quaque hora* Because the drug is given every hour, it will be given 24 times in one day.	
at bedtime	At bedtime, hour of sleep	Latin, *hora somni*.	hs
		Sample Time 10 PM	
stat	Immediately	Latin, *statim*	
		Sample Time Now!	

The time abbreviations in the following table are based on a 24-hour day. To determine the number of times a medication is given in a day, divide 24 by the number given in the abbreviation.

Time Abbreviation	Meaning	Explanation
q2h	Every 2 hours	The drug will be given 12 times in a 24-hour period (24 ÷ 2).
		Sample Times even hours at 2 AM, 4 AM, 6 AM, 8 AM, 10 AM, 12 noon, 2 PM, 4 PM, 6 PM, 8 PM, 10 PM, 12 midnight
q4h	Every 4 hours	The drug will be given six times in a 24-hour period (24 ÷ 4)
		Sample Times 2 AM, 6 AM, 10 AM, 2 PM, 6 PM, 10 PM
q6h	Every 6 hours	The drug will be given four times in a 24-hour period (24 ÷ 6)
		Sample Times 6 AM, 12 noon, 6 PM, 12 midnight
q8h	Every 8 hours	The drug will be given three times in a 24-hour period (24 ÷ 8)
		Sample Times 6 AM, 2 PM, 10 PM
q12h	Every 12 hours	The drug will be given twice in a 24-hour period (24 ÷ 12)
		Sample Times 6 AM, 6 PM

There are three additional time abbreviations that require explanation. They are as follows:

Time Abbreviation	Meaning	Explanation	Do Not Use
every other day	Every other day	Latin, *quaque otra die*	qod

This abbreviation is interpreted by the days of the **month:** the nurse writes on the medication record: odd days of the month

Sample Time	10 AM on the first, third, fifth day, and so on

The nurse might write: even days of the month

Sample Time	10 AM on the second, fourth, sixth day, and so on

prn	As needed

Latin, *pro re nata*

This abbreviation is usually combined with a time abbreviation.

Example	q4h prn (every 4 hours as needed)

This permits the nurse to assess the patient and make a nursing judgment about whether to administer the medication.

Sample	acetaminophen 650 mg po q4h prn (650 milligrams acetaminophen by mouth, every 4 hours as needed for pain)

The nurse assesses the patient for pain every 4 hours. If the patient has pain, the nurse may administer the drug. This abbreviation has three administration implications:

1. The nurse **must wait** 4 hours before giving the next dose.
2. Once 4 hours have elapsed, the dose may be given any time thereafter.
3. Sample times are not given because the nurse does not know when the patient will need the drug.

3 times weekly	Three times per week

Latin, *ter in vicis*

Time relates to days of the **week.**

Sample Time	10 AM on Monday, Wednesday, Friday

Do not confuse with tid (three times per **day**).

SELF TEST 1 Abbreviations

After studying the abbreviations for times of administration, give the meaning of the following terms.
Include sample times. Indicate if the abbreviation is "Do Not Use" and which words to substitute for it.
The correct answers are given at the end of the chapter.

1. tid _3 times day_
2. pc _after meal_
3. qod _every other day_
4. bid _2 day_
5. hs _at bedtime_
6. stat _immediately_
7. qid _4 time day_

8. q4h _every 4 hours_
9. ac _before meals_
10. qd _every day_
11. q8h _8 times day_
12. qh _every hour_
13. prn _as needed_
14. q4h prn _every 4 as needed_

Military Time: The 24-Hour Clock

If a handwritten prescription does not clearly distinguish "AM" from "PM," confusion about times of administration can arise. To prevent error, many institutions have converted from the traditional 12-hour clock to a 24-hour clock, referred to as *military time*.

The 24-hour clock begins at midnight as 0000. The hours from 1 AM to 12 noon are the same as traditional time; colons and the terms AM and PM are omitted (Fig. 2-1). Examples:

Traditional	Military
12 midnight	0000
1 AM	0100
5 AM	0500
7:30 AM	0730
11:45 AM	1145
12:00 noon	1200

The hours from 1 PM continue numerically; 1 PM becomes 1300. To change traditional time to military time from 1 PM on, add 12. Examples:

Traditional	Military
1 PM	1300
2:30 PM	1430
5 PM	1700
7:15 PM	1915
10:45 PM	2245
11:59 PM	2359

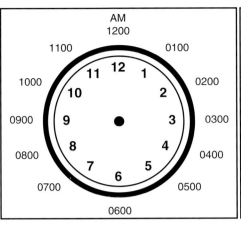
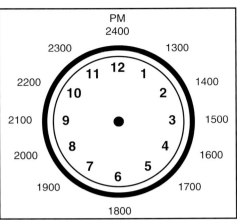

Example of a military, or 24-hour, clock.

SELF TEST 2 | **Military Time**

A. Change these traditional times to military time. Answers are given at the end of the chapter.

1. 2 PM _____

2. 9 AM _____

3. 4 PM _____

4. 12 noon _____

5. 1:30 AM _____

6. 9:15 PM ___2115 hrs._____

7. 4:50 AM _____

8. 6:20 PM _____

B. Change these military times to traditional times. Answers are given at the end of the chapter.

1. 0130 _____

2. 1745 _____

3. 1100 _____

4. 2015 _____

5. 1910 _____

6. 0600 _____

7. 0050 _____

8. 1000 _____

Routes of Administration

Of the following abbreviations, some are based on Latin words and some are not. Note the Latin words and also the alternative abbreviations, which are given in parentheses. Figure 2-2 shows the use of several abbreviations for routes of administration.

Route Abbreviation	Meaning	Origin and Explanation	Do Not Use
Write out	Right ear	Latin, *aures dextra*	AD
Write out	Left ear	Latin, *aures laeva*	AL
Write out	Each ear	Latin, *aures utrae*	AU
HHN	Hand-held nebulizer	Medication is placed in a device that produces a fine spray for inhalation.	
IM	Intramuscularly	The injection is given at a 90° angle into a muscle.	
IV	Intravenously	The injection is given into a vein.	
IVP	Intravenous push	Medication is injected directly in a vein.	

(continued)

Route Abbreviation	Meaning	Origin and Explanation	Do Not Use
IVPB	Intravenous piggyback	Medication prepared in a small volume of fluid is attached to an IV (which is already infusing fluid into a patient's vein) at specified times.	
MDI	Metered-dose inhaler	An aerosol device delivers medication by inhalation.	
NEB	Nebulizer	Medication is placed in a device that produces a fine spray for inhalations.	
NGT (ng)	Nasogastric tube	Medication is placed in the stomach through a tube in the nose.	
Write out	In the right eye	Latin, *oculus dextra*	OD
Write out	In the left eye	Latin, *oculus sinister*	OS
Write out	In both eyes	Latin, *oculi utrique*	OU
po (PO)	By mouth	Latin, *per os*	
pr (PR)	In the rectum	Latin, *per rectum*	
Sub-Q or Sub Q	Subcutaneously	The injection is usually given at a 45° angle into subcutaneous tissue.	sc sq s.c. s.q.
SL	Sublingual, under the tongue	Latin, *sub lingua*	

SELF TEST 3   Abbreviations (Routes)

After studying the abbreviations for routes of administration, give the meaning of the following terms. Indicate if the abbreviation is "Do Not Use" and which words substitute for it. The correct answers are given at the end of the chapter.

1. SL _____
2. OU _____
3. NGT _____
4. IV _____
5. po _____

6. OD _____
7. IVPB _____
8. OS _____
9. IM _____
10. pr _____

11. SC _____
12. AU _____
13. AL _____

1 mL   **Carpuject®**
with Luer Lock

Demerol®
meperidine
hydrochloride
injection, USP

Warning: May be habit forming.

75 mg/mL
For IM, SC or Slow IV Use
Sterile Aqueous Injection 7.5%
pH adjusted with NaOH or HCl.
For usual dosage and route of administration, see package insert.
Store at room temperature up to 25°C (77°F).
Caution: Federal (USA) law prohibits dispensing without prescription.
Demerol® is a registered trademark of Sanofi Pharmaceuticals, Inc.

©Abbott 1997   08-8409-2/R1-11/97   Printed in USA
Abbott Laboratories, North Chicago, IL 60064, USA

FIGURE 2-2

Label states the routes of administration. Meperidine HCL may be administered intramuscularly (IM), subcutaneously, or slowly intravenous (IV). (Courtesy of Abbott Laboratories.)

Metric and SI Abbreviations

Metric abbreviations in dosage relate to a drug's weight or volume and are the most common measures in dosage. The International System of Units (Système International d'Unités; SI) was adapted from the metric system in 1960. Most developed countries except the United States have adopted SI nomenclature to provide a standard language of measurement.

Differences between metric and SI systems do not occur in dosage. The meaning and abbreviations for weight and volume are the same. Weight measures are based on the gram; volume measures are based on the litre.

Study the meaning of the abbreviations listed in the following table. Under "Explanation," you'll see one equivalent for each abbreviation, to help you understand what kinds of quantities are involved.

Metric Abbreviation	Meaning	Explanation	Do Not Use
cc	Cubic centimetre	This is a measure of volume usually reserved for measuring gases. However, you may still find it used as a liquid measure. (One cubic centimetre is approximately equal to 16 drops from a medicine dropper.)	cc
g	gram	This is a solid measure of weight. (One gram is approximately equal to the weight of two small paper clips.)	
kg	kilogram	This is a weight measure. (One kilogram equals 2.2 pounds.)	
L	litre	This is a liquid measure. (One litre is a little more than a quart.)	
mcg	Microgram	This is a measure of weight. (One thousand micrograms make up 1 milligram: 1000 mcg = 1 mg.)	μg
mEq	Milliequivalent	No equivalent necessary. Drugs are prepared and ordered in this weight measure.	
mg	Milligram	This is a measure of weight. (One thousand milligrams make up 1 gram: 1000 mg = 1 g.)	
mL	Millilitre	This is a liquid measure. The terms *cubic centimetre* (cc) and *millilitre* (mL) are interchangeable in dosage (1 cc = 1 mL).	
unit	Unit	This is a measure of biologic activity. Nurses do not calculate this measure.	U

> **Example**   penicillin potassium 300,000 units
>
> *Important:* It is considered safer to write the word *unit* rather than use the abbreviation, because the *U* could be read as a zero and a medication error might result.

SELF TEST 4   Abbreviations (Metric)

After studying metric abbreviations, write the meaning of the following terms. Indicate if the abbreviation is not to be used and the words to substitute for it. The correct answers are given at the end of the chapter.

1. 0.3 g _____

2. 150 mcg _____

3. 80 U __*Unit*_____

4. 0.5 mL _____

5. 0.25 mg _____

6. 14 kg _____

7. 20 mEq _____

8. 1.5 L _____

9. 50 μg __*mcy*_____

Apothecary Abbreviations

The apothecaries system of measurement was the first system used to measure medication amounts. Today apothecary measures are obsolete, for several reasons: 1) Equivalency with the metric system is not exact. 2) The system requires roman numerals and fractions. 3) Apothecary symbols can easily be misinterpreted. Tables 2-2 and 2- 3 contain a brief overview of the apothecary system and the roman numerals used in that system.

TABLE 2-2   Apothecary Abbreviations

Apothecary Abbreviation	Meaning	Explanation
ʒ	Dram	This is a liquid measure. It is slightly less than a household teaspoon. (One dram equals 4 millilitres; ʒi = 4 mL.)
ʒ	Ounce	This is a liquid measure. It is slightly more than a household ounce. (One ounce equals 32 millilitres: ʒi = 32 mL.)
gr	Grain	Latin, *granum.* This solid measure was based on the weight of a grain of wheat in ancient times. There is no commonly used equivalent to the grain in the metric system.
gtt	Drop	Latin, *guttae.* This liquid measure was based on a drop of water. (One drop equals 1 minim.)
m (M, Mₓ)	Minim	Latin, *minim.* (One minim equals one drop: 1 m = 1 gtt.)
ṡṡ	One half	Latin, *semis*

TABLE 2-3   Roman Numerals and Arabic Numbers

Arabic	Roman
1	I *or* i
2	II *or* ii
3	III *or* iii
4	IV *or* iv
5	V *or* v
6	VI *or* vi
7	VII *or* vii
8	VIII *or* viii
9	IX *or* ix
10	X *or* x
15	XV *or* xv
20	XX *or* xx
40	XL *or* xl
50	L *or* l
60	LX *or* lx
100	C *or* c

Household Abbreviations

Household measures were previously used by physicians and healthcare providers to order and administer medications at home. However, as can be seen in Table 2-4, household measures are not exact and are considered only equivalent measures. Physicians in Canada no longer prescribe medications using household measures. Nurses must seek clarification for all orders not written using the metric system.

TABLE 2-4

Apothecary Measure	U.S. Household Measure	Canadian Household Measure	Standard Metric Equivalent	Exact Metric Conversion
15 or 16 m	15 or 16 drops	¼ teaspoon	1 mL	1.23 mL
1 fl dr	1 teaspoonful	1 tsp	5 mL	4.92 mL
2 fl dr	1 dessertspoon	2 tsp	10 mL	9.86 mL
4 fl dr	1 tablespoonful	1 Tbsp	15 mL	14.7 mL
8 fl dr	1 fluid ounce	2 Tbsp	30 mL	29.6 mL
4 fl oz	1 teacupful	½ cup	125 mL	118 mL
8 fl oz	1 glassful	1 cup	250 mL	236 mL
16 fl oz	1 pint	2 cups	500 mL	473 mL
32 fl oz	1 quart	4 cups	1 L	946 mL
15,360 gr	32 ounces	2 pounds	1 kg	0.91 kg

◼◻ Terms and Abbreviations for Drug Preparations

The following abbreviations and terms are used to describe selected drug preparations. Some of these abbreviations are rarely used, yet are included here for reference.

Term Abbreviation	Meaning	Explanation
cap, caps	Capsule	Medication is encased in a gelatin shell.
CR	Controlled release	
LA	Long acting	These abbreviations indicate that the drug has been prepared in a form that allows extended action. Therefore, the drug is given less frequently.
SA	Sustained action	
SR	Slow release	
DS	Double strength	
EC	Enteric coated	The tablet is coated with a substance that will not dissolve in the acid secretions of the stomach; instead, it dissolves in the more alkaline secretions of the intestines.
el, elix	Elixir	A drug is dissolved in a hydroalcoholic sweetened base.
sol	Solution	The drug is contained in a clear liquid preparation.
sp	Spirit	This is an alcoholic solution of a volatile substance (e.g., spirit of ammonia).
sup, supp	Suppository	This is a solid, cylindrically shaped drug that can be inserted into a body opening (e.g., the rectum or vagina).
susp	Suspension	Small particles of drug are dispersed in a liquid base and must be shaken before being poured; gels and magmas are also suspensions.
syr	Syrup	A sugar is dissolved in a liquid medication and flavoured to disguise the taste.
tab, tabs	Tablet	Medication is compressed or molded into a solid form; additional ingredients are used to shape and colour the tablet.
tr, tinct.	Tincture	This is a liquid alcoholic or hydroalcoholic solution of a drug.
ung, oint.	Ointment	This is a semisolid drug preparation that is applied to the skin (for external use only).
KVO	Keep vein open	**Example Order** 1000 mL dextrose 5% in water IV KVO. The nurse is to continue infusing this fluid.
TKO	To keep open	
Discontinue	Discontinue	**Example Order** Discontinue ampicillin (do not use D/C)
NKA	No known allergies	This is an important assessment that is noted on the medication record of a patient.
NKDA	No known drug allergies	This is an important assessment that is noted on the medication record of a patient.

SELF TEST 5   Abbreviations (Drug Preparations)

After studying the abbreviations for drug preparations, write out the meaning of the following terms. The correct answers are given at the end of the chapter.

1. elix _elixir_
2. DS _double strength_
3. NKA _no known allergy_
4. caps _capsule_
5. susp _suspension_

6. tab _tablet_
7. SR _____
8. LA _____
9. supp _____
10. tr _____

Now consider the formerly confusing orders that appeared at the beginning of this chapter.

Original: Morphine sulfate 15 mg Sub Q stat and 10 mg q4h prn

Interpretation: Morphine sulfate 15 mg subcutaneously immediately and 10 mg every 4 hours as needed.

Original: Chloromycetin 0.01% Opth Oint left eye bid

Interpretation: Chloromycetin 0.01% ophthalmic ointment left eye twice a day.

Original: Ampicillin 1 g IVPB q6h

Interpretation: Ampicillin 1 gram intravenous piggyback every 6 hours.

tbsp =
3 tsp = 1 tbsp
1 tbsp = 15ml

1 fl oz = 2 tbsp = 30 ml

1 gr = 60 mg
15 gr = 1 gram

PROFICIENCY TEST 1   Abbreviations

Name: _____

There are 50 items and each is worth 2 points. Indicate if the abbreviation is "Do Not Use" and which words to substitute for it. See Appendix A for answers.

1. bid _____
2. hs _____
3. prn _____
4. OU _____
5. po _____
6. pr _____
7. SL _____
8. mL _____
9. q4h _____
10. SC _____
11. AU _____
12. g _____
13. PC _____
14. qd _____
15. stat _____

16. q12h _____
17. tid _____
18. OS _____
19. kg _____
20. qn _____
21. qh _____
22. OD _____
23. mEq _____
24. AC _____
25. qid _____
26. mg _____
27. IM _____
28. qod _____
29. NGT _____
30. q8h _____

31. L _____
32. mcg _____
33. q6h _____
34. μg _____
35. U _____
36. tsp _____
37. AD _____
38. gr _____
39. IV _____
40. susp _____
41. tbsp _____
42. IVPB _____
43. m _____
44. q2h _____
45. q3h _____

Name: _____

Now that you have studied the language of prescriptions, you are ready to interpret medication orders.
Write the following orders in longhand. Give sample times. The correct answers are given in Appendix A.

1. Nembutal 100 mg at bedtime prn po _____

_____

2. Propranolol hydrochloride 40 mg po bid _____

_____

3. Ampicillin 1 g IVPB q6h _____

_____

4. Demerol 50 mg IM q4h prn for pain _____

_____

5. Tylenol 325 mg tabs ii po stat _____

_____

6. Pilocarpine gtt ii OU q3h _____

_____

7. Scopolamine 0.8 mg subcutaneously stat _____

_____

8. Digoxin el 0.25 mg po qd _____

_____

9. Kaochlor 30 mEq po bid _____

_____

10. Liquaemin sodium 6000 units subcutaneously q4h _____

_____

11. Tobramycin 70 mg IM q8h _____

_____

12. Prednisone 10 mg po every other day _____

_____

13. Milk of magnesia 1 tbsp po at bedtime daily _____

_____

14. Septra DS tab i every day po_____

_____

15. Morphine sulfate 15 mg subcutaneously stat and 10 mg q4h prn _____

_____

PROFICIENCY TEST 3 Interpreting Written Prescription Orders

Name: _____

Below are actual prescriptions written by physicians and other healthcare providers. Interpret each in longhand. In a real life situation, if the order is not clear, check with the person who wrote the order. Note any "Do Not Use" abbreviations. The correct answers are given in Appendix A.

1. *Calace 100 mg po ПD*	1.
2. *Ativan 1mg IVP x 1 now*	2.
3. *10 meq KCl in 100cc NS over 1h x 1*	3.
4. *Tylenol #3 tt tabs po q4° for Pai*	4.
5. *Heparin 25,000 IU in 250a D5W @ 500 u/Hr.*	5.
6. *Ticlid 250mg t PO BID.*	6.
7. *Lopresor 25 mg po BID.*	7.
8. *Benadryl 25 mg po qhs*	8.

Answers to Self Tests

Self Test 1 Abbreviations

1. Three times a day (**sample times:** 10 AM, 2 PM, 6 PM)
2. After meals (**sample times:** 10 AM, 2 PM, 6 PM)
3. Every other day (**sample times:** odd days of month at 10 AM). Do not use "qod" (write out "every other day").
4. Twice a day (**sample times:** 10 AM, 6 PM)
5. Do not use hs. Use "at bedtime." (**sample time:** 10 PM)
6. Immediately (**sample time:** whatever the time is now)
7. Four times a day (**sample times:** 10 AM, 2 PM, 6 PM, 10 PM)
8. Every 4 hours (**sample times:** 2 AM, 6 AM, 10 AM, 2 PM, 6 PM, 10 PM)
9. Before meals (**sample times:** 7:30 AM, 11:30 AM, 4:30 PM)
10. Do not use qd; use "every day." (**sample time:** 10 AM)
11. Every 8 hours (**sample times:** 6 AM, 2 PM, 10 PM)
12. Every hour
13. Whenever necessary (**sample times:** No time routine can be written.)
14. Every 4 hours as needed (**sample times:** No time routine is written because we do not know when the drug will be needed.)

Self Test 2 Military Time

A.
1. 1400
2. 0900
3. 1600
4. 1200
5. 0130
6. 2115
7. 0450
8. 1820

B.
1. 1:30 AM
2. 5:45 PM
3. 11 AM
4. 8:15 PM
5. 7:10 PM
6. 6 AM
7. 12:50 AM
8. 10 AM

Self Test 3 Abbreviations (Routes)

1. Sublingual; under the tongue
2. Do not use OU; use "both eyes"
3. Nasogastric tube
4. Intravenously
5. By mouth
6. Do not use OD; use "right eye"
7. Intravenous piggyback
8. Do not use OS; use "left eye"
9. Intramuscularly
10. Rectally
11. Do not use SC; use "subcutaneously."
12. Do not use au; use "both ears."
13. Do not use al; use "left ear."

Self Test 4 Abbreviations (Metric)

1. Three tenths of a gram
2. One hundred fifty micrograms
3. Eighty units. Do not use U; use "unit."
4. Five tenths of a millilitre
5. Twenty-five hundredths of a milligram
6. Fourteen kilograms
7. Twenty milliequivalents
8. One and five tenths of a litre
9. Fifty micrograms. Do not use μg; use "microgram."

Self Test 5 Abbreviations (Drug Preparations)

1. Elixir
2. Double strength
3. No known allergies
4. Capsules

5. Suspension
6. Tablet
7. Slow release
8. Long acting

9. Suppository
10. Tincture

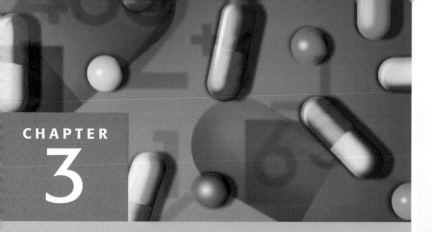

CHAPTER 3

Metric System of Measurement

Medication orders are written in metric terms. In this chapter, you will learn solid and liquid measures in the metric system.

Medicine cups are marked in metric, apothecary, and household measures; syringes are marked in metric lines.

Solid Measures in the Metric System

Measures of Weight

These are the solid measures in the metric system and their abbreviations:

Gram: g

Milligram: mg

Microgram: mcg (μg, which uses the Greek letter mu [μ], is no longer accepted by the ISMP for its approved abbreviation list)

Kilogram: kg

Weight Equivalents

These are the basic weight equivalents in the metric system:

1 g = 1000 mg

1 mg = 1000 mcg

As you can see, the gram is the largest of these.

To equal the weight of a single gram, you need 1000 mg.

To equal the weight of a single milligram, you need 1000 mcg.

The symbol >, which means "greater than," indicates these relationships:

g > mg > mcg

Read this notation as "A gram is greater than a milligram, which is greater than a microgram."

Converting Solid Equivalents

If the available supply is not in the same weight measure as the medication order, you will have to calculate how much of a drug to give.

Example

Order: 0.25 g

Supply: tablets labeled 125 mg

Since 1 g = 1000 mg, you change 0.25 g to milligrams by multiplying the number of grams by 1000.

$$
\begin{array}{r}
0.25 \\
\times\,1000 \\
\hline
250.00
\end{array}
$$

To convert the order, you use 0.25 g = 250 mg.

Here's an easy rule to help you remember this type of conversion:

Large to small—multiply by 1000

Small to large—divide by 1000

Following this rule, if you are converting grams to milligrams (a larger measurement to a smaller one), multiply the original number by 1000. If you are converting from micrograms to milligrams (a smaller measurement to a larger one), divide the original number by 1000.

There's another method of conversion as well. In decimals, the thousandth place is three numbers after the decimal point. You can change grams to milligrams by moving the decimal point three places to the *right*, which produces the same answer as multiplying by 1000. You can also change milligrams to grams by moving the decimal point three places to the *left*, which is the same as dividing by 1000. You'll be using this method in some of the calculations to come.

RULE   **CHANGING GRAMS TO MILLIGRAMS**

To multiply by 1000, move the decimal point three places to the right. ▪

Example

EXAMPLE 1

0.25 g = _____ mg

0.250 = 250

0.25 g = 250 mg

EXAMPLE 2

0.1 g = _____ mg

0.100 = 100

0.1 g = 100 mg

Grams to Milligrams Quick Method: Should you move the decimal point to the left or to the right? This Quick Method can help you decide.

1. First, write the order.

2. Write the equivalent measure you need.

3. Show which way the decimal point should move by drawing an *arrow*.

4. Make sure the open part of your arrow always faces the larger measure.

5. Remember that in the equivalent 1 g = 1000 mg, the gram is the larger measure, with 1000 mg equaling the weight of 1 gram.

Example

EXAMPLE 1

Order: 0.25 g

Supply: 125 mg

You want to convert grams to milligrams.

0.25 g > _____ mg

The arrow tells you to move the decimal point three places to the *right*.

0.250 = 250

Therefore, 0.25 g = 250 mg

EXAMPLE 2

Order: 1.5 g

Supply: 500 mg

You want to convert grams to milligrams.

1.5 g > _____ mg

1.500 = 1500

Therefore, 1.5 g = 1500 mg

SELF TEST 1 | **Grams to Milligrams**

Convert from grams to milligrams. For correct answers, see the end of the chapter.

1. 0.3 g = _____300_____ mg

2. 0.001 g = _____1 mg_____ mg

3. 0.02 g = _____20_____ mg

4. 1.2 g = _____1200_____ mg

5. 5 g = _____5000_____ mg

6. 0.4 g = _____ mg

7. 0.08 g = _____ mg

8. 0.275 g = _____275_____ mg

9. 0.04 g = _____ mg

10. 0.325 g = _____ mg

11. 2 g = _____2000_____ mg

12. 0.0004 g = _____0·4_____ mg

RULE	**CHANGING MILLIGRAMS TO GRAMS**

To divide by 1000, move the decimal point three places to the left. ▣

Example

EXAMPLE 1

100 mg = _____ g

100. = 0.1

100 mg = 0.1 g

EXAMPLE 2

8 mg = _____ g

008. = 0.008

8 mg = 0.008 g

Milligrams to Grams Quick Method: The arrow method also works to convert milligrams to grams.

1. First, write the order.

2. Write the equivalent measure you need.

3. Show which way the decimal point should move by drawing an *arrow*.

4. Make sure the open part of your arrow always faces the larger measure.

5. Remember that in the equivalent 1 g = 1000 mg, the gram is the larger measure.

Example

EXAMPLE 1

Order: 15 mg

Supply: 0.03 g

You want to convert milligrams to grams.

15 mg < g

The arrow tells you to move the decimal point three places to the *left*.

015. = 0.015

15 mg = 0.015 g

EXAMPLE 2

Order: 500 mg

Supply: 1 g

You want to convert milligrams to grams.

500 mg = _____ g

500 mg < g

The arrow tells you to move the decimal point three places to the *left*.

500. = 0.5

500 mg = 0.5 g

SELF TEST 2 Milligrams to Grams

Convert from milligrams to grams. For correct answers, see the end of the chapter.

1. 4 mg = _0.004_____ g

2. 120 mg = _____ g

3. 40 mg = _____ g

4. 75 mg = _____ g

5. 250 mg = _____ g

6. 1 mg = _____ g

7. 50 mg = _0.05_____ g

8. 600 mg = _0.6_____ g

9. 5 mg = _____ g

10. 360 mg = _____ g

11. 10 mg = _____ g

12. 0.1 mg = _____ g

RULE **CHANGING MILLIGRAMS TO MICROGRAMS**

The second major weight equivalent in the metric system is

1 mg = 1000 mcg.

Some medications are so powerful that smaller microgram doses are sufficient to produce a therapeutic effect. Rather than using milligrams written as decimals, it's easier to write orders in micrograms as whole numbers.

To multiply by 1000, move the decimal point three places to the right.

Example

EXAMPLE 1

0.1 mg = _____ mcg

$0.100 = 100$

0.1 mg = 100 mcg

EXAMPLE 2

0.25 mg = _____ mcg

$0.250 = 250$

0.25 mg = 250 mcg

Milligrams to Micrograms Quick Method: Should you move the decimal point to the left or to the right? Here are the steps:

1. First, write the order.

2. Write the equivalent measure you need.

3. Show which way the decimal point should move by drawing an *arrow.*

4. Make sure the open part of your arrow faces the larger measure.

5. Remember that in the equivalent 1 mg = 1000 mcg, the milligram is the larger measure, with 1000 mcg equaling the weight of 1 mg.

Example

EXAMPLE 1

Order: 0.1 mg

Supply: 200 mcg

You want to convert milligrams to micrograms.

0.1 mg > _____ mcg

The arrow is telling you to move the decimal point three places to the *right*.

0.100 = 100

Therefore, 0.1 mg = 100 mcg

EXAMPLE 2

Order: 0.3 mg

Supply: 600 mcg

You want to convert milligrams to micrograms.

0.3 mg > _____ mcg

0.300 = 300

Therefore, 0.3 mg = 300 mcg

SELF TEST 3   Milligrams to Micrograms

Convert from milligrams to micrograms. For correct answers, see the end of the chapter.

1. 0.3 mg = _____ mcg

2. 0.001 mg = _____ mcg

3. 0.02 mg = _____ mcg

4. 0.08 mg = _____ mcg

5. 1.2 mg = _____ mcg

6. 0.4 mg = _____ mcg

7. 5 mg = _____ mcg

8. 0.7 mg = _____ mcg

9. 0.04 mg = _____ mcg

10. 10 mg = _____ mcg

11. 0.9 mg = _____ mcg

12. 0.01 mg = _____ mcg

RULE   **CHANGING MICROGRAMS TO MILLIGRAMS**

To divide by 1000, move the decimal point three places to the left. ■

Example

EXAMPLE 1

300 mcg = _____ mg

300. = 0.3

300 mcg = 0.3 mg

EXAMPLE 2

50 mcg = _____ mg

050. = 0.05

50 mcg = 0.05 mg

Micrograms to Milligrams Quick Method: The arrow method also converts micrograms to milligrams.

1. First, write the order.

2. Write the equivalent measure you need.

3. Show which way the decimal point should move by drawing an *arrow*.

4. Make sure the open part of your arrow faces the larger measure.

5. Remember that in the equivalent 1 mg = 1000 mcg, the milligram is the larger measure.

Example

EXAMPLE 1
Order: 100 mcg

Supply: 0.1 mg

You want to convert micrograms to milligrams.

100 mcg < mg

The arrow tells you to move the decimal point three places to the *left*.

100. = 0.1

100 mcg = 0.1 mg

EXAMPLE 2
Order: 50 mcg

Supply: 0.1 mg

You want to convert micrograms to milligrams.

50 mcg = ___·05___ mg

mcg < mg

The arrow tells you to move the decimal point three places to the *left*.

050. = 0.05

50 mcg = 0.05 mg

SELF TEST 4   Micrograms to Milligrams

Convert from micrograms to milligrams. For correct answers, see the end of the chapter.

1. 800 mcg = _____ mg

2. 4 mcg = _____ mg

3. 14 mcg = _____ mg

4. 25 mcg = _____ mg

5. 1 mcg = _____ mg

6. 200 mcg = _____ mg

7. 50 mcg = _____ mg

8. 750 mcg = _____ mg

9. 325 mcg = _____ mg

10. 75 mcg = _____ mg

11. 0.1 mcg = _____ mg

12. 150 mcg = _____ mg

SELF TEST 5 — Mixed Conversions

Convert mixed metric weight measures. For correct answers, see the end of the chapter.

1. 0.3 mg = _____ g
2. 0.03 g = _____ mg
3. 15 mcg = _____ mg
4. 0.1 g = _____ mg
5. 100 mcg = _____ mg

6. 50 mg = _____ g
7. 0.014 g = _____ mg
8. 200 mg = _____ g
9. 0.2 mg = _____ mcg
10. 0.65 mg = _____ mcg

SELF TEST 6 — Common Equivalents

Fill in the blanks to convert mg to g or to mcg.

1. 1000 mg = _____ g
2. 600 mg = _____ g
3. 500 mg = _____ g
4. 300 mg = _____ g
5. 200 mg = _____ g
6. 100 mg = _____ g
7. 60 mg = _____ g

8. 30 mg = _0.03_ g
9. 15 mg = _0.015_ g
10. 10 mg = _0.01_ g
11. 0.6 mg = _600_ mcg
12. 0.4 mg = _400_ mcg
13. 0.3 mg = _300_ mcg
14. 0.25 mg = _250_ mcg

SELF TEST 7 — Review of Grams to Milligrams

1. What are the methods for converting grams to milligrams? _____
_____
_____

2. 1 g = _____ mg
3. 0.01 g = _____ mg
4. 0.2 g = _____ mg
5. 0.12 g = _____ mg
6. 0.6 g = _____ mg
7. 0.5 g = _____ mg
8. 0.3 g = _____ mg

9. 0.2 g = _____ mg
10. 0.1 g = _____ mg
11. 0.06 g = _____ mg
12. 0.03 g = _____ mg
13. 0.015 g = _____ mg
14. 0.01 g = _____ mg

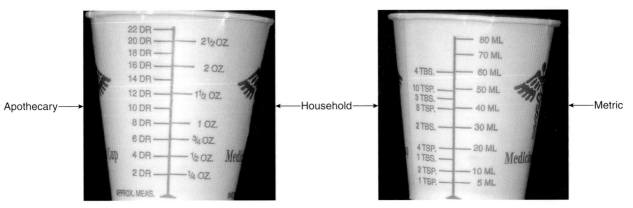

Apothecary→ ←Household→ ←Metric

A medicine cup with metric, household, and apothecary equivalents. Two sides of the cup are shown. (© 2004 Lacey-Bordeaux Photography.)

Liquid Measures in the Metric System

Liquid Measures and Equivalents

These are the liquid measures in the metric system and their abbreviations:

Litre: L

Millilitre: mL

Liquid equivalents in the metric system are:

1 L = 1000 mL

Apothecary and Household Systems of Measurement

Although some equipment used to administer medications may contain apothecary and/or household measurement lines, you must use the metric measurement lines, which correspond to how medications are prescribed and distributed in Canada (Figures 3-1 and 3-2).

Milliunit and Milliequivalent

A unit is a standard of measurement, and a milliunit is one-thousandth of a unit. A drug used in obstetrics, Pitocin (oxytocin), is administered in milliunits per minute (see Chapter 9).

A milliequivalent is used to measure the amount of solute per litre. It is used when measuring different substances found in biological fluids, such as the amount of potassium in blood (normal value: 3.5 to 5.0 milliequivalents per litre). Some medications are administered in milliequivalents. Milliequivalents is abbreviated mEq.

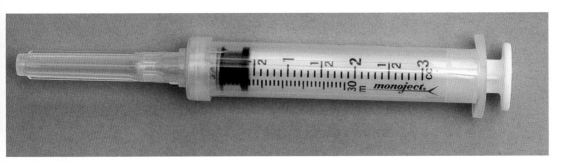

A 3-mL syringe with metric and apothecary measures. (© 2004 Lacey-Bordeaux Photography.)

PROFICIENCY TEST 1   Exercises in Equivalents and Mixed Conversions

Name: _____

Aim for 100% accuracy on this test. See Appendix A for answers.

1. 100 mg = _____ g
2. 1 L = _____ mL
3. 0.015 g = _____ mg
4. 10 mg = _____ g
5. 0.2 g = _____ mg
6. 30 mg = _____ g
7. 500 mg = _____ g
8. 1 g = _____ mg
9. 60 mg = _____ g
10. 0.1 g = _____ mg

11. 600 mg = _____ g
12. 10 mcg = _____ mg
13. 0.5 mcg = _____ mg
14. 0.6 mg = _____ g
15. 250 mcg = _____ mg
16. 1 mg = _____ g
17. 0.125 mg = _____ mcg
18. 0.01 mg = _____ mcg
19. 0.001 mg = _____ mcg

Answers to Self Tests

Self Test 1 Grams to Milligrams

1. 300	**4.** 1200	**7.** 80	**10.** 325
2. 1	**5.** 5000	**8.** 275	**11.** 2000
3. 20	**6.** 400	**9.** 40	**12.** 0.4

Self Test 2 Milligrams to Grams

1. 0.004	**4.** 0.075	**7.** 0.05	**10.** 0.36
2. 0.12	**5.** 0.25	**8.** 0.6	**11.** 0.01
3. 0.04	**6.** 0.001	**9.** 0.005	**12.** 0.0001

Self Test 3 Milligrams to Micrograms

1. 300	**4.** 80	**7.** 5000	**10.** 10000
2. 1	**5.** 1200	**8.** 700	**11.** 900
3. 20	**6.** 400	**9.** 40	**12.** 10

Self Test 4 Micrograms to Milligrams

1. 0.8	**4.** 0.025	**7.** 0.05	**10.** 0.075
2. 0.004	**5.** 0.001	**8.** 0.75	**11.** 0.0001
3. 0.014	**6.** 0.2	**9.** 0.325	**12.** 0.15

Self Test 5 Mixed Conversions

1. 0.0003	**4.** 100	**7.** 14	**9.** 200
2. 30	**5.** 0.1	**8.** 0.2	**10.** 650
3. 0.015	**6.** 0.05		

Self Test 6 Common Equivalents

1. 1	**5.** 0.2	**9.** 0.015	**12.** 400
2. 0.6	**6.** 0.1	**10.** 0.01	**13.** 300
3. 0.5	**7.** 0.06	**11.** 600	**14.** 250
4. 0.3	**8.** 0.03		

Self Test 7 Review of Grams to Milligrams

1. Multiply grams by 1000, move decimal point three places to the right, or use an arrow with the open part toward gram to show movement of decimal point three places.	**7.** 500
	8. 300
	9. 200
	10. 100
2. 1000	**11.** 60
3. 10	**12.** 30
4. 200	**13.** 15
5. 120	**14.** 10
6. 600	

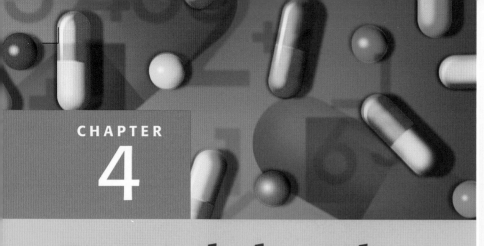

CHAPTER
4

Drug Labels and Packaging

Drug Labels

An understanding of drug labels and the ways in which drugs are packaged provides a background for dosage and administration.

Labels contain specific facts and appear on drugs intended to be administered as packaged: either in solid form or in liquid form. Occasionally, the label does *not* include some details—such as route of administration, usual dose, and storage—because the container is too small. When you need more information than the label provides, consult a professional reference. Figure 4-1 shows a sample drug label.

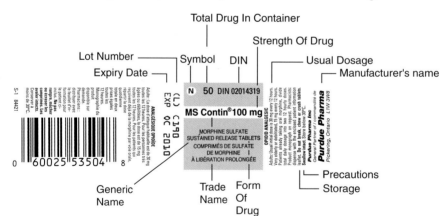

FIGURE 4-1

Label of MS Contin. (Courtesy of Purdue Pharma Inc.)

DIN. The Drug Identification Number (DIN) is an eight-digit numerical code located on the label of prescription and over-the-counter drug products that have been evaluated by the Therapeutic Products Directorate (TPD) and approved for sale in Canada under the *Food and Drugs Act* and *Regulations.*

• In Figure 4-1, the DIN is 02014319.

SYMBOLS

Pr - identifies the product as a prescription drug.

C – identifies the product as a controlled drug.

N – identifies a narcotic as defined under the Narcotic Control Regulations.

Sterile/Stérile – identifies that the drug is required to be sterile by *Food and Drugs Regulations.*

TOTAL AMOUNT OF DRUG IN CONTAINER. The net amount of the drug in the container in terms of weight, measure, or number.

- Figure 4-1 indicates 50 tablets.

TRADE NAME. The name that is assigned to the drug by its manufacturer under which the drug is sold or advertised and is used to distinguish the drug. Several companies may manufacture the same drug, using different trade names.

- In Figure 4-1, the trade name is MS Contin.

GENERIC NAME. Also known as the common or proper name of the drug, the generic name is the official accepted name of a drug. A drug may have several trade names but only one official generic name.

- In Figure 4-1, the generic name is morphine sulfate.

STRENGTH OF THE DRUG. For solid drugs, the label shows metric weights; for liquid drugs, the label states the solution of the drug in a solvent.

- In Figure 4-1, the strength of the drug is 100 mg.

FORM OF THE DRUG. The label specifies the type of preparation in the container.

- Figure 4-1 indicates that the drug is dispensed in sustained release tablets.

USUAL DOSAGE. The dosage information states how much drug is administered at a single time or during a 24-hour period. It also identifies who should receive the drug.

- Figure 4-1 indicates the usual dosage is 30 mg every 12 hours with suggested modifications for very elderly or debilitated patients.

ROUTE OF ADMINISTRATION. The label specifies how the drug is to be given: orally, parenterally, or topically. If the label does not specify the route, the drug is in an oral form.

- In Figure 4-1, the route is oral.

CLASSIFICATION. A system to categorize drugs into groups with similar activities and uses.

- In Figure 4-1, the therapeutic classification is opioid analgesic.

STORAGE. Certain conditions are necessary to protect the drug from losing its potency (effectiveness), so this information is crucial. Some drugs come in a dry form and must be dissolved, i.e., reconstituted. The drug may need one kind of storage when it's dry and another kind after reconstitution.

- Figure 4-1 specifies storing the drug below 30°C

PRECAUTIONS. The label may include specific instructions related to safety, effectiveness, and/or administration that the nurse must note and follow.

- Figure 4-1 shows these precautions: "Do not break, chew, or crush tablet. Swallow intact."

MANUFACTURER'S NAME AND ADDRESS. If you have any questions about the drug, direct them to this company.

- In Figure 4-1, the company is Purdue Pharma.

EXPIRY DATE. A drug expires on the last day of the indicated month. After that date, the manufacturer recommends that the drug not be used.

- In Figure 4-1 the expiration date is October 2010.

LOT NUMBER. This number indicates the batch of drug from which this stock came.

- In Figure 4-1, the lot number is C190.

ACTIVE INGREDIENTS. Active Pharmaceutical Ingredients (API) are active chemicals used in the manufacturing of drugs. In addition, a quantitative list of any preservatives present must be listed. Information may appear on the outer label or in the literature accompanying the drug.

RECONSTITUTION. Some drugs that are typically dispensed in a dry (powder) form need to be reconstituted. The drug label or drug insert provides specific directions about the amount and type of liquid (diluent) to use for dissolving the drug as well as the resulting concentration.

Example   Amoxicillin (Polymox) comes in powder form. Prepare suspension at time of dispensing. Add 88 mL water to the bottle. For ease in preparation, add the water in two portions. Shake well after each addition. This provides 150 mL suspension. Dosage is 125 mg amoxicillin per 5 mL solution.

SELF TEST 1   **Drug Labels**

Read the label in Figure 4-2 and fill in the blanks. Answers are given at the end of the chapter.

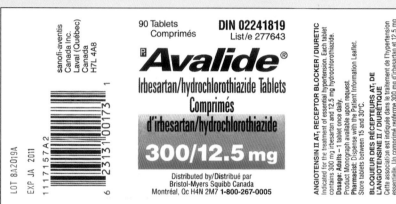

FIGURE 4-2

Label of Avalide. (Courtesy of Bristol-Meyers Squibb Canada.)

1. DIN _____

2. Total amount of drug in the container _____

3. Trade name _____

4. Generic name _____

5. Strength of the drug _____

6. Form of the drug _____

7. Usual dosage _____

8. Route of administration _____

9. Storage _____

_____

10. Precautions _____

_____

11. Manufacturer _____

12. Expiration date _____

(continued)

SELF TEST 1 Drug Labels *(Continued)*

Read the label in Figure 4-3 and fill in the blanks. Answers are given at the end of the chapter.

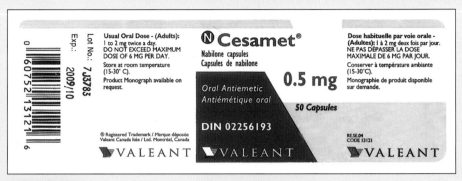

FIGURE 4-3

Label of Cesamet (Courtesy of Valeant.)

13. What is the trade name? _____

14. What is the generic name? _____

15. By what route(s) may this drug be given? _____

16. In what form is the drug dispensed? _____

17. What is the strength of the drug? _____

18. What is the total amount of drug in the container? _____

19. What is the usual adult dose? _____

    _____

20. List precautions. _____

    _____

When a medication container holds a single drug, the written prescription indicates the dose in milligrams or grams, and calculation may be necessary.

Example

   a. Tylenol 0.6 g po q4h prn for temperature ↑ 38.5°C

      Label: Tylenol 325 mg tablets

   b. Prednisone 20 mg po bid

      Label: Prednisone 10 mg tablets

   c. Digoxin 0.5 mg po daily

      Label: Digoxin 0.25 mg

   d. Cefozil 0.5 g po q8h

      Label: 125 mg/5 mL

Some medication labels indicate more than one drug in the dose form. These combination drugs are ordered according to the number of tablets to give or the amount of liquid to pour.

Example

  a. Order: Tylenol #3 tabs 2 tabs po q4h prn for pain

      Label: acetaminophen 300 mg/codeine 30 mg tablet

  b. Order: Robitussin DM 10 mg po qid

      Label: guaifenesin 100 mg/dextromethorphan 10 mg per 5 mL

  c. Order: Talwin Compound 1 tab po q6h

      Label: aspirin 325 mg/pentazocine 12.5 mg

Drug Packaging

Drugs come in two types of packaging: *unit-dose* and *multidose.* Each type may contain a solid or liquid form of the drug for oral, parenteral, or topical use. Most institutions use a combination of unit-dose and multidose.

Unit-Dose Packaging

In an institutional setting, each dose is individually wrapped and labelled, and a 24-hour supply is prepared by the pharmacy and dispensed. A major value of unit-dose packaging is that two professionals—the pharmacist and the nurse—check the drug and the dose, thereby decreasing the possibility of error.

    The medication may be stored in a medication cart, in a locked cabinet at the patient's bedside, or in a locked medication dispensing system.

    Unit-dose packaging does not relieve the nurse from responsibility to check the label three times and to calculate the amount of drug needed. Be aware that unit-dose drugs come in different strengths, and when trade names are ordered instead of generic names, there is always a chance of error. A dose may consist of one unit packet, two or more unit packets, or a fraction of one packet. Skilled-care nursing facilities often use a system that dispenses the unit-dose medication for one month (Fig. 4-4).

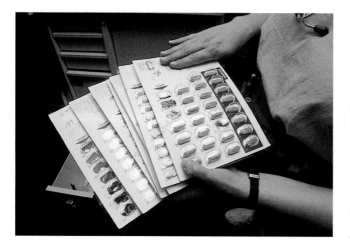

FIGURE 4-4

In long-term care settings, where medication prescriptions remain the same over weeks or months, "bingo" cards are a cost-effective method of dispensing medications. Each bubble contains one dose for the client. (Used with permission from Craven/Hirnle. [2007]. *Fundamentals of nursing.* Philadelphia: Lippincott Williams & Wilkins, p. 551.)

Example   A nurse has a unit-dose 100-mg tablet. If an order calls for 50 mg, only half the tablet should be administered.

If a nurse has an order for 75 mg, and each unit packets contain 25-mg tablets, the nurse administers three tablets.

FOR THE ORAL ROUTE. For oral administration, unit-dose packaging comes in a number of forms:

1. Plastic bubble, foil, or paper wrappers containing tablets or capsules (Fig. 4-5A).

2. Plastic or glass containers that hold a single dose of a liquid or a powder. The powder is reconstituted to a liquid form by following the directions given on the label (Fig. 4-5B).

3. A sealed medication cup containing a liquid. Once the nurse removes the cover, the medication is ready to administer; the amount administered depends on the correct calculation of the dose (Fig. 4-5C).

FOR THE PARENTERAL ROUTE. These drugs—which may come in a powder or a liquid form—are given by injection, via the route specified in the order (e.g., intramuscular [IM], subcutaneous, intravenous piggy-back [IVPB]). Drugs packaged in the containers described below are sterile, and sterile technique is essential in their preparation and administration.

1. An *ampoule* (ampule) is a glass container that holds a single sterile dose of drug—either a liquid, a powder, or a crystal (Fig. 4-6). The container has a narrow neck that must be broken to reach the drug. Then the nurse uses a sterile syringe and needle to withdraw the medication. Directions tell how to reconstitute the powder forms. Once the glass is broken, the drug cannot be kept sterile, so the nurse must be sure to discard any portion of the drug not immediately used.

2. A *vial* is a glass or plastic container with a sealed rubber top (see Fig. 4-6). Medication in the container can be kept sterile. The container may have a sterile liquid or a sterile powder that the nurse

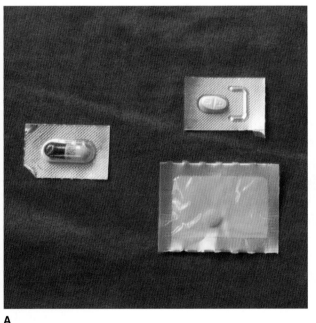
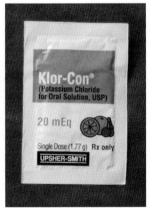
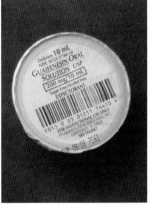

A   B   C

FIGURE 4-5

(**A**) Unit-dose tablets and capsules in foil wrappers. (**B**) Unit-dose powder in a sealed packet; it is placed in a container and diluted before giving. (**C**) Sealed cup containing a liquid medication. (Copyright © 2008 Lacey-Bordeaux Photography.)

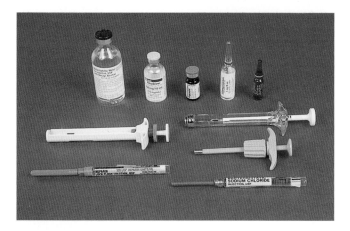

FIGURE 4-6

Parenteral route: (*top row*) vials and ampoules; (*middle and bottom rows*) prefilled cartridges and holders.

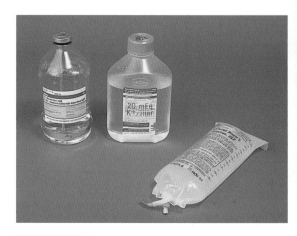

FIGURE 4-7

Plastic or glass containers hold medication for IV use.

must reconstitute with a sterile diluent. Since *single-dose vials* do not contain a preservative or a bacteriostatic agent, the nurse must discard any medication remaining after the dose is prepared.

3. Flexible *plastic bags* or *glass vials* may hold sterile medication for intravenous use (Fig. 4-7). The nurse administers the fluid via IV tubing connected to a needle or catheter placed in the patient's blood vessel.

4. *Prefilled syringes* contain sterile liquid medication that is ready to administer without further preparation.

5. *Prefilled cartridges* are actually small vials with a needle attached. They fit into a metal or plastic holder and eject one unit-dose of a sterile drug in liquid form (Fig. 4-8).

FOR TOPICAL ADMINISTRATION. Drugs applied to the skin or mucous membranes can achieve a local effect. They can also achieve a systemic effect because they can be absorbed into the circulation.

1. *Transdermal patches* or *pads* are adhesive bandages placed on the skin (Fig. 4-9). They hold a drug form that is slowly absorbed into the circulation over a period ranging from hours to several days.

2. *Lozenges (pastilles)* are disklike solids that slowly dissolve in the mouth (e.g., cough drops). Some drugs are prepared in a gum and are released by chewing (e.g., nicotine).

3. *Suppositories* in foil or plastic wrappers are molded forms that can be inserted into the rectum or vagina (Fig. 4-10). They hold medication in a substance (such as cocoa butter) that melts at body temperature and releases the drug. Suppositories may be used for unconscious patients or those unable to swallow.

4. *Plastic, disposable, squeezable containers* hold either prepared solutions for the vagina (douches) or enema solutions that are administered rectally (Fig. 4-11). To ease insertion, the containers for enemas have a lubricated nozzle. Squeezing the container forces the solution out.

Multidose Packaging

Within an institutional setting, such as a hospital, the nursing floor or unit may receive large stock containers of medications from which doses are poured. Although this type of packaging reduces the pharmacy's workload, it adds to preparation time and increases the possibility of error.

FOR THE ORAL ROUTE. Stock bottles contain a liquid or a solid form such as tablets, capsules, or powders. Large stock bottles hold medication that is dispensed over a period of days. When reconstituting the powders, the nurse must write the date and time of preparation on the container's label and must carefully note storage directions and expiration date. Caution: Powders, once dissolved, begin losing potency (Fig. 4-12A).

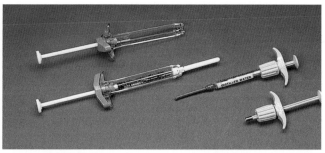

A

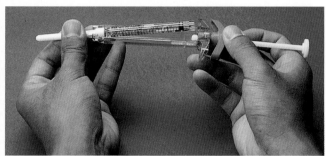

B

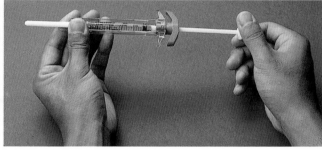

C

FIGURE 4-8

(**A**) Prefilled cartridges. (**B**) Inserting cartridge into injector device. (**C**) Cartridge is screwed into device, ready to administer drug.

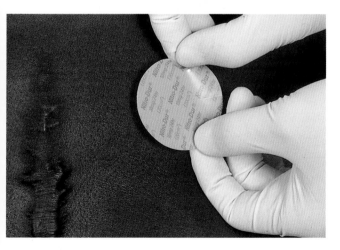

FIGURE 4-9

Transdermal patches or pads are placed on the skin. Drugs prepared in this manner include estrogen, fentanyl, testosterone, and nitroglycerin.

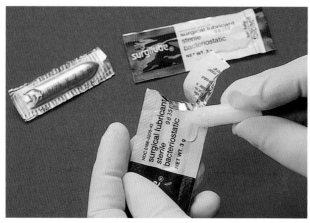

A

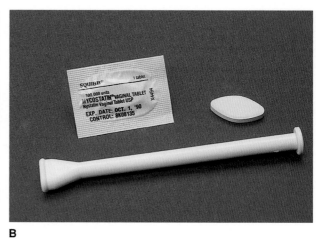

B

FIGURE 4-10

(**A**) Rectal suppository. (**B**) Vaginal suppository and applicator.

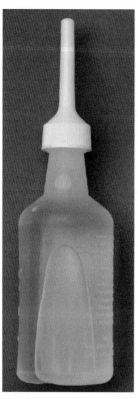

A

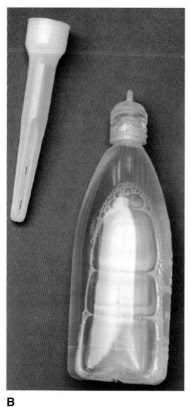

B

FIGURE 4-11

Unit-dose containers for rectal enema (**A**) and vaginal irrigation (**B**). (© 2004 Lacey-Bordeaux Photography.)

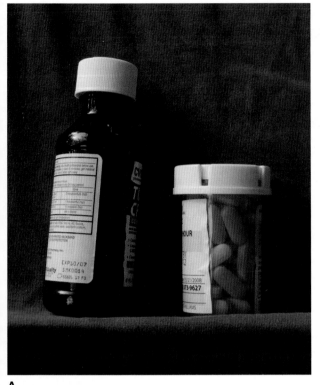

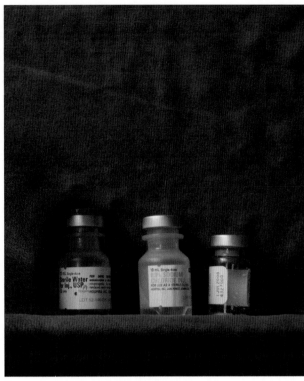

A   **B**

FIGURE 4-12

Multidose containers: (**A**) for the oral route; (**B**) for the parenteral route. (Copyright © 2008 Lacey-Bordeaux Photography.)

FOR THE PARENTERAL ROUTE. Multidose vials contain either a sterile liquid or a powder to be reconstituted using sterile technique. The nurse must write the date and time of preparation on the label and must note the expiration date and storage (Fig. 4-12B).

FOR TOPICAL ADMINISTRATION. Since these containers are used over an extended period of time, it's important to avoid contaminating them. The nurse should label the container with the patient's name and reserve the container's use for only that patient. Here are some guidelines on using containers for topical medication:

1. Metal or plastic tubes often contain ointments or creams for application to the skin or mucous membranes. Squeezing the tubes releases the medication (Fig. 4-13A).

2. To avoid contamination of medicated creams, ointments, and pastes in jars, always use a sterile tongue blade or sterile glove to remove the medication.

3. When using dropper bottles for eye, ear, or nose medications, prevent cross-contamination by labelling each container with the patient's name and using the container only for that patient. The nurse must be careful to avoid touching mucous membranes with the dropper, because contamination of the dropper can cause pathogens to grow. Droppers come in two forms: monodrop containers, which are squeezed to release the medication, and containers with removable droppers. Separate, packaged droppers are also available to administer medications; these are sometimes calibrated (i.e., is, marked in millilitres; Fig. 4-13B, C).

   Eye medications are labelled "ophthalmic" or "for the eye." Ear drugs are labelled "otic" or "auric" or "for the ear." Drugs for nasal administration are labelled "nose drops." Do not interchange these routes.

4. Lozenges and pastilles may be packaged in multidose as well as unit-dose containers.

5. Metered-dose inhalers (MDIs; Fig. 4-14) are aerosol devices with two parts: a canister under pressure and a mouthpiece. The canister contains multiple drug doses in either a liquid form or a microfine powder or crystal. The mouthpiece fits on the canister, and finger pressure on the mouthpiece opens a valve on the

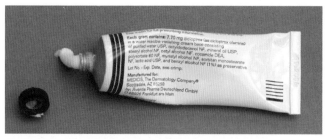

A

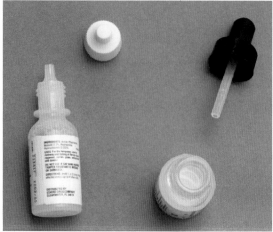

B   **C**

FIGURE 4-13

Topical multidose containers. (**A**) Tubes for creams or ointments. (**B**) Monodrop containers—the dropper is attached. (**C**) Removable dropper is sometimes calibrated for liquid measures. (© 2004 Lacey-Bordeaux Photography.)

canister that discharges one dose. The physician's or healthcare provider's order states the number of inhalations or "puffs" to be taken. Medications for inhalation also may be packaged as liquids in vials or bottles or as capsules containing powder for use with either a hand-held nebulizer (HHN) or an intermittent positive-pressure breathing apparatus (IPPB). Dry powder inhalers (DPI), such as Advair, contain a set number of doses and are administered in a way similar to that for metered-dose inhalers (see Fig. 4-14).

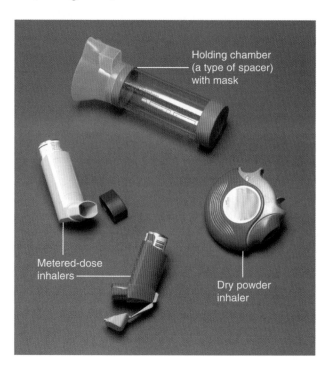

Holding chamber (a type of spacer) with mask

Metered-dose inhalers

Dry powder inhaler

FIGURE 4-14

Examples of metered-dose inhalers and spacers. (Used with permission from Taylor, C. [2008]. *Fundamentals of nursing*. Philadelphia: Lippincott Williams & Wilkins, p. 810.)

SELF TEST 2 Drug Packaging

Match Column A with the letters in Column B to identify the meaning of terms used in drug packaging. Answers are given at the end of the chapter.

Column A

1. _____ Unit-dose
2. _____ Ampoule
3. _____ Parenteral
4. _____ Prefilled cartridge
5. _____ Reconstitution
6. _____ Topical
7. _____ Transdermal patch
8. _____ Vial
9. _____ Lozenge
10. _____ Cocoa butter

Column B

a. Dissolving a powder into solution

b. Glass or plastic container with a sealed rubber top

c. Route of administration to skin or mucous membranes

d. Individually wrapped and labelled drugs

e. Disklike solid that dissolves in the mouth

f. Suppository ingredient that melts at body temperature

g. General term for an injection route

h. Adhesive bandage applied to the skin that gradually releases a drug

i. Small vial, with a needle attached, that fits into a syringe holder

j. Glass container that must be broken to obtain the drug

Complete these statements related to drug packaging. Answers are given at the end of the chapter.

11. Date and time of reconstitution must be written _____ _____ _____

12. The best way to avoid cross-contamination of a multidose tube of ointment is to _____ _____

13. To remove medication from a jar of paste, the nurse should use _____ _____

14. Dropper bottles for eye medications will be labelled _____ _____

15. Doses of medication that require use of a metered-dose inhaler are ordered in _____ _____

16. Medications for the ear will be labelled _____ _____

17. The term *multidose* refers to _____ _____

(continued)

SELF TEST 2 **Drug Packaging** *(Continued)*

18. The type of drug packaging that decreases the possibility of error is termed _____

    _____

19. Drugs administered topically for a local effect may be absorbed and produce another effect
    that is called _____

    _____

    _____

20. The word *lozenge* describes _____

    _____

    _____

PROFICIENCY TEST 1 Labels and Packaging

Name: _____

Complete these questions. See Appendix A for answers.

1. Explain the difference between each of these pairs.
   a. 1. Unit-dose _____
      2. Multidose _____
   b. 1. Ampoule _____
      2. Vial_____
   c. 1. Topical _____
      2. Parenteral _____
   d. 1. Trade name_____
      2. Generic name _____
   e. 1. Prefilled _____
      2. Reconstituted _____

2. Choose the correct answer.
   _____ a. A major advantage of the unit-dose system of drug administration is that
      1. the drug supply is always available
      2. no error is possible
      3. drugs are less expensive than stock bottles
      4. the pharmacist provides a second professional check
   _____ b. A major disadvantage of ampoules over vials is that ampoules
      1. are only glass
      2. when opened cannot be kept sterile
      3. contain only liquids
      4. cannot be used for injections
   _____ c. An order reads Valium 5 mg po now. A nurse correctly chooses diazepam. What name does
      diazepam represent?
      1. Generic
      2. Chemical
      3. Trade
      4. Proprietary
   _____ d. Which drug form is safest to administer to an unconscious patient?
      1. Suppository
      2. Syrup
      3. Capsule
      4. Aerosol

(continued)

PROFICIENCY TEST 1 Labels and Packaging *(Continued)*

3. Match the following:

   1. _____ Avoid cross-contamination   **a.** Topical application

   2. _____ Removing medication from a jar   **b.** Auric

   3. _____ Eye medication   **c.** Slow absorption over time

   4. _____ Puffs ordered   **d.** Reconstitution

   5. _____ Date and time label   **e.** Use a tongue blade

   6. _____ Lozenge   **f.** Cough drop

   7. _____ Parenteral   **g.** Individual nose droppers

   8. _____ Local effect   **h.** Ophthalmic

   9. _____ Transdermal   **i.** Inhalation

   10. _____ Ear medication   **j.** IM, subcutaneous, IV

PROFICIENCY TEST 2   Interpreting a Label

*Name:*_____

Read the label and answer the questions. See Appendix A for answers.

DIN 02231893
STERILE/STÉRILE

**METHYLPREDNISOLONE
SODIUM SUCCINATE
FOR INJECTION, USP**
Succinate sodique de
méthylprednisolone
pour injection, USP

40 mg   per vial/
par fiole

Anti-inflammatory/Anti-inflammatoire
Glucocorticoid/Glucocorticoïde
For I.V. or I.M. use/
Pour usage i.v. ou i.m.

novopharm

Lot: 8740606

Exp: 06.2008

Courtesy of Novopharm
Limited.

1. Generic name _____

2. Route(s) of administration _____

3. Therapeutic classification _____

4. Total volume when reconstituted _____

5. Strength of reconstituted solution _____

6. Directions to reconstitute _____

   _____

7. Drug form as dispensed _____

8. Storage _____

   _____

9. Expiration date _____

10. Precautions _____

    _____

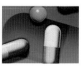

Answers to Self Tests

Self Test 1 Drug Labels

1. 02241819
2. 90 tablets
3. Avalide
4. Irbesartan/hydrochlorothiazide
5. 300/12.5 mg
6. tablets
7. 1 tablet once daily
8. Oral
9. Store between 15° and 30°C.
10. Pharmacist: Dispense with the Patient Information Leaflet.

11. Bristol-Meyers Squibb, Canada
12. January 2011
13. Cesamet
14. Nabilone
15. Oral
16. Capsules
17. 0.5 mg
18. 50 capsules
19. 1 to 2 mg twice a day
20. Do not exceed maximum dose of 6 mg per day. Store at room temperature 15°−30°C.

Self Test 2 Drug Packaging

1. d
2. j
3. g
4. i
5. a
6. c
7. h
8. b
9. e
10. f
11. On the label of any powder that nurse dissolves. Powders begin to lose their potency as soon as they are placed in solution. By writing the date and time on the label, the nurse will be able to check for expiration time.

12. Label the tube with one patient's name and restrict its use to that one patient.
13. A sterile tongue blade or sterile gloves to prevent contamination of the jar contents.
14. "Ophthalmic" or "for the eye"
15. Number of inhalations or puffs
16. "Otic" or "auric"
17. Large stock containers that hold many doses of a drug
18. Unit-dose
19. A systemic effect; the drug reaches the circulation and is carried to other parts of the body.
20. A disklike solid that is slowly dissolved in the mouth (e.g., a cough drop)

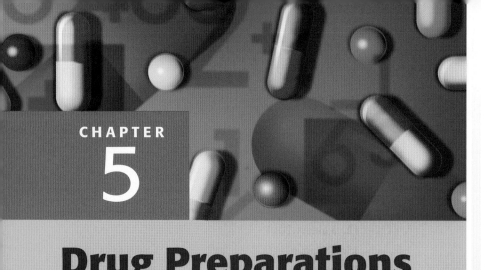

CHAPTER
5

Drug Preparations and Equipment to Measure Doses

Drugs are manufactured in different forms for oral, parenteral, and topical administration. This chapter focuses on the more common drug preparations used in the clinical area and on the equipment that nurses use to prepare accurate doses. (For more information on medication administration, see Chapter 13.)

Drug Preparations

Oral Route

Oral drug forms are generally the easiest for the patient to take and the most convenient for the nurse to administer.

Tablets

- Tablets are made from powdered drugs that have been compressed or molded into solid shapes.
- Tablets may contain ingredients that bind the powder or aid in its gastrointestinal absorption (Fig. 5-1A).
- For a patient who has difficulty swallowing, you can crush plain tablets for oral administration. Several types of pill or tablet crushers are available.

Scored Tablets

- Scored tablets contain a line across the centre, so you can easily break them into two halves.
- Do not break *unscored* tablets, because you can't be certain that the drug is evenly distributed (see Fig. 5-1A).
- When in doubt about whether it's okay to break a tablet, check with the pharmacist.

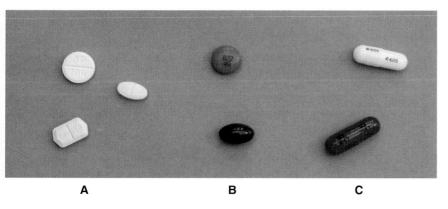

FIGURE 5-1
(**A**) Tablets that may be crushed or broken on the scored line. (**B**) Tablets that may not be crushed. (**C**) Capsules. (© 2004 Lacey-Bordeaux Photography.)

Coated Tablets

- The coating makes these tablets smooth and easy to swallow.
- If necessary, you can crush some coated tablets.
- When in doubt about whether it's okay to break a coated tablet, check with the pharmacist.

Enteric-coated Tablets

- The enteric coating on these tablets protects the drug from being inactivated in the stomach. It also reduces the chance that the drug will irritate the gastric mucosa.
- Enteric-coated tablets dissolve in the more alkaline secretions of the intestine, rather than in the highly acidic stomach juices.
- Do not crush enteric-coated tablets (Fig. 5-1B).

Prolonged-release or Extended-release Tablets

- These tablets come in three types, with these abbreviations: XL, for extended length; CD, for controlled dose; SR, for sustained release.
- All three types disintegrate more slowly and have a longer duration of action than other tablets.
- With these tablets, a patient needs fewer doses: only one or two tablets each day.
- Do not crush prolonged-release tablets.

Sublingual Tablets

- Placed under the tongue, these tablets dissolve quickly.
- The patient absorbs the medication through the capillaries, so it reaches the patient's circulation without passing through the gastrointestinal tract.

Coded Tablets

- These tablets are easy to identify, because on their surface you can see either a number, a letter, or both (Fig. 5-1).

Capsules

- Capsules are gelatin containers that hold a drug in solid or liquid form.
- Avoid opening capsules. The drug is encased in the capsule for a good reason—possibly because contact with gastric juices will decrease the drug's potency or because the drug could irritate the stomach lining.

- Occasionally, if a patient has difficulty swallowing, you may open a capsule and combine its contents with a semisolid such as applesauce or custard. *But be sure to take these precautions:*
  - Before deciding to mix a capsule's contents into food, *always check with the pharmacist* to find out whether the drug is available as a liquid or whether an alternative drug exists (Fig. 5-1C).
  - Do not open capsules called *spansule, timespan, time release,* or *sustained release.* They are long-acting, and contain particles of the drug that are coated to dissolve at different times.

Lozenges

- These are small, solid tablets with medication.
- They dissolve slowly in the mouth.
- Many contain sugar or syrup and may be contraindicated (inappropriate) for patients with diabetes mellitus.
- They are often used for throat irritation.

Syrups

- Syrups are solutions of sugar in water, which disguise the medication's unpleasant taste.
- Because of the sugar they contain, syrups may be contraindicated for patients with diabetes mellitus.

Elixirs

- Elixirs are clear hydroalcoholic liquids that are sweetened.
- They may be contraindicated for patients with a history of alcoholism or diabetes mellitus.

Fluidextracts and Tinctures

- Fluidextracts and tinctures are alcoholic, liquid concentrations of a drug.
- Because these are very potent, they are ordered in small amounts.
- Tinctures are ordered in drops.
- Fluidextracts are the most concentrated of all liquids. The average dose of a fluidextract is 10 mL or less.

Solutions

- Solutions are clear liquids that contain a drug dissolved in water.

Suspensions

- A suspension consists of solid particles of a drug, dispersed in a liquid.
- Because the particles settle to the bottom of the container upon standing, you must resuspend them to obtain an accurate dose.
- Therefore, before you pour any oral preparation, be sure to shake the bottle.

Magmas

- Magmas—for example, milk of magnesia—contain large, bulky particles.

Gels

- Gels—for example, magnesium hydroxide gel—contain small particles.

Emulsions

- Emulsions are creamy, white suspensions of fats or oils in an agent that reduces surface tension and thus makes the oil easier to swallow—for example, emulsified castor oil.

Powders

- Powders are dry, finely ground drugs, reconstituted according to directions.
- Oral antibiotics are frequently supplied as powders.
- In liquid form, powders become oral suspensions.
- Powders must be dissolved according to the manufacturer's instructions.
- When you reconstitute a powder, write these four facts on the label: the date, the time, your initials, and the solution you made.

Parenteral Route

The term *parenteral* does not actually indicate a specific route; rather, it's a general term meaning "by injection." The drug forms for parenteral administration include solutions, suspensions, and powders (as defined above). These are four common parenteral routes:

- ID (intradermal)
- Sub Q (subcutaneous)
- IM (intramuscular)
- IV (intravenous) and IVPB (intravenous piggyback)

Drug forms for parenteral use are sterile. To prepare and administer them, you need to use aseptic technique.

Topical Route

These are the commonly ordered preparations:

Aerosol Powders or Liquids

- Combined with a propellant, these are sprayed onto the skin.
- In nebulizers and inhalers, these are used in the mucous membranes of the respiratory tract.

Powders

- Powders, in dry form, may be applied to the skin.

Creams

- Creams are semisolid drug preparations.
- You can apply them externally to the skin or mucous membranes.
- Vaginal creams use a special applicator for insertion.

Ointments

- Ointments are semisolid preparations in a petroleum or lanolin base for topical use.
- Ointments used for the eye must be labelled "ophthalmic."

Pastes

- Pastes are thick ointments used to protect the skin.
- They absorb secretions and soften the skin.

Suppositories

- Suppositories are medication molded together with a firm base, such as cocoa butter, that melts at body temperature.
- They are shaped for insertion into the rectum, the vagina, and less commonly, the urethra.

Transdermal Medications

- These medications consist of drug molecules contained in a unique polymer patch that is applied to the skin just like an ordinary plastic bandage.
- Easy to apply, the patch is effective for hours or days at a time, because it is slowly released and absorbed through the skin.

Topical Drops (eye drops, nose drops, ear drops)

- These are water or saline drops.
- Medication is added for specific conditions.
- They are used in topical treatment of eyes, ears, or nose.
- Specific techniques are used for administration.

The health provider's orders will indicate whether the topical medication should be applied to the skin, eye, ear, nose, vagina, or rectum.

SELF TEST 1 Terms

Match Column A with the letters in Column B to identify the meaning of the terms used for drug preparations. For correct answers, see the end of the chapter.

Column A

1. _____ Scored tablet
2. _____ Enteric coated
3. _____ Spansule
4. _____ Sublingual tablet
5. _____ Capsule
6. _____ Syrup
7. _____ Elixir
8. _____ Fluidextract
9. _____ Tincture
10. _____ Magma
11. _____ Gel
12. _____ Topical
13. _____ Suppository

Column B

a. Coated drug particles dissolve at different times

b. The most concentrated of all liquids

c. Hydroalcoholic liquid ordered in drops

d. Large particles suspended in a liquid

e. A solid that can be broken in half

f. Route applied to skin or mucous membrane

g. Small particles suspended in a liquid

h. Medication that dissolves under the tongue

i. Gelatin containers for a solid or liquid drug

j. Molded solid inserted into the rectum

k. Drug dissolves in the more alkaline secretions of the intestine

l. Sweetened hydroalcoholic liquid

m. Solution of sugar in water to improve the taste of a drug

Equipment to Measure Doses

Solids for oral administration come in tablets and capsules. Once you calculate the number to give, you pour the amount needed into a small container or cup and then discard the container after you've given the medication.

Liquids may be prepared as unit doses, ready for you to administer, or they may be stored in stock bottles, thus requiring calculation and measurement. Two practices will help you measure liquids accurately:

1. Pour liquids to a line. Never estimate a dose between two lines.

2. Pour liquids at eye level and on a flat surface (Fig. 5-2). The surface of the liquid has a natural curve called the meniscus. At eye level, the centre of the curve should be on the measurement line, while the fluid at the sides of the container will appear to be above the line (Fig. 5-3).

To measure liquids, nurses typically use a medicine cup or a syringe.

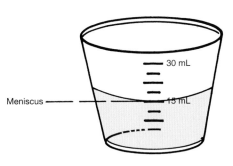

FIGURE 5-2

Liquids are poured at eye level. (Used with permission from Evans-Smith, P. [2005]. *Taylor's clinical nursing skills*. Philadelphia: Lippincott Williams & Wilkins, p. 117.)

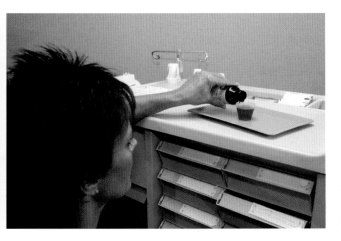

FIGURE 5-3

When viewing the liquid from eye level, the meniscus (lower curve of the fluid) should be on the line.

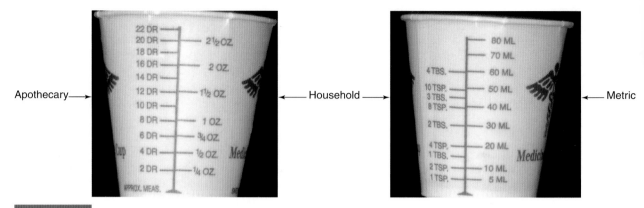

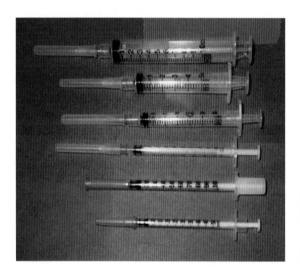

FIGURE 5-4

A medicine cup showing apothecary, household, and metric dose units. (© 2004 Lacey-Bordeaux Photography.)

Medicine Cup

The medicine cup is a disposable container—made of plastic or paper—with markings that show equivalent measures for metric doses in millilitres, for apothecary doses in drams, and for household doses in tablespoons and teaspoons (Fig. 5-4).

Syringes

Nurses use several different types of syringes to prepare routine parenteral doses. Each one serves a different purpose (Fig. 5-5).

Here are explanations for four types: the 3-mL syringe, the 1-mL syringe, and the insulin syringe—either the 100-units insulin syringe or low-dose 50-units insulin syringe.

FIGURE 5-5

(*Top to bottom*) 12-mL syringe, 6-mL syringe, 3-mL syringe, 1-mL syringe (often called a *tuberculin syringe*), insulin 100-units syringe, and insulin 50-units syringe.

SYRINGE. The syringe shown in Figure 5-6 is routinely used for injections. It has a 22-gauge needle, and the needle is 1½ inches long. The term *gauge* indicates the diameter (width) of the needle.

How to use a 3-mL syringe:

- The markings on one side are in mL to the nearest tenth. Each line indicates 0.1 mL.

- When you're preparing a dose, hold the syringe with the needle up, and draw down the medication into the barrel. Suppose you're preparing a dose calculated to be 1.1 mL. Looking at Figure 5-6, count the lines to reach the correct dose.

The 3-mL syringe shows markings for 0.7 mL and 0.8 mL. What would you do if a dosage answer were 0.75 mL? Although you must not approximate doses between lines, you can handle the problem in two other ways.

1st way: Round off 0.75 mL to the nearest tenth. The answer would be 0.8 mL, which can be drawn up to a line. (For details about rounding off numbers, see Chapter 1 and also later in this chapter.)

2nd way: Instead, use a *precision syringe,* which shows markings to the nearest hundredth.

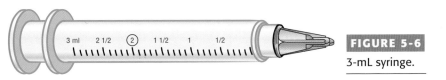

FIGURE 5-6

3-mL syringe.

SELF TEST 2 **3-mL Syringe Amounts**

Use an arrow to indicate these amounts on the 3-mL syringe in Figure 5-6. Check your answers at the end of this chapter.

0.3 mL

1.2 mL

½ mL

2.7 mL

PRECISION SYRINGE. The 1-mL precision syringe has a 25-gauge needle that is ⅝-inch long. Of all the syringes nurses use, this one is the most accurate. It is sometimes called a tuberculin syringe. This syringe is marked in hundredths of a millilitre (Fig. 5-7).

How to use a 1-mL precision syringe:
The markings on one side are in minims. There is a short line between each half minim, and a long line indicating a whole minim.

- Markings are in millilitres. There are nine lines before 0.10. Each line is 0.01 mL.

- To prepare an injection, hold the syringe with the needle up, then draw down the medication into the barrel. Suppose you're preparing a dose calculated to be 0.25 mL. Looking at Figure 5-7, count the lines to reach the dose.

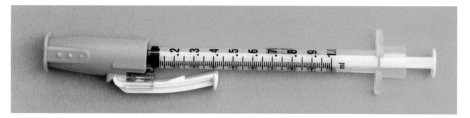

SELF TEST 3   1-mL Syringe Amounts

Use arrows to mark the following doses on the 1-mL precision syringe in Figure 5-7. Check your answers at the end of this chapter.

0.3 mL

0.45 mL

0.61 mL

0.95 mL

Rounding Off Numbers in Liquid Dosage Answers

When you're solving liquid injection problems, the answers are in millilitres. Sometimes the answer is not an even number—and if so, you must decide the degree of accuracy you can obtain. The degree of accuracy depends on the syringe you choose for giving the dose.

RULE   **ROUNDING OFF NUMBERS**

1. **When the last number is 5 or more, add 1 to the previous number.**
2. **When the number is 4 or less, drop the number.**

Example

0.864 becomes 0.86	4.562 becomes 4.56
1.55 becomes 1.6	2.38 becomes 2.4
0.33 becomes 0.3	0.25 becomes 0.3

If you're using the 3-mL syringe, carry out decimals two places and then round off to the nearest tenth for millilitres.

If you're using the 1-mL precision syringe, carry out decimals three places and then round off to the nearest hundredth for millilitres.

Note: Pediatric dosing may not use rounding, because these young patients need the exact dose. Always check with institutional policy and use correct pediatric equipment.

SELF TEST 4 3-mL Syringe—Rounding Answers

The following are possible answers to dosage problems that require use of a 3-mL syringe. Put a check (✓) next to the answer if it is acceptable. If it is not acceptable, change the answer to a correct form. Check your answers at the end of this chapter.

a. 0.1 mL _____

b. 1½ mL _____

c. 0.83 mL _____

d. 0.2 mL _____

e. 1.7 mL _____

f. ½ mL _____

g. 0.4 mL _____

h. 0.65 mL _____

SELF TEST 5 1-mL Syringe—Rounding Answers

The following are possible answers to dosage problems that require the use of a 1-mL precision syringe. Put a check (✓) next to the answer if it is acceptable. If not acceptable, change the answer to a correct form. Check your answers at the end of this chapter.

a. 0.65 mL _____

b. 0.04 mL _____

c. 0.346 mL _____

d. 0.290 mL _____

e. 0.758 mL _____

FIGURE 5-8

A 1-mL insulin syringe (© 2004 Lacey-Bordeaux Photography.)

INSULIN SYRINGE. The 1-mL syringe (100-units) is marked in *units* rather than in millilitres. Use it only to prepare insulin. The physician or healthcare provider orders the type of insulin, the strength of insulin, and the number of units (Fig. 5-8).

Example Order: 20 units NPH insulin every day subcutaneous.

Look at Figure 5-8. Between every 10 units, you'll see four short lines. These markings indicate that each line equals 2 units on this syringe. *Always check the markings on a syringe to be certain you understand what each line equals.*

Example Order: 20 units NPH (unit-100) insulin every morning subcutaneous.

To prepare this injection, hold the syringe with the needle up, then draw 20 units of insulin into the barrel.

For odd-numbered insulin doses, do not use the syringe in Figure 5-8. Instead use a low-dose insulin syringe. Make sure the doses are exact, not approximate.

SELF TEST 6 1-mL Insulin Syringe

Use arrows on the insulin syringe in Figure 5-8 to indicate the following amounts. Check your answers at the end of this chapter.

22 units

34 units

50 units

LOW-DOSE INSULIN SYRINGE. The low-dose 50-units insulin syringe has a 28-gauge needle that is ½-inch long (Fig. 5-9). Notice that between every 5 units, the syringe shows four short lines. These markings indicate that each line equals 1 unit. The syringe is marked for 50-units, so you can use this syringe to draw up any dose of insulin up to 50 units.

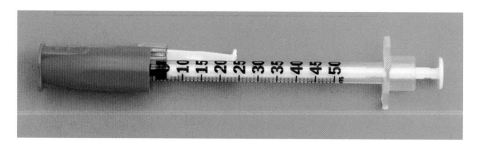

FIGURE 5-9

A ½-mL (low-dose) insulin syringe for 50 units or less. (© 2004 Lacey-Bordeaux Photography.)

SELF TEST 7 0.5-mL Insulin Syringe

Use arrows on the insulin syringe in Figure 5-9 to indicate the following amounts. Answers are given at the end of this chapter.

33 units

12 units

40 units

Needles for Intramuscular and Subcutaneous Injections

Each of the four syringes described above has a different injection needle.

Syringe	Gauge	Length, in.
3 mL	22	1½–3
1 mL	25	⅝–⅞
1 mL insulin	25–26	½–⅝
½ mL low-dose insulin	25–28	½–⅝

The term *gauge* (G) indicates the needle's diameter or width. The higher the gauge number, the finer or smaller the needle's diameter. In the gauges directly above, the low-dose insulin syringe needle has the smallest diameter (28 gauge), which makes it the finest needle in this group. A 16-gauge needle, used to transfuse blood cells, would be very wide and would have a wide opening.

The length of the needle you use depends on the route of injection. For deep intramuscular injections, you use a long needle. For subcutaneous injections, you use a short needle.

Choosing which type of needle to use for an adult or a child depends on three factors: the route of administration, the size and condition of the patient, and the amount of adipose tissue present at the site (Fig. 5-10).

Most hospitals use needleless systems to draw up parenteral medications and for intravenous therapy (Fig. 5-11). This helps to prevent accidental needle-sticks.

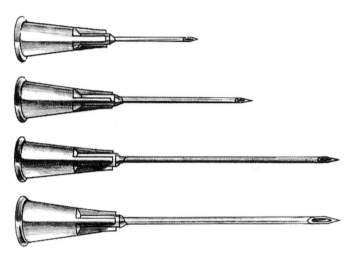

Needles usually used for **intradermal** injections are ⅜" to ⅝" (1 to 1.5 cm) long and are 25G. Such needles usually have short bevels.

Needles for **subcutaneous** injections are ⅝" to ⅞" (1.5 to 2 cm) long, have medium bevels, and are 25G to 23G.

Needles for **intramuscular** use are 1" to 3" (2.5 to 7.5 cm) long, have medium bevels, and are 23G to 18G.

Needles for **intravenous** use are 1" to 3" long, have long bevels, and are 25G to 14G.

FIGURE 5-10

When choosing a needle, the nurse must consider the needle gauge, bevel, and length. Gauge refers to the inside diameter of the needle; the smaller the gauge, the larger the diameter. Bevel refers to the angle at which the needle tip is opened. Length is the distance from the tip to the hub of the needle.

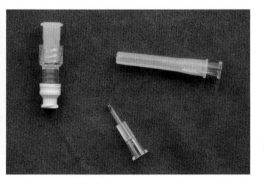

FIGURE 5-11

Needleless system. (Copyright © 2008 Lacey-Bordeaux Photography.)

PROFICIENCY TEST 1 Drug Preparations and Equipment

Name: _____

Complete these statements. See Appendix A for answers.

1. Elixirs may be contraindicated for patients with a history of _____

   or _____

2. The average dose of a fluidextract is _____

3. In giving medications parenterally, four common routes are _____ ,

   _____ , _____ , and _____

4. When a powder is reconstituted, what four facts must the nurse write on the label?

   a. _____

   b. _____

   c. _____

   d. _____

5. What route(s) require(s) aseptic technique in preparing and administering drugs?

   _____

6. An example of a drug listed as a magma is _____

7. What must you always do before pouring an oral suspension?

   _____

8. List six drug preparations that can be administered topically.

   _____   _____

   _____   _____

   _____   _____

9. List two advantages in using transdermal medications.

   _____

   _____

10. Define an ointment. _____

    _____

11. List two practices that help you pour oral liquids accurately.

    a. _____

    b. _____

12. Define the following:

    a. Meniscus _____

    _____

    b. Needle gauge _____

    _____

(continued)

13. What factors determine the needle length chosen for an injection?

_____

_____

_____

14. List two rules for rounding off numbers.

   a. _____

       _____

   b. _____

       _____

15. What determines how dosage answers are rounded off?

_____

_____

_____

Answers to Self Tests

Self Test 1 Terms

1. e	**5.** i	**8.** b	**11.** g
2. k	**6.** m	**9.** c	**12.** f
3. a	**7.** l	**10.** d	**13.** j
4. h			

Self Test 2 3-mL Syringe Amounts

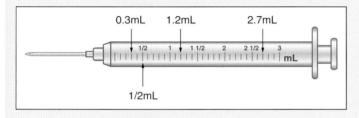

Self Test 3 1-mL Syringe Amounts

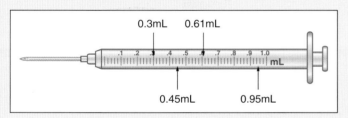

Self Test 4 3-mL Syringe—Rounding Answers

a. 0.1 mL ✓	**d.** 0.2 mL ✓	**g.** 0.4 mL ✓
b. 1½ mL ✓	**e.** 1.7 mL ✓	**h.** 0.65 mL 0.7 mL
c. 0.83 mL 0.8 mL	**f.** ½ mL ✓	

Self Test 5 1-mL Syringe—Rounding Answers

a. 0.65 mL ✓	**d.** 0.290 mL 0.29 mL
b. 0.04 mL ✓	**e.** 0.758 mL 0.76 mL
c. 0.346 mL 0.35 mL	

Self Test 6 1-mL Insulin Syringe

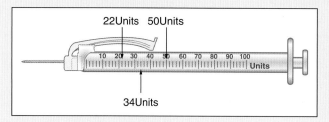

Self Test 7 0.5-mL Insulin Syringe

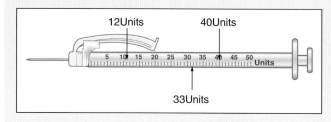

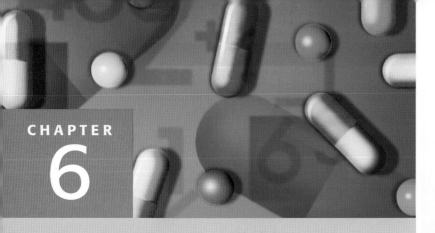

LEARNING OBJECTIVES

1. Using proportion expressed as two ratios

2. Using proportion expressed as two fractions

3. Using the formula method

4. Converting order and supply to the same weight measure

5. Clearing decimal points before solving a problem

6. Using equivalents when conversions are needed

7. Interpreting special types of oral solid and liquid orders that do not require calculation

CHAPTER 6

Calculation of Oral Medications— Solids and Liquids

Drugs for oral administration are prepared by pharmaceutical companies as solids (tablets, capsules) and liquids. When the dose ordered by the physician or healthcare provider differs from the supply, the nurse calculates the amount to give the patient. The calculations can be solved in several ways. This chapter shows how to do the math in three ways: by two ratios, two fractions, and the formula method. Chapter 11 shows another way: dimensional analysis.

In dosage calculations, you start with three pieces of information:

1. The doctor's or healthcare provider's order

2. The quantity or strength of drug on hand

3. The solid or liquid form of the supply drug (i.e., the form the drug arrives in)

The unknown is the amount of drug to administer, usually designated as X or x. These letters represent the above information:

    D = desired dose (order)

    H = on hand or have

    S = supply

    X or x = unknown or answer (amount of drug to give)

Proportions Expressed as Two Fractions

Using fractions, set up proportions so that like units are across from each other (the units and the numerators match and the units and denominators match). The first fraction is the known equivalent.

| Example | To express "One tablet is equal to 50 mg" write $\dfrac{1 \text{ tablet}}{50 \text{ mg}}$ |

The second fraction is the unknown, the desired (ordered) dose. Example: x tablets is equal to 100 mg, written as $\dfrac{\text{x tablets}}{100 \text{ mg}}$

The completed proportion looks like

$$\frac{S}{H} = \frac{x}{D} \left(\frac{\text{Supply}}{\text{Have}} = \frac{x}{\text{Desire}} \right)$$

For the previous example, it would look like this: $\dfrac{1 \text{ tablet}}{50 \text{ mg}} = \dfrac{\text{x tablets}}{100 \text{ mg}}$

Next, solve for x. (For a review of how to solve proportions, refer to Chapter 1.) In our current example, solving for x follows this process:

1. $\dfrac{1 \text{ tablet}}{50 \text{ mg}} = \dfrac{\text{x tablets}}{100 \text{ mg}}$

   $\dfrac{1 \text{ tablet}}{50 \text{ mg}} \diagdown \dfrac{\text{x tablets}}{100 \text{ mg}}$

   $100 \times 1 = 50\text{x}$

2. $\dfrac{100 \times 1}{50} = \text{x}$

3. $\dfrac{100}{50} = \text{x}$

Answer: 2 tablets = x

Proportions Expressed as Two Ratios

You can set up a ratio by using colons. Double colons separate the two ratios. The first ratio is the known equivalent; the second ratio is the desired (ordered) dose, the unknown. The ratio must always follow the same sequence.

The ratio will look like this:

S : H : : x : D   Supply : Have : : x : Desire

For the previous example, your ratio would look like this:

1 tablet : 50 mg : : x : 100 mg

Next, solve for x. (For a review of how to solve ratios, refer to Chapter 1.)

1. 1 tablet : 50 mg : : x : 100 mg

2. $1 \times 100 = 50x$

3. $\dfrac{100}{50} = \dfrac{50\,x}{50}$

4. $\dfrac{100}{50} = x$

Answer: 2 tablets = x

Formula Method

The formula method is simpler than either of the above methods. Here's how the formula method is set up:

$$\frac{D}{H} \times S = x \qquad \frac{\text{Desire}}{\text{Have}} \times \text{Supply} = x$$

Using a formula eliminates the need for cross-multiplying, a potential source of error in calculation. When you use this method with oral solids, the supply is typically either 1 tablet or 1 capsule.

For the purposes of this book, we'll use these three methods—the formula method, the proportion method expressed as two fractions, and the proportion method expressed as two ratios. You just need to see which method makes the most sense to you, then learn it thoroughly and use it. If you want to look ahead to the method of dimensional analysis, see Chapter 11. Answers for the proficiency tests in each chapter will include our three methods plus dimensional analysis.

Oral Solids

Application of the Rule for Oral Solids

RULE   **FORMULA METHOD**

$$\frac{\textbf{Desire}}{\textbf{Have}} \times \textbf{Supply} = \textbf{x}$$

RULE   **PROPORTION EXPRESSED AS TWO RATIOS**

Supply : Have : : x : Desire

RULE   **PROPORTION EXPRESSED AS TWO FRACTIONS**

$$\frac{\textbf{Supply}}{\textbf{Have}} = \frac{\textbf{x}}{\textbf{Desire}}$$

Example   Order: APO-CAPTO (captopril) 6.25 mg po bid

Supply: Read the label

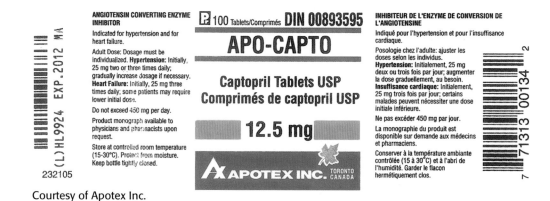

Courtesy of Apotex Inc.

Desire: The order. In this example, desired is 6.25 mg.

Have: The strength of the drug supplied in the container. In the example, the label says that each tablet contains 12.5 mg.

Supply: The unit form in which the drug comes. APO-CAPTO comes in tablet form. Because tablets and capsules are single entities, the supply for oral solid drugs is always one.

Amount: How much supply to give. For oral solids, the answer will be the number of tablets or capsules to administer.

When you're solving any problem, first check that the order and the supply are in the same weight measure. If they are not, you must convert one or the other amount to its equivalent. In this example, no equivalent is needed; both the order and the supply are in milligrams.

Example   Desire: APO-CAPTO (captopril) 6.25 mg po

Have: 12.5 mg

Supply: 1 tablet

RULE   **FORMULA METHOD**

$$\frac{D}{H} \times S = x$$

$$\frac{1}{2} \frac{6.25 \text{ mg}}{12.5 \text{ mg}} \times 1 \text{ tablet} = x$$

$$\frac{1}{2} \text{ tablet} = x$$

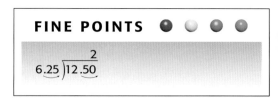

FINE POINTS ● ○ ● ●

$$6.25 \overline{\smash{)}12.50} 2$$

RULE   **PROPORTION EXPRESSED AS TWO RATIOS**

S : H : : x : D

1 tablet : 12.5 mg : : x : 6.25 mg

6.25 × 1 = 12.5x

$$\frac{6.25}{12.5} = x$$

$\frac{1}{2}$ **tablet = x**

RULE   **PROPORTION EXPRESSED AS TWO FRACTIONS**

$$\frac{S}{H} = \frac{x}{\textbf{Desire}}$$

$$\frac{\textbf{1 tablet}}{\textbf{12.5 mg}} \times \frac{x}{\textbf{6.25 mg}}$$

6.25 × 1 = 12.5x

$$\frac{6.25}{12.5} = x$$

$\frac{1}{2}$ **tablet = x**

> **FINE POINTS**
>
> Note that the ratio and proportion methods end with the same equation—in this case,
>
> $$\frac{6.25}{12.5} = x$$
>
> When illustrating these two methods, one combined final equation will be shown.

Clearing Decimals When Using the Formula Method

When the numerator and denominator in $\frac{D}{H}$ are decimals, add zeros to make the number of decimal places the same. Then drop the decimal points. This short arithmetic operation replaces long division:

$$\frac{\overset{\text{added}}{\downarrow}}{0.5\underset{\frown}{0}\text{mg}} \quad \text{numerator}$$
$$\overline{0.2\underset{\frown}{5}\text{mg}} \quad \text{denominator or divisor}$$

In division, you must clear the denominator (divisor) of decimal points before you can carry out the arithmetic. Then you move the decimal point in the numerator the same number of places. (For further help in dividing decimals, refer to Chapter 1.)

Example

Order: Lanoxin (digoxin) 0.125 mg po every day

Supply: Read the label

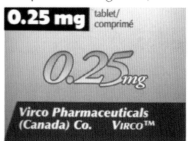

DIN 0224 2323

250 TABLETS COMPRIMÉS

Pr

Lanoxin®

Digoxin Tablets, C.S.D.
Comprimés de digoxine, D.N.C.

0.25 mg tablet/comprimé

0.25 mg

Virco Pharmaceuticals
(Canada) Co. VIRCO™

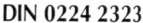

Courtesy of Virco Pharmaceuticals (Canada) Co.

No equivalent is needed. It is stated on the label: 0.25 mg.

Formula Method	*Proportion Expressed as Two Ratios*	*Proportion Expressed as Two Fractions*
$\dfrac{\overset{1}{\cancel{0.125}} \text{ mg}}{\underset{2}{\cancel{0.250}} \text{ mg}} \times 1 \text{ tablet} = \dfrac{1}{2} \text{ tablet}$	1 tablet : 0.25 mg :: x : 0.125 mg	$\dfrac{1 \text{ tablet}}{0.25 \text{ mg}} \times \dfrac{\text{x}}{0.125 \text{ mg}}$

$$0.125 = 0.25x$$

$$\dfrac{\overset{1}{\cancel{0.125}} \text{ mg}}{\underset{2}{\cancel{0.250}} \text{ mg}} = x$$

$$\tfrac{1}{2} \text{ tablet} = x$$

Example

Order: Valtrex (valacyclovir) 1 g po q6h

Supply: 1 caplet equals 500 mg

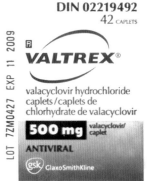

DIN 02219492

42 CAPLETS

Pr

VALTREX®

valacyclovir hydrochloride
caplets/caplets de
chlorhydrate de valacyclovir

500 mg valacyclovir/caplet

ANTIVIRAL

gsk GlaxoSmithKline

LOT 7ZM0427 EXP 11 2009

ADULT DOSAGE: Herpes Zoster: 1000 mg three times daily for 7 days. **Herpes Labialis:** 2000 mg twice daily for 1 day. **Genital Herpes: Initial Episode:** 1000 mg twice daily for 10 days. **Recurrences:** 500 mg twice daily for 3 days. **Suppression:** 500 or 1000 mg once daily based on number of recurrences per year, or 500 mg twice daily in HIV infected patients. **Reduction of Transmission:** 500 mg once daily. Safety and efficacy in children have not been adequately studied. Product Monograph available to physicians and pharmacists on request. Store between 15° C and 30° C. Protect from light. **PHARMACIST:** Dispense with patient leaflet provided to you.

POSOLOGIE – ADULTES : Zona : 1000 mg 3 fois par jour pendant 7 jours. **Herpès labial :** 2 000 mg 2 fois par jour pendant 1 journée. **Herpès génital : Épisode initial :** 1 000 mg 2 fois par jour pendant 10 jours. **Récurrences :** 500 mg 2 fois par jour pendant 3 jours. **Suppression :** 500 ou 1 000 mg 1 fois par jour selon le nombre de récurrences par année, ou 500 mg 2 fois par jour chez les patients infectés par le VIH. **Réduction de la transmission :** 500 mg 1 fois par jour. L'innocuité et l'efficacité chez l'enfant n'ont pas été établies. Monographie du produit fournie sur demande aux médecins et aux pharmaciens. Conserver à une température de 15 à 30 °C, à l'abri de la lumière. **PHARMACIEN :** Remettre au patient le feuillet de renseignements fourni.

® GlaxoSmithKline Inc., licensee / licencié

GlaxoSmithKline Inc.
Mississauga, Ontario
Montreal, Quebec

A013293

Courtesy of GlaxoSmithKline.

Equivalent: 1 g = 1000 mg

Formula Method	Proportion Expressed as Two Ratios	Proportion Expressed as Two Fractions
$\dfrac{\overset{2}{\cancel{1000}\ \text{mg}}}{\underset{1}{\cancel{500}\ \text{mg}}} \times 1\ \text{cap} = 2\ \text{caps}$	$1\ \text{cap} : 500\ \text{mg} :: x : 1000\ \text{mg}$	$\dfrac{1}{500\ \text{mg}} \times \dfrac{x}{1000\ \text{mg}}$ $1000 = 500$

$$\frac{1000}{500} = x$$

$$2\ \text{caps} = x$$

Example

Order: Synthroid (levothyroxine) 75 mcg po every day

Supply: Read the label

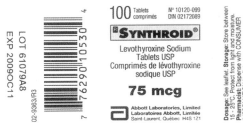

Courtesy of Abbott Laboratories.

75 mcg = 0.075 mg

Because the order and the supply are in the same weight measure, no calculation is necessary. Give 1 tablet.

Example

Order: GlucoNorm (repaglinide) 7.3 mg po every day

Supply: Read the label

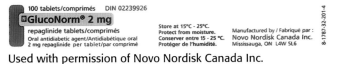

Used with permission of Novo Nordisk Canada Inc.

No equivalent is needed.

Formula Method	Proportion Expressed as Two Ratios	Proportion Expressed as Two Fractions
$\dfrac{\overset{1.5}{\cancel{3}\,mg}}{\underset{1}{\cancel{2}\,mg}} \times 1\ tablet$ $= 1\frac{1}{2}\ tablets$	$1\ tablet : 2\ mg :: x : 3\ mg$	$\dfrac{1\ tablet}{2\ mg} \times \dfrac{x}{3\ mg}$ $3 = 2x$ $\dfrac{3}{2} = x$ $1\frac{1}{2}\ tablets = x$

Because the supply is scored, you can administer $1\frac{1}{2}$ tablets.

Example   Order: Bonefos (clodronate disodium) 800 mg po bid

Supply: Read the label

Chaque capsule de gélatine dure contient : 400 mg de clodronate disodique anhydre (sous forme de tétrahydrate).
POSOLOGIE CHEZ L'ADULTE :
Hypercalcémie néoplasique : À la suite d'un traitement intraveineux, la dose orale d'entretien quotidienne recommandée se situe entre 1600 mg et 2400 mg (4 à 6 capsules) administrés en 1 ou 2 prises. La dose quotidienne maximale recommandée est de 3200 mg (8 capsules).
Métastases osseuses ostéolytiques d'origine tumorale : La dose de départ recommandée est de 1600 mg/jour. Cette dose peut être augmentée; toutefois, la dose quotidienne ne devrait pas dépasser 3200 mg.
Réduire la dose chez les patients atteints d'insuffisance rénale grave.
Voir le dépliant pour des instructions détaillées.
Conserver entre 15 et 30 °C.
* Bayer et la croix Bayer sont des marques déposées de Bayer AG, Bonefos est une marque déposée, utilisées sous licence par Bayer Inc. Monographie fournie sur demande.

LOT 73390A
EXP. 11SE

DIN 01984845

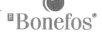

®Bonefos®

Clodronate disodium capsules / Capsules de clodronate disodique

400 mg

Bone metabolism regulator / Régulateur du métabolisme osseux

120 capsules

Each hard gelatin capsule contains: 400 mg of anhydrous clodronate disodium (as the tetrahydrate).
ADULT DOSAGE:
Hypercalcemia due to malignancy: Following intravenous therapy, the oral recommended daily maintenance dose is in the range of 1600 mg to 2400 mg (4 to 6 capsules) given in single or 2 divided doses. Maximum recommended daily dose is 3200 mg (8 capsules).
Osteolytic bone metastases due to malignancy: The recommended starting dose is 1600 mg/day. The dose may be increased, however the daily dose should not exceed 3200 mg.
Reduce dose in patients with severe renal impairment.
See package insert for detailed directions.
Store between 15°C and 30°C.
*Bayer and Bayer Cross are registered trademarks of Bayer AG, Bonefos is a registered trademark, used under license by Bayer Inc. Product Monograph available on request.

Bayer Inc.
Toronto, ON M9W 1G6
www.bayer.ca

80362545

Courtesy of Bayer.

No equivalent is needed.

Formula Method	Proportion Expressed as Two Ratios	Proportion Expressed as Two Fractions
$\dfrac{\overset{2}{\cancel{800}} \text{ mg}}{\underset{1}{\cancel{400}} \text{ mg}} \times 1 \text{ cap} = 2 \text{ tablets}$	$1 \text{ tablet} : 400 \text{ mg} :: x : 800 \text{ mg}$	$\dfrac{1 \text{ cap}}{400 \text{ mg}} \times \dfrac{x}{800 \text{ mg}}$

$$800 = 400x$$

$$\frac{800}{400} = x$$

$$2 \text{ caps} = x$$

Example Order: OxyContin (oxycodone) 80 mg po every 12 hours

Supply: Read the label

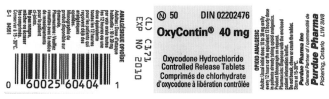

Courtesy of Purdue Pharma.

No equivalent is needed.

Formula Method	Proportion Expressed as Two Ratios	Proportion Expressed as Two Fractions
$\dfrac{\overset{2}{\cancel{80}} \text{ mg}}{\underset{1}{\cancel{40}} \text{ mg}} \times 1 \text{ tablet} = 2 \text{ tablets}$	$1 \text{ tablet} : 40 \text{ mg} :: x : 80 \text{ mg}$	$\dfrac{1 \text{ tablet}}{40 \text{ mg}} \times \dfrac{x}{80 \text{ mg}}$

$$80 = 40x$$

$$\frac{80}{40} = x$$

$$2 \text{ tablets} = x$$

Give 2 tablets.

| **Example** | Order: Lipitor (atorvastatin calcium) 20 mg po every day |
| | Supply: Read the label |

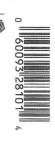 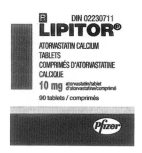

Courtesy of Pfizer Co.

Formula Method	**Proportion Expressed as Two Ratios**	**Proportion Expressed as Two Fractions**
$\dfrac{\overset{2}{\cancel{20}} \text{ mg}}{\underset{1}{\cancel{10}} \text{ mg}} \times 1 \text{ tablet} = 2 \text{ tablets}$	$1 \text{ tablet} : 10 \text{ mg} :: x : 20 \text{ mg}$	$\dfrac{1 \text{ tablet}}{10 \text{ mg}} \times \dfrac{x}{20 \text{ mg}}$

$$20 = 10x$$

$$\frac{20}{10} = x$$

$$2 \text{ tablets} = x$$

| **Example** | Order: Avapro (irbesartan) 0.3 g po once a day |
| | Supply: Read the label |

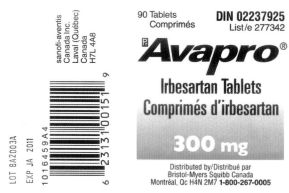

Courtesy of Bristol-Meyers Squibb.

Equivalent: 0.3 g = 300 mg

Formula Method	*Proportion Expressed as Two Ratios*	*Proportion Expressed as Two Fractions*
$\frac{300 \text{ mg}}{300 \text{ mg}} \times 1 \text{ tablet} = 1 \text{ tablet}$	1 tablet : 300 mg : : x : 300 mg	$\frac{1 \text{ tablet}}{300 \text{ mg}} \times \frac{x}{300 \text{ mg}}$

$$300 = 300\,x$$

$$\frac{300}{300} = x$$

$$1 \text{ tablet} = x$$

Example Order: Lyrica (pregabalin) 150 mg po twice a day

Supply: Read the label

 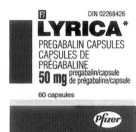 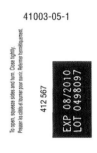

Courtesy of Pfizer.

Formula Method	*Proportion Expressed as Two Ratios*	*Proportion Expressed as Two Fractions*
$\frac{150 \text{ mg}}{50 \text{ mg}} \times 1 \text{ capsule} = 3 \text{ capsules}$	1 cap : 50 mg : : x : 150 mg	$\frac{1 \text{ cap}}{50 \text{ mg}} \times \frac{x}{150 \text{ mg}}$

$$150 = 50\,x$$

$$\frac{150}{50} = x$$

$$3 \text{ capsules} = x$$

SELF TEST 1   Oral Solids

Solve these practice problems. Answers are given at the end of the chapter. Remember the three methods:

Formula Method	Proportion Expressed as Two Ratios	Proportion Expressed as Two Fractions
$\dfrac{D}{H} \times S = x$	$S : H :: x : D$	$\dfrac{S}{H} \times \dfrac{x}{D}$

1. Order: Decadron (phenytoin) 1.5 mg po bid   *2*
   Supply: tablets labelled 0.75 mg

2. Order: Lanoxin (digoxin) 0.25 mg po every day   *1/2*
   Supply: scored tablets labelled 0.5 mg

3. Order: Omnipen (ampicillin) 0.5 g po q6h   *2*
   Supply: capsules labelled 250 mg

4. Order: Deltasone (prednisone) 10 mg po tid   *4*
   Supply: tablets labelled 2.5 mg

5. Order: aspirin 650 mg po stat   *2*
   Supply: tablets labelled 325 mg

6. Order: Procardia (nifedipine) 20 mg po bid   *2*
   Supply: capsules labelled 10 mg

7. Order: Prolixin (fluphenazine) 10 mg po daily   *4*
   Supply: tablets labelled 2.5 mg

8. Order: penicillin G potassium 200,000 units po q8h   *1/2*
   Supply: scored tablets labelled 400,000 units

9. Order: Lanoxin (digoxin) 0.5 mg po every day   *2*
   Supply: scored tablets labelled 0.25 mg

10. Order: Capoten (captopril) 18.75 mg po tid   *1 1/2*
    Supply: scored tablets labelled 12.5 mg

11. Order: Seroquel (quetiapine) 300 mg po bid   *1 1/2*
    Supply: tablets labelled 200 mg

12. Order: Catapres (clonidine) 0.3 mg po hs   *3*
    Supply: tablets labelled 0.1 mg

13. Order: Capoten (captopril) 6.25 mg po bid   *1/4*
    Supply: scored tablets labelled 25 mg

14. Order: Catapres (clonidine) 400 mcg po every day
    Supply: tablets labelled 0.2 mg   *2*

(continued)

SELF TEST 1 Oral Solids *(Continued)*

15. Order: Coumadin (warfarin) 7.5 mg po every day
    Supply: scored tablets labelled 5 mg

16. Order: Micronase (glyburide) 0.625 mg every day
    Supply: scored tablets labelled 1.25 mg

17. Order: Naprosyn (naproxen) 0.5 g po every day   *0.500*
    Supply: scored tablets labelled 250 mg

18. Order: Hydrodiuril (hydrochlorothiazide) 37.5 mg po every day
    Supply: scored tablets labelled 25 mg

19. Order: Keflex (cephalexin) 1 g po q6h
    Supply: capsules labelled 500 mg

20. Order: Lioresal (baclofen) 25 mg po tid   *2.5*
    Supply: scored tablets labelled 10 mg

Special Types of Oral Solid Orders

Drugs that contain a number of active ingredients are ordered by the number to be administered and do not require calculation. Similarly, over-the-counter (OTC) medications are often ordered by how many are to be administered.

Example   *EXAMPLE 1*
Vitamin B_{12} 1 tablet po every day

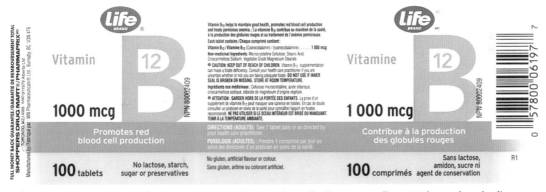

©Shoppers Drug Mart Inc. Shoppers Drug Mart is a trademark of 911979 Alberta Ltd., used under license.

Interpret as: Give 1 tablet by mouth every day.

EXAMPLE 2

Amoxicillin and clavulanate 500 mg/
125 mg tablets

1 tablet every 8 hours po
Interpret as: Give 1 tablet every 8 hours.

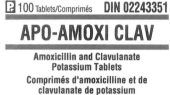
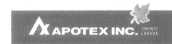

ANTIBIOTIC AND ß-LACTAMASE INHIBITOR

Each tablet contains amoxicillin trihydrate
equivalent to 500 mg of amoxicillin and
clavulanate potassium equivalent to
125 mg of clavulanic acid.

Usual Adult Dosage: 1 tablet every 8 hours.

**Do not substitute two 250/125 mg tablets
for one 500/125 mg tablet. The ratio of
amoxicillin to clavulanic acid is different.**

Product monograph available to physicians
and pharmacists upon request.

Store at room temperature 15–30°C.
Protect from light and humidity.
Keep bottle tightly closed at all times.
Do not remove dessicant.

℗ 100 Tablets/Comprimés   **DIN 02243351**

APO-AMOXI CLAV

**Amoxicillin and Clavulanate
Potassium Tablets**

**Comprimés d'amoxicilline et de
clavulanate de potassium**

Norme Apotex Standard

500/125 mg

⬥**APOTEX INC.** TORONTO CANADA

ANTIBIOTIQUE ET INHIBITEUR DE ß-LACTAMASES

Chaque comprimé contient du trihydrate d'amoxicilline
équivalent à 500 mg d'amoxicilline, et du clavulanate de
potassium équivalent à 125 mg d'acide clavulanique.

Posologie pour adultes: Un comprimé toutes les 8 heures.

**Ne pas remplacer un comprimé 500/125 mg par deux
comprimé 250/125 mg. La proportion de l'amoxicilline
par rapport à l'acide clavulanique est différente.**

La monographie du produit est disponible
sur demande aux médecins et pharmaciens.

Entreposer à la température ambiante
de 15 à 30°C. Protéger de la lumière et
de l'humidité. Tenir le flacon bien fermé
en tout temps. Ne pas enlever
le dessiccatif.

Courtesy of Apotex Inc.

 ## Oral Liquids

For liquids, the three methods are set up just as for oral solids, except the supply will include a liquid
measurement, usually millilitres (mL).

Formula Method	Proportion Expressed as Two Ratios	Proportion Expressed as Two Fractions
$\dfrac{\text{Desire}}{\text{Have}} \times \text{Supply} = \text{Amount (x)}$	Supply : Have : : x : Desire	$\dfrac{\text{Supply}}{\text{Have}} = \dfrac{x}{\text{Desire}}$

Example

Order: Lactulose oral solution 10 g po
every day

Supply: Read the label

Equivalent: 10 g = 10,000 mg

COLONIC CONTENT ACIDIFIER - LAXATIVE

Each mL contains : Lactulose 667 mg

FOR OCCASIONAL USE ONLY

LAXATIVE : Usual Adult dose : 10 to 20 g (15 to 30 mL) per day; dosage
may be increased up to 40 g (60 mL) per day. May be mixed with liquid.

PEDIATRIC : Consult a doctor for pediatric use.

CAUTION : Diabetics should use only on the advice of a physician. Do not
use in the presence of abdominal pain, nausea, fever or vomiting. Overuse
or extended use may cause dependence for bowel function. Do not take
any type of laxative for more than one week unless under the advice of a
physician. A laxative should not be taken within 2 hours of another
medicine because the desired effect of the other medicine may be reduced.

LOT6M39C EXP DE2009

15 mL   **DIN 00703486**

pms-LACTULOSE

Lactulose
Solution
USP

667 mg/mL

**pharma
science**

ACIDIFIANT DU CONTENU
DU CÔLON - LAXATIF

Chaque mL contient : 667 mg de lactulose

POUR USAGE OCCASIONNEL SEULEMENT

LAXATIF : Posologie habituelle (adulte) : 10 à 20 g (15 à
30 mL) par jour; la dose peut être augmentée jusqu'à 40 g
(60 mL) par jour. Peut être mélangé avec du liquide.

PÉDIATRIQUE : Consulter un médecin pour un usage
pédiatrique.

Solution de
Lactulose
USP

Courtesy of Pharmascience.

Formula Method	Proportion Expressed as Two Ratios	Proportion Expressed as Two Fractions
$\dfrac{10000 \text{ mg}}{667 \text{ mg}} \times 1 \text{ mL} = 14.99 \text{ mL}$ $= 15 \text{ mL}$	$1 \text{ mL} : 667 \text{ mg} :: x : 10000 \text{ mg}$	$\dfrac{1 \text{ mL}}{667 \text{ mg}} \times \dfrac{x}{10000 \text{ mg}}$

$$1 \times 10000 = 667x$$

$$\frac{10000}{667} = x$$

$$14.99 = x$$

$$15 \text{ mL} = x$$

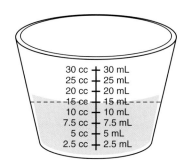

Administer 15 mL of Lactulose everyday.

Before solving each problem, check to be certain that the order and your supply are in the same measure. If they are not, you must convert one or the other to its equivalent. Convert whichever one is easier for you to solve.

Example   Order: Lanoxin (digoxin) 0.375 mg po every day
Supply: Read the label

DIN 111333222   5mL

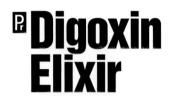
Digoxin
Elixir

Each mL contains **50** mcg
(0.05 mg) digoxin

EXP DEC.2009

No equivalent is needed.

Formula Method	Proportion Expressed as Two Ratios	Proportion Expressed as Two Fractions
$\dfrac{\overset{1.5}{\cancel{0.375}\text{ mg}}}{\underset{1}{\cancel{0.25}\text{ mg}}} \times 5 \text{ mL} = 1.5 \times 5 = 7.5 \text{ mL}$	$5 \text{ mL} : 0.25 \text{ mg} :: x : 0.375 \text{ mg}$	$\dfrac{5 \text{ mL}}{0.25 \text{ mg}} = \dfrac{x}{0.375 \text{ mg}}$

$$5 \times 0.375 = 0.25x$$

$$\frac{1.875}{0.25} = x$$

$$7.5 \text{ mL} = x$$

Use an oral syringe to draw up 7.5 mL.

Example   Order: amoxicillin oral suspension 500 mg po q8h

Supply: Read the label

DIRECTIONS FOR RECONSTITUTION:

For ease in preperations; add water to the bottle in two portions and shake well after each addition.

Add total of **116 mL** water for reconstitution

Each 5 mL = 125 mg amoxiciliin

Usual Adult Dosage: 250–500 mg every 8 hours

Usual Child Dosage:
20–40 mg/kg in divided doses every 8 hrs.

See accompanying prescribing information.

DIN 02262894   150 mL

Pr **Amoxicillin**®
125mg/5mL
Oral Suspension from Powder

Storage: The reconstituted formulation is stable for 14 days under refrigeration (6°c) or 7 days at room temperature (25°c).

DATE / TIME:

INITIALS:

LOT #97103   EXP JUL.2012

Formula Method	*Proportion Expressed as Two Ratios*	*Proportion Expressed as Two Fractions*
$\dfrac{\overset{4}{\cancel{500}}\ mg}{\underset{1}{\cancel{125}}\ mg}\times 5\ mL = 4\times 5 = 20\ mL$	$5\ mL : 125\ mg :: x : 500\ mg$	$\dfrac{5\ mL}{125\ mg}\times\dfrac{x}{500\ mg}$

$$5\times 500 = 125x$$

$$\frac{2500}{125} = x$$

$$20\ mL = x$$

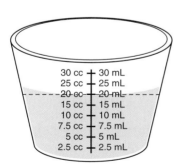

30 cc — 30 mL
25 cc — 25 mL
20 cc — 20 mL
15 cc — 15 mL
10 cc — 10 mL
7.5 cc — 7.5 mL
5 cc — 5 mL
2.5 cc — 2.5 mL

Administer 20 mL of amoxicillin po every 8 hours

SELF TEST 2   Oral Liquids

Solve these oral liquid problems. Answers are given at the end of the chapter.

1. Order: EES (erythromycin) suspension 0.75 g po qid
   Supply: liquid labelled 250 mg/mL

2. Order: ampicillin suspension 500 mg po q8h
   Supply: liquid labelled 250 mg/5 mL

3. Order: Keflex (cephalexin) in oral suspension 0.35 g po q6h
   Supply: liquid labelled 125 mg/5 mL

4. Order: Sandimmune (cyclosporine) 150 mg po stat and every day
   Supply: liquid labelled 100 mg/mL in a bottle with a calibrated dropper

5. Order: Stelazine (trifluoperazine) 5 mg po bid
   Supply: liquid labelled 10 mg/mL

6. Order: Lanoxin (digoxin) 0.02 mg po every day
   Supply: pediatric elixir 0.05 mg/mL in a bottle with a dropper marked in tenths of a millilitre

7. Order: potassium chloride 30 mEq po every day
   Supply: liquid labelled 20 mEq/15 mL

8. Order: Lanoxin (digoxin) elixir 0.25 mg via nasogastric tube every day
   Supply: liquid labelled 0.25 mg/mL

9. Order: Risperdal (risperidone) 3 mg po bid
   Supply: liquid labelled 1 mg/mL

10. Order: Phenergan (promethazine) HCl syrup 12.5 mg po tid
    Supply: liquid labelled 6.25 mg/5 mL

11. Order: Vistaril (hydroxyzine) 50 mg po qid
    Supply: syrup labelled 10 mg per 5 mL

12. Order: Lasix (furosemide) 40 mg po q12h
    Supply: liquid labelled 10 mg/mL

13. Order: potassium chloride 10 mEq po bid
    Supply: liquid labelled 20 mEq/30 mL

14. Order: Compazine (prochlorperazine) 10 mg po tid
    Supply: syrup labelled 5 mg/5 mL

15. Order: phenobarbital 100 mg po hs
    Supply: elixir labelled 20 mg/5 mL

16. Order: Tylenol (acetaminophen) 650 mg po q4h prn
    Supply: elixir labelled 160 mg/5 mL

17. Order: Benadryl (diphenhydramine) 25 mg po q4h
    Supply: liquid labelled 12.5 mg/5 mL

18. Order: Thorazine (chlorpromazine) 50 mg po tid
    Supply: syrup labelled 10 mg/5 mL

19. Order: Colace (docusate) 100 mg po every day
    Supply: syrup labelled 50 mg/15 mL

20. Order: codeine 0.06 g po q4–6h prn
    Supply: liquid labelled 15 mg/5 mL

Special Types of Oral Liquid Orders

Some liquids, including OTC preparations and multivitamins, are ordered in the amount to be poured and administered. No calculation is required.

Example

EXAMPLE 1

Order: Robitussin (dextromethorphan) syrup 10 mL q4h prn po

Supply: liquid labelled Robitussin syrup

No calculation is needed. Pour 10 mL and take every 4 hours by mouth as necessary.

EXAMPLE 2

Order: milk of magnesia 30 mL tonight po

Supply: liquid labelled milk of magnesia

No calculation is required. Pour 30 mL milk of magnesia and give tonight by mouth.

Oral Solid and Liquid Problems Without Written Calculations

As you develop proficiency in solving problems, you will be able to calculate many answers "in your head" without written work.

SELF TEST 3 **Mental Drill: Oral Solids**

Solve the problems "in your head" and write the amount to be given. Answers appear at the end of the chapter.

Order	Supply (scored tablets)	Answer
1. 20 mg	10 mg	2
2. 0.125 mg	0.25 mg	½
3. 0.25 mg	0.125 mg	
4. 200,000 units	100,000 units	
5. 0.5 mg	0.25 mg	
6. 0.2 g 0.200	400 mg	2
7. 1 g	1000 mg	1
8. 0.1 g	100 mg	1
9. 0.01 g	20 mg	½
10. 650 mg	325 mg	2
11. 500 mg	250 mg	
12. 50 mg	0.1 g	½
13. 4 mg	2 mg	

SELF TEST 4 | Mental Drill: Oral Liquids

Solve the problems "in your head" and write the amount to be given. Answers appear at the end of the chapter.

Order	Supply	Answer
1. 20 mg	10 mg/5 mL	_____
2. 10 mg	2 mg/5 mL	_____
3. 0.5 g	250 mg/5 mL	_____
4. 0.1 g	200 mg/10 mL	_____
5. 250 mg	0.1 g/6 mL	_____
6. 100 mg	50 mg/10 mL	_____
7. 12 mg	4 mg/5 mL	_____
8. 15 mg	30 mg/10 mL	_____
9. 15 mg	10 mg/4 mL	_____
10. 0.25 mg	0.5 mg/5 mL	_____

Putting It Together

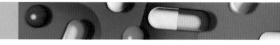

Ms. CM is an 86-year-old female who is being admitted with rapid atrial fibrillation that started about 2300h yesterday. No shortness of breath. Admitted for evaluation.

Past Medical History: hypertension, intermittent atrial fibrillation 3-4 years, chronic aortic insufficiency with dilated left ventricle; previous hospitalization several weeks ago with atrial fibrillation with a rapid ventricular rate. Other medical problems include moderate varicose veins, early dementia, and chronic tobacco use.

No known drug allergies

Current Vital Signs: Blood pressure is 172/58, pulse 120-140/min, respirations 20/min, oxygen saturation 96% on 2 L via nasal prongs, afebrile

Medication Orders

Coumadin (warfarin) *anticoagulant* 7.5 mg po daily

Prinivil (lisinopril) *antihypertensive* 20 mg po q12

Lanoxin (digoxin) *antiarrhythmic, increases cardiac contractility*

> **Loading dose:** 0.75 mg po × 1; 0.25 mg po in 6 hours and 12 hours then
>
> 0.125 mg po daily, hold if HR < 60

(continued)

Putting It Together

K-Dur (potassium chloride) *potassium supplement* 30 mEq po qd

Xanax (alprazolam) *antianxiety* 0.25-0.5 mg q6h prn anxiety

Pepcid (famotidine) *histamine 2 blocker, decreases gastric acid* 20 mg po

Tylenol (acetaminophen) *anti-inflammatory* 650 mg q4h prn mild pain

Tums (calcium carbonate) *mineral supplement, antacid* 1 g po daily

Calculations

1. Calculate how many tablets of Coumadin to administer. Available supply is 5 mg scored tablets.

2. Calculate how many tablets of Prinivil to administer. Available supply is 10 mg.

3. Calculate the loading dose of 0.75 mg of digoxin. Available supply is 500 mcg scored tablets and 250 mcg scored tablets. What are two options of administration?

4. Calculate the loading dose of 0.25 mg of digoxin. Available supply is 500 mcg scored tablets and 250 mcg scored tablets. What are two options of administration?

5. Calculate the maintenance dose of 0.125 mg of digoxin. Available supply is 500 mcg scored tablets and 250 mcg scored tablets. What are two options of administration?

6. K-Dur 10 mEq is equal to 750 mg of potassium. How many mg of potassium would be in 15 mEq?

7. Calculate how many tablets of Xanax to administer with the range ordered. Available supply is 125 mcg tablets.

8. Calculate how many tsp of Pepcid to administer. Available supply is 40 mg in 5 mL.

9. Calculate how many tablets of Tylenol to administer. Available supply is 325 mg tablets.

10. Calculate how many tablets of Tums to administer. Available supply is 200 mg tablets.

Critical Thinking Questions

1. What medications would have a higher potential for error in calculation and why?

2. What medications have parameters for administration? Should any of these medications be held, given the above scenario?

3. What are some alternatives to giving several tablets of a specific medication, i.e., 4 tablets, to equal the ordered dose?

4. Are any orders written incorrectly and why? What should you do to correct these?

5. This patient has difficulty with taking medications. What are some alternatives to administration?

Answers in Appendix B.

Name: _____

For liquid answers, draw a line on the medicine cup indicating the amount you would pour.
Answers are given in Appendix A.

1. Order: KCl elixir 20 mEq po bid
 Supply: liquid labelled 30 mEq/15 mL
 Answer   _____

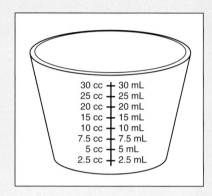

2. Order: Dilantin (phenytoin) suspension 150 mg po tid
 Supply: liquid labelled 75 mg/7.5 mL
 Answer   _____

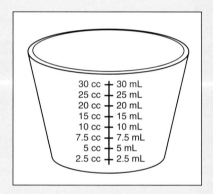

3. Order: Lanoxin (digoxin) elixir 0.125 mg po every day
 Supply: liquid labelled 0.25 mg/10 mL
 Answer   _____

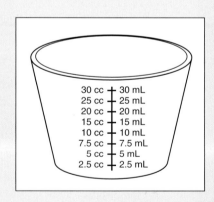

(continued)

Name: _____

For liquid answers, draw a line on the medicine cup indicating the amount you would pour. Answers are given in Appendix A.

4. Order: Dilantin (phenytoin) oral suspension 375 mg po tid
       Supply: liquid labelled 125 mg/5 mL
       Answer   _____

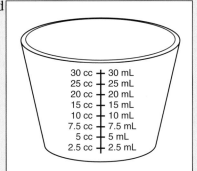

5. Order: Tagamet (famotidine) 40 mg
       Supply: suspension labelled 20 mg/2.5 mL
       Answer   _____

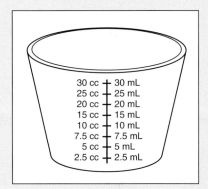

6. Order: Lanoxin (digoxin) 0.5 mg po every day
       Supply: tablets labelled 0.25 mg
       Answer   _____

7. Order: Lanoxin (digoxin) 100 mcg po every day
       Supply: 0.1-mg capsules
       Answer   _____

8. Order: Zyloprim (allopurinol) 250 mg po every day
       Supply: scored tablets 100 mg
       Answer   _____

9. Order: ampicillin 0.5 g po q6h
       Supply: capsules labelled 250 mg
       Answer   _____

10. Order: Synthroid (levothyroxine) 0.3 mg po every day
        Supply: tablets labelled 300 mcg scored
        Answer   _____

PROFICIENCY TEST 2 Calculation of Oral Doses

Name: _____

For liquid answers, draw a line on the medicine cup indicating the amount you would pour. Answers are given in Appendix A.

1. Order: Advil (ibuprofen) 0.8 g po tid
   Supply: tablets labelled 400 mg
   Answer _____

2. Order: Niazid (isoniazid) 0.3 g po every day
   Supply: tablets labelled 300 mg
   Answer _____

3. Order: Tenormin (atenolol) 75 mg po bid
   Supply: 50 mg tablets
   Answer _____

4. Order: Tylenol (acetaminophen) 0.65 g po q4h
   Supply: tablets labelled 325 mg
   Answer _____

5. Order: Altace (ramipril) 10 mg po daily
   Supply: tablets labelled 2.5 mg
   Answer _____

6. Order: Mycostatin (nystatin) oral suspension 750,000
   units po tid
   Supply: liquid labelled 100,000 units/mL
   Answer _____

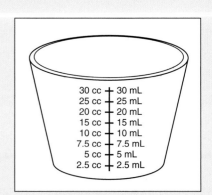

7. Order: oxacillin sodium 0.75 g po q6h
   Supply: liquid labelled 250 mg/5 mL
   Answer _____

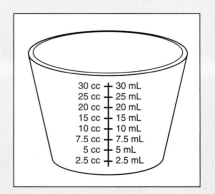

(continued)

Name: _____

For liquid answers, draw a line on the medicine cup indicating the amount you would pour.
Answers are given in Appendix A.

8. Order: penicillin V potassium 500 mg po q6h
  Supply: liquid labelled 250 mg/5 mL
  Answer _____

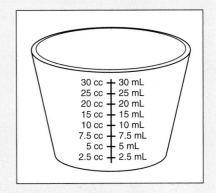

9. Order: Mylanta II 30 mL q4h prn
  Supply: liquid labelled Mylanta II
  Answer _____

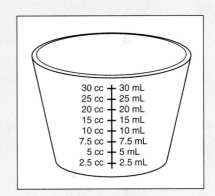

10. Order: Theo-Dur (theophylline) 160 mg po q6h
  Supply: liquid labelled 80 mg/15 mL
  Answer _____

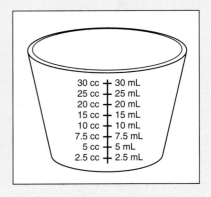

Name: _____

For each question, determine the amount to be given. Answers are given in Appendix A.

1. Order: potassium chloride 20 mEq po in juice bid
    Supply: liquid in a bottle labelled 30 mEq/15 mL

2. Order: syrup of Sumycin (tetracycline) hydrochloride 80 mg po q6h
    Supply: liquid in a dropper bottle labelled 125 mg/5 mL

3. Order: Inderal (propranolol) 0.02 g po bid
    Supply: scored tablets labelled 10 mg

4. Order: ampicillin sodium 0.5 g po q6h
    Supply: capsules of 250 mg

5. Order: Lanoxin (digoxin) 0.5 mg po every day
    Supply: scored tablets of 0.25 mg

6. Order: Deltasone (prednisone) 40 mg po every day
    Supply: liquid in a bottle labelled 5 mg/5 mL

7. Order: Hydrodiuril (hydrochlorothiazide) 75 mg po every day
    Supply: scored tablets 50 mg

8. Order: Lasix (furosemide) 40 mg po every day
    Supply: scored tablets of 80 mg

9. Order: Lanoxin (digoxin) 0.125 mg po
    Supply: liquid in a dropper bottle labelled 500 mcg/10 mL

10. Order: Dilantin (phenytoin) suspension 75 mg po tid
    Supply: liquid in a bottle labelled 50 mg/10 mL

11. Order: Valium (diazepam) 5 mg po q4h prn
    Supply: scored tablets 2 mg

12. Order: Synthroid (levothyroxine) 0.15 mg po every day
    Supply: scored tablets 300 mcg

13. Order: Antabuse (disulfiram) 375 mg po today
    Supply: scored tablets 250 mg

14. Order: Advil (ibuprofen) 0.6 g po q4h prn
    Supply: film-coated tablets 300 mg

15. Order: Chlor-Trimeton (chlorpheniramine maleate) syrup 1.5 mg po bid
    Supply: liquid in a bottle 1 mg/8 mL

16. Order: Benadryl (diphenhydramine maleate) syrup 25 mg po q4h while awake
    Supply: liquid labelled 12.5 mg/5 mL

17. Order: Mylicon (simethicone) liq 60 mg po in $\frac{1}{2}$ glass H_2O
    Supply: liquid in a dropper bottle labelled 40 mg/0.6 mL

18. Order: Diuril (chlorothiazide) oral suspension 0.5 g via NGT po every day
    Supply: liquid labelled 250 mg/5 mL

19. Order: Demerol (meperidine HCl) syrup 15 mg po q4h prn
    Supply: liquid labelled 50 mg/5 mL

20. Order: Vistaril (hydroxyzine) suspension 50 mg q6h po
    Supply: liquid labelled 25 mg/5 mL

Answers to Self Tests

Self Test 1 Oral Solids

Formula Method	Proportion Expressed as Two Ratios	Proportion Expressed as Two Fractions
$\dfrac{D}{H} \times S = x$	$S : H : : x : D$	$\dfrac{S}{H} = \dfrac{x}{D}$

1. No equivalent is needed.

Formula Method	Proportion Expressed as Two Ratios	Proportion Expressed as Two Fractions
$\dfrac{\overset{2}{\cancel{1.50}}\ \text{mg}}{\underset{1}{\cancel{0.75}}\ \text{mg}} \times 1\ \text{tablet} = 2\ \text{tablets}$	1 tablet : 0.75 mg : : x : 1.5 mg	$\dfrac{1\ \text{tablet}}{0.75\ \text{mg}} \diagdown \dfrac{x}{1.5\ \text{mg}}$

$$1.5 = 0.75x$$

$$\frac{1.5}{0.75} = x$$

$$2\ \text{tablets} = x$$

2. No equivalent is needed.

Formula Method	Proportion Expressed as Two Ratios	Proportion Expressed as Two Fractions
$\dfrac{\overset{1}{\cancel{0.25}}\ \text{mg}}{\underset{2}{\cancel{0.50}}\ \text{mg}} \times 1\ \text{tablet} = \frac{1}{2}\ \text{tablet}$	1 tablet : 0.5 mg : : x : 0.25 mg	$\dfrac{1\ \text{tablet}}{0.5\ \text{mg}} \diagdown \dfrac{x}{0.25\ \text{mg}}$

$$0.25 = 0.5x$$

$$\frac{0.25}{0.5} = x$$

$$0.5\ \text{or}\ \tfrac{1}{2}\ \text{tablet} = x$$

Formula Method	Proportion Expressed as Two Ratios	Proportion Expressed as Two Fractions
$\dfrac{\overset{2}{\cancel{500}}\ \text{mg}}{\underset{1}{\cancel{250}}\ \text{mg}} \times 1\ \text{capsule} = 2\ \text{capsules}$	1 capsule : 250 mg : : x : 500 mg	$\dfrac{1\ \text{capsule}}{250\ \text{mg}} \diagdown \dfrac{x}{500\ \text{mg}}$

3. Equivalent 0.5 g = 500 mg

$$\frac{500}{250} = x$$

$$2\ \text{capsules} = x$$

4. No equivalent is needed.

Formula Method	Proportion Expressed as Two Ratios	Proportion Expressed as Two Fractions
$\dfrac{\overset{4}{10.0}\ \text{mg}}{\underset{1}{2.5}\ \text{mg}} \times 1\ \text{tablet} = 4\ \text{tablets}$	1 tablet : 2.5 mg : : x : 10 mg	$\dfrac{1\ \text{tablet}}{2.5\ \text{mg}} \times \dfrac{\text{x}}{10}$

$$10 = 2.5\text{x}$$
$$\frac{10}{2.5} = \text{x}$$
$$4\ \text{tablets} = \text{x}$$

5. No equivalent is needed.

Formula Method	Proportion Expressed as Two Ratios	Proportion Expressed as Two Fractions
$\dfrac{\overset{2}{650}\ \text{mg}}{\underset{1}{325}\ \text{mg}} \times 1\ \text{tablet} = 2\ \text{tablets}$	1 tablet : 325 mg : : x : 650 mg	$\dfrac{1\ \text{tablet}}{325\ \text{mg}} \times \dfrac{\text{x}}{650\ \text{mg}}$

$$650 = 325\text{x}$$
$$\frac{650}{325} = \text{x}$$
$$2\ \text{tablets} = \text{x}$$

6. No equivalent is needed.

Formula Method	Proportion Expressed as Two Ratios	Proportion Expressed as Two Fractions
$\dfrac{20\ \text{mg}}{10\ \text{mg}} \times 1\ \text{capsule} = 2\ \text{capsules}$	1 capsule : 10 mg : : x : 20 mg	$\dfrac{1\ \text{capsule}}{10\ \text{mg}} \times \dfrac{\text{x}}{20\ \text{mg}}$

$$20 = 10\text{x}$$
$$\frac{20}{10} = \text{x}$$
$$2\ \text{capsules} = \text{x}$$

7. No equivalent is needed.

Formula Method	Proportion Expressed as Two Ratios	Proportion Expressed as Two Fractions
$\dfrac{\overset{4}{10}\ \text{mg}}{\underset{1}{2.5}\ \text{mg}} \times 1\ \text{tablet} = 4\ \text{tablets}$	1 tablet : 2.5 mg : : x : 10 mg	$\dfrac{1\ \text{tablet}}{2.5\ \text{mg}} \times \dfrac{\text{x}}{10\ \text{mg}}$

$$10 = 2.5\text{x}$$
$$\frac{10}{2.5} = \text{x}$$
$$4\ \text{tablets} = \text{x}$$

8. No equivalent is needed.

Formula Method	Proportion Expressed as Two Ratios	Proportion Expressed as Two Fractions
$\dfrac{\overset{1}{\cancel{200{,}000 \text{ units}}}}{\underset{2}{\cancel{400{,}000 \text{ units}}}} \times 1 \text{ tablet} = \frac{1}{2} \text{ tablet}$	1 tablet : 400,000 units : : x : 200,000	$\dfrac{1 \text{ tablet}}{400{,}000 \text{ units}} \times \dfrac{x}{200{,}000 \text{ units}}$

$$200{,}000 = 400{,}000x$$

$$\frac{200{,}000}{400{,}000} = x$$

$$0.5 \text{ or } \tfrac{1}{2} \text{ tablet} = x$$

Formula Method	Proportion Expressed as Two Ratios	Proportion Expressed as Two Fractions
$\dfrac{\overset{2}{\cancel{0.50 \text{ mg}}}}{\underset{1}{\cancel{0.25 \text{ mg}}}} \times 1 \text{ tablet} = 2 \text{ tablets}$	1 tablet : 0.25 mg : : x : 0.5 mg	$\dfrac{1 \text{ tablet}}{0.25 \text{ mg}} \times \dfrac{x}{0.5 \text{ mg}}$

9. No equivalent is needed.

$$0.5 = 0.25x$$

$$\frac{0.50}{0.25} = x$$

$$2 \text{ tablets} = x$$

10. No equivalent is needed.

Formula Method	Proportion Expressed as Two Ratios	Proportion Expressed as Two Fractions
$\dfrac{\overset{1.5}{\cancel{18.75 \text{ mg}}}}{\underset{1}{\cancel{12.5 \text{ mg}}}} \times 1 \text{ tablet} = 1.5 \text{ tablets}$ or $1\frac{1}{2}$ tablets	1 tablet : 12.5 mg : : x : 18.75 mg	$\dfrac{1 \text{ tablet}}{12.5 \text{ mg}} \times \dfrac{x}{18.75 \text{ mg}}$

$$18.75 = 12.5x$$

$$\frac{18.75}{12.5} = x$$

$$1.5 \text{ or } 1\tfrac{1}{2} \text{ tablets} = x$$

11. No equivalent is needed.

Formula Method	Proportion Expressed as Two Ratios	Proportion Expressed as Two Fractions
$\dfrac{\cancel{300 \text{ mg}}}{\cancel{200 \text{ mg}}} \times 1 \text{ tablet} = 1\frac{1}{2} \text{ tablets}$	1 tablet : 200 mg : : x : 300 mg	$\dfrac{1 \text{ tablet}}{200 \text{ mg}} \times \dfrac{x}{300 \text{ mg}}$

$$300 = 200x$$

$$\frac{300}{200} = x$$

$$1\tfrac{1}{2} \text{ tablets} = x$$

12. No equivalent is needed.

Formula Method	Proportion Expressed as Two Ratios	Proportion Expressed as Two Fractions
$\dfrac{0.3 \text{ mg}}{0.1 \text{ mg}} \times 1 \text{ tablet} = x$ $3 \text{ tablets} = x$	$1 \text{ tablet} : 0.1 \text{ mg} :: x : 0.3 \text{ mg}$	$\dfrac{1 \text{ tablet}}{0.1 \text{ mg}} \times \dfrac{x}{0.3 \text{ mg}}$

$$0.3 = 0.1x$$
$$\frac{0.3}{0.1} = x$$
$$3 \text{ tablets} = x$$

13. No equivalent is needed.

Formula Method	Proportion Expressed as Two Ratios	Proportion Expressed as Two Fractions
$\dfrac{\overset{0.25}{\cancel{6.25} \text{ mg}}}{\underset{1}{\cancel{25} \text{ mg}}} \times 1 \text{ tablet} = 0.25 \text{ tablet}$ (tablets can be quartered)	$1 \text{ tablet} : 25 \text{ mg} :: x : 6.25 \text{ mg}$	$\dfrac{1 \text{ tablet}}{25 \text{ mg}} \times \dfrac{x}{6.25 \text{ mg}}$

$$6.25 \text{ mg} = 25x$$
$$\frac{6.25}{25} = x$$
$$0.25 \text{ or } \tfrac{1}{4} \text{ tablet} = x$$

14. Equivalent: 0.2 mg = 200 mcg

Formula Method	Proportion Expressed as Two Ratios	Proportion Expressed as Two Fractions
$\dfrac{\overset{2}{\cancel{400} \text{ mcg}}}{\underset{1}{\cancel{200} \text{ mcg}}} \times 1 \text{ tablet} = 2 \text{ tablets}$	$1 \text{ tablet} : 200 \text{ mcg} :: x : 400 \text{ mcg}$	$\dfrac{1 \text{ tablet}}{200 \text{ mcg}} \times \dfrac{x}{400 \text{ mcg}}$

$$400 = 200x$$
$$\frac{400}{200} = x$$
$$2 \text{ tablets} = x$$

15. No equivalent is needed.

Formula Method	Proportion Expressed as Two Ratios	Proportion Expressed as Two Fractions
$\dfrac{\overset{1.5}{\cancel{7.5} \text{ mg}}}{\cancel{5} \text{ mg}} \times 1 \text{ tablet} = 1.5 \text{ tablets}$ or $1\tfrac{1}{2}$ tablets	$1 \text{ tablet} : 5 \text{ mg} :: x : 7.5 \text{ mg}$	$\dfrac{1 \text{ tablet}}{5 \text{ mg}} \times \dfrac{x}{7.5 \text{ mg}}$

$$7.5 \text{ mg} = 5x$$
$$\frac{7.5}{5} = x$$
$$1.5 \text{ or } 1\tfrac{1}{2} \text{ tablets} = x$$

16. No equivalent is needed.

Formula Method	Proportion Expressed as Two Ratios	Proportion Expressed as Two Fractions
$\dfrac{\overset{0.5}{\cancel{0.625} \text{ mg}}}{\cancel{1.25} \text{ mg}} \times 1 \text{ tablet} = 0.5 \text{ tablet}$ or ½ tablet	1 tablet : 1.25 mg : : x : 0.625 mg	$\dfrac{1 \text{ tablet}}{1.25 \text{ mg}} \times \dfrac{\text{x}}{0.625 \text{ mg}}$

$$0.625 = 1.25\text{x}$$

$$\frac{0.625}{1.25} = \text{x}$$

$$0.5 \text{ or } ½ \text{ tablet} = \text{x}$$

17. Equivalent: 0.5 g = 500 mg

Formula Method	Proportion Expressed as Two Ratios	Proportion Expressed as Two Fractions
$\dfrac{\overset{2}{\cancel{500} \text{ mg}}}{\underset{1}{\cancel{250} \text{ mg}}} \times 1 \text{ tablet} = 2 \text{ tablets}$	1 tablet : 250 mg : : x : 500 mg	$\dfrac{1 \text{ tablet}}{250 \text{ mg}} \times \dfrac{\text{x}}{500 \text{ mg}}$

$$500 = 250\text{x}$$

$$\frac{500}{250} = \text{x}$$

$$2 \text{ tablets} = \text{x}$$

18. No equivalent is needed.

Formula Method	Proportion Expressed as Two Ratios	Proportion Expressed as Two Fractions
$\dfrac{\overset{1.5}{\cancel{37.5} \text{ mg}}}{\underset{1}{\cancel{25} \text{ mg}}} \times 1 \text{ tablet} = 1.5 \text{ tablets}$ or 1½ tablets	1 tablet : 25 mg : : x : 37.5 mg	$\dfrac{1 \text{ tablet}}{25 \text{ mg}} \times \dfrac{\text{x}}{37.5 \text{ mg}}$

$$37.5 = 25\text{x}$$

$$\frac{37.5}{25} = \text{x}$$

$$1.5 \text{ or } 1½ \text{ tablets} = \text{x}$$

19. Equivalent: 1 g = 1000 mg

Formula Method	Proportion Expressed as Two Ratios	Proportion Expressed as Two Fractions
$\dfrac{\overset{2}{\cancel{1000} \text{ mg}}}{\underset{1}{\cancel{500} \text{ mg}}} \times 1 \text{ capsule} = 2 \text{ capsules}$	1 capsule : 500 mg : : x : 1000 mg	$\dfrac{1 \text{ capsule}}{500 \text{ mg}} \times \dfrac{\text{x}}{1000 \text{ mg}}$

$$1000 = 500\text{x}$$

$$\frac{1000}{500} = \text{x}$$

$$2 \text{ capsules} = \text{x}$$

20. No equivalent is needed.

Formula Method	Proportion Expressed as Two Ratios	Proportion Expressed as Two Fractions
$\dfrac{\overset{2.5}{\cancel{25}}\ \cancel{mg}}{\underset{1}{\cancel{10}}\ \cancel{mg}} \times 1 \text{ tablet} = 2.5 \text{ tablets}$ or $2\frac{1}{2}$ tablets	$1 \text{ tablet} : 10 \text{ mg} :: x : 25 \text{ mg}$	$\dfrac{1 \text{ tablet}}{10 \text{ mg}} \diagdown \dfrac{x}{25 \text{ mg}}$

$$25 = 10x$$
$$\frac{25}{10} = x$$
$$2.5 \text{ or } 2\tfrac{1}{2} \text{ tablets} = x$$

Self Test 2 Oral Liquids

> **FINE POINTS**
>
> Calculations may be done in different ways. Answers should be the same regardless of the method chosen to solve the problem.

Formula Method	Proportion Expressed as Two Ratios	Proportion Expressed as Two Fractions
$\dfrac{D}{H} \times S = X$	$S : H :: x : D$	$\dfrac{S}{H} = \dfrac{x}{D}$

1. Equivalent 0.75 g = 750 mg

Formula Method	Proportion Expressed as Two Ratios	Proportion Expressed as Two Fractions
$\dfrac{\overset{3}{\cancel{750}}\ \cancel{mg}}{\underset{1}{\cancel{250}}\ \cancel{mg}} \times 1 \text{ mL} = 3 \text{ mL}$	$1 \text{ mL} : 250 \text{ mg} :: x : 750 \text{ mg}$	$\dfrac{1 \text{ mL}}{250 \text{ mg}} \diagdown \dfrac{x}{750 \text{ mg}}$

$$750 = 250x$$
$$\frac{750}{250} = x$$
$$3 \text{ mL} = x$$

2. No equivalent is needed.

Formula Method	Proportion Expressed as Two Ratios	Proportion Expressed as Two Fractions
$\dfrac{\overset{2}{\cancel{500}}\ \cancel{mg}}{\underset{1}{\cancel{250}}\ \cancel{mg}} \times 5 \text{ mL} = 10 \text{ mL}$	$5 \text{ mL} : 250 \text{ mg} :: x : 500 \text{ mg}$	$\dfrac{5 \text{ mL}}{250 \text{ mg}} \diagdown \dfrac{x}{500 \text{ mg}}$

$$2500 = 250x$$
$$\frac{2500}{250} = x$$
$$10 \text{ mL} = x$$

3. Equivalent 0.35 g = 350 mg

Formula Method	Proportion Expressed as Two Ratios	Proportion Expressed as Two Fractions
$\dfrac{\overset{14}{\overset{70}{\cancel{350}}} \text{ mg}}{\underset{25}{\underset{5}{\cancel{125}}} \text{ mg}} \times \overset{1}{\cancel{5}} \text{ mL} = 14 \text{ mL}$	5 mL : 125 mg : : x : 350 mg	$\dfrac{5 \text{ mL}}{125 \text{ mg}} \diagdown \dfrac{x}{350 \text{ mg}}$

$$1750 = 125x$$
$$\frac{1750}{125} = x$$
$$14 \text{ mL} = x$$

4. No equivalent is needed.

Formula Method	Proportion Expressed as Two Ratios	Proportion Expressed as Two Fractions
$\dfrac{\overset{3}{\cancel{150}} \text{ mg}}{\underset{2}{\cancel{100}} \text{ mg}} \times 1 \text{ mL} = \tfrac{3}{2} = 1.5 \text{ mL}$	1 mL : 100 mg : : x : 150 mg	$\dfrac{1 \text{ mL}}{100 \text{ mg}} \diagdown \dfrac{x}{150 \text{ mg}}$

$$150 = 100x$$
$$\frac{150}{100} = x$$
$$1.5 \text{ mL} = x$$

5. No equivalent is needed.

Formula Method	Proportion Expressed as Two Ratios	Proportion Expressed as Two Fractions
$\dfrac{5 \text{ mg}}{10 \text{ mg}} \times 1 \text{ mL} = x$ $\tfrac{1}{2} \text{ or } 0.5 \text{ mL} = x$	1 mL : 10 mg : : x : 5 mg	$\dfrac{1 \text{ mL}}{10 \text{ mg}} \diagdown \dfrac{x}{5 \text{ mg}}$

$$5 = 10x$$
$$\frac{5}{10} = x$$
$$\tfrac{1}{2} \text{ or } 0.5 \text{ mL} = x$$

6. No equivalent is needed.

Formula Method	Proportion Expressed as Two Ratios	Proportion Expressed as Two Fractions
$\dfrac{0.02 \text{ mg}}{0.05 \text{ mg}} \times 1 \text{ mL} = \tfrac{2}{5} = 0.4 \text{ mL}$	1 mL : 0.05 mg : : x : 0.02 mg	$\dfrac{1 \text{ mL}}{0.05 \text{ mg}} \diagdown \dfrac{x}{0.02 \text{ mg}}$

$$0.02 = 0.05x$$
$$\frac{0.02}{0.05} = x$$
$$0.4 \text{ mL} = x$$

7. No equivalent is needed.

Formula Method	Proportion Expressed as Two Ratios	Proportion Expressed as Two Fractions
$\dfrac{30 \text{ mEq}}{20 \text{ mEq}} \times 15 \text{ mL} = \dfrac{3 \times 15}{2}$ $= \dfrac{45}{2} = 22.5 \text{ mL}$	$15 \text{ mL} : 20 \text{ mEq} :: x : 30 \text{ mEq}$	$\dfrac{15 \text{ mL}}{20 \text{ mEq}} \times \dfrac{x}{30 \text{ mEq}}$

$$15 \times 30 = 20x$$
$$\frac{450}{20} = x$$
$$22.5 \text{ mL} = x$$

8. No equivalent is needed.

Formula Method	Proportion Expressed as Two Ratios	Proportion Expressed as Two Fractions
$\dfrac{0.25 \text{ mg}}{0.25 \text{ mg}} \times 1 \text{ mL} = 1 \text{ mL}$	$1 \text{ mL} : 0.25 \text{ mg} :: x : 0.25 \text{ mg}$	$\dfrac{1 \text{ mL}}{0.25 \text{ mg}} \times \dfrac{x}{0.25 \text{ mg}}$

$$0.25 = 0.25x$$
$$\frac{0.25}{0.25} = x$$
$$1 \text{ mL} = x$$

9. No equivalent is needed.

Formula Method	Proportion Expressed as Two Ratios	Proportion Expressed as Two Fractions
$\dfrac{3 \text{ mg}}{1 \text{ mg}} \times 1 \text{ mL} = x$ $3 \text{ mL} = x$	$1 \text{ mL} : 1 \text{ mg} :: x : 3 \text{ mg}$	$\dfrac{1 \text{ mL}}{1 \text{ mg}} \times \dfrac{x}{3 \text{ mg}}$

$$3 = 1x$$
$$\frac{3}{1} = x$$
$$3 \text{ mL} = x$$

10. No equivalent is needed.

Formula Method	Proportion Expressed as Two Ratios	Proportion Expressed as Two Fractions
$\dfrac{\overset{10}{\cancel{12.5}} \text{ mg}}{\underset{1}{\cancel{\underset{1.25}{6.25}}} \text{ mg}} \times \overset{1}{\cancel{5}} \text{ mL} = 10 \text{ mL}$	$5 \text{ mL} : 6.25 \text{ mg} :: x : 12.5 \text{ mg}$	$\dfrac{5 \text{ mL}}{6.25 \text{ mg}} \times \dfrac{x}{12.5 \text{ mg}}$

$$62.5 = 6.25x$$
$$\frac{62.5}{6.25} = x$$
$$10 \text{ mL} = x$$

FINE POINTS

Alternate arithmetic

$12.5 \times 5 = 62.5$

$$6.25 \overline{)62.50} \atop \begin{array}{r}10.\\ \underline{62\ 5}\\ 0\end{array}$$

11. No equivalent is needed.

Formula Method	Proportion Expressed as Two Ratios	Proportion Expressed as Two Fractions
$\dfrac{\overset{5}{\cancel{50}}\ \text{mg}}{\underset{1}{\cancel{10}}\ \text{mg}} \times 5\ \text{mL} = 25\ \text{mL}$	$5\ \text{mL} : 10\ \text{mg} :: x : 50\ \text{mg}$	$\dfrac{5\ \text{mL}}{10\ \text{mg}} \times \dfrac{x}{50\ \text{mg}}$

$$5 \times 50 = 10x$$

$$\frac{250}{10} = x$$

$$25\ \text{mL} = x$$

12. No equivalent is needed.

Formula Method	Proportion Expressed as Two Ratios	Proportion Expressed as Two Fractions
$\dfrac{\overset{4}{\cancel{40}}\ \text{mg}}{\underset{1}{\cancel{10}}\ \text{mg}} \times 1\ \text{mL} = 4\ \text{mL}$	$1\ \text{mL} : 10\ \text{mg} :: x : 40\ \text{mg}$	$\dfrac{1\ \text{mL}}{10\ \text{mg}} \times \dfrac{x}{40\ \text{mg}}$

$$40 = 10x$$

$$\frac{40}{10} = x$$

$$4\ \text{mL} = x$$

13. No equivalent is needed.

Formula Method	Proportion Expressed as Two Ratios	Proportion Expressed as Two Fractions
$\dfrac{\overset{1}{\cancel{10}}\ \text{mEq}}{\underset{2}{\cancel{20}}\ \text{mEq}} \times 30\ \text{mL} = \dfrac{30}{2} = 15\ \text{mL}$	$30\ \text{mL} : 20\ \text{mEq} :: x : 10\ \text{mEq}$	$\dfrac{30\ \text{mL}}{20\ \text{mEq}} \times \dfrac{x}{10\ \text{mEq}}$

$$30 \times 10 = 20x$$

$$\frac{300}{20} = x$$

$$15\ \text{mL} = x$$

14. No equivalent is needed.

Formula Method	Proportion Expressed as Two Ratios	Proportion Expressed as Two Fractions
$\dfrac{\overset{2}{\cancel{10}} \text{ mg}}{\underset{1}{\cancel{5}} \text{ mg}} \times 5 \text{ mL} = 10 \text{ mL}$	$5 \text{ mL} : 5 \text{ mg} :: x : 10 \text{ mg}$	$\dfrac{5 \text{ mL}}{5 \text{ mg}} \times \dfrac{x}{10 \text{ mg}}$

$$10 \times 5 = 5x$$
$$\frac{50}{5} = x$$
$$10 \text{ mL} = x$$

15. No equivalent is needed.

Formula Method	Proportion Expressed as Two Ratios	Proportion Expressed as Two Fractions
$\dfrac{\overset{5}{\cancel{100}} \text{ mg}}{\underset{1}{\cancel{20}} \text{ mg}} \times 5 \text{ mL} = 25 \text{ mL}$	$5 \text{ mL} : 20 \text{ mg} :: x : 100 \text{ mg}$	$\dfrac{5 \text{ mL}}{20 \text{ mg}} \times \dfrac{x}{100 \text{ mg}}$

$$5 \times 100 = 20x$$
$$\frac{500}{20} = x$$
$$25 \text{ mL} = x$$

16. No equivalent is needed.

Formula Method	Proportion Expressed as Two Ratios	Proportion Expressed as Two Fractions
$\dfrac{650 \text{ mg}}{160 \text{ mg}} \times 5 \text{ mL} = \dfrac{3250}{160} = 20.31$ or 20 mL	$5 \text{ mL} : 160 \text{ mg} :: x : 650 \text{ mg}$	$\dfrac{5 \text{ mL}}{160 \text{ mg}} \times \dfrac{x}{650 \text{ mg}}$

$$650 \times 5 = 160x$$
$$\frac{3250}{160} = x$$
$$20.31 \text{ or } 20 \text{ mL} = x$$

17. No equivalent is needed.

Formula Method	Proportion Expressed as Two Ratios	Proportion Expressed as Two Fractions
$\dfrac{\overset{2}{\cancel{25}} \text{ mg}}{\underset{1}{\cancel{12.5}} \text{ mg}} \times 5 \text{ mL} = 10 \text{ mL}$	$5 \text{ mL} : 12.5 \text{ mg} :: x : 25 \text{ mg}$	$\dfrac{5 \text{ mL}}{12.5 \text{ mg}} \times \dfrac{x}{25 \text{ mg}}$

$$5 \times 25 = 12.5x$$

$$\frac{125}{12.5} = x$$

$$10 \text{ mL} = x$$

18. No equivalent is needed.

Formula Method	Proportion Expressed as Two Ratios	Proportion Expressed as Two Fractions
$\dfrac{\overset{5}{\cancel{50}} \text{ mg}}{\underset{1}{\cancel{10}} \text{ mg}} \times 5 \text{ mL} = 25 \text{ mL}$	$5 \text{ mL} : 10 \text{ mg} :: x : 50 \text{ mg}$	$\dfrac{5 \text{ mL}}{10 \text{ mg}} \times \dfrac{x}{50 \text{ mg}}$

$$5 \times 50 = 10x$$

$$\frac{250}{10} = x$$

$$25 \text{ mL} = x$$

19. No equivalent is needed.

Formula Method	Proportion Expressed as Two Ratios	Proportion Expressed as Two Fractions
$\dfrac{\overset{2}{\cancel{100}} \text{ mg}}{\underset{1}{\cancel{50}} \text{ mg}} \times 15 \text{ mL} = 30 \text{ mL}$	$15 \text{ mL} : 50 \text{ mg} :: x : 100 \text{ mg}$	$\dfrac{15 \text{ mL}}{50 \text{ mg}} \times \dfrac{x}{100 \text{ mg}}$

$$15 \times 100 = 50x$$

$$\frac{1500}{50} = x$$

$$30 \text{ mL} = x$$

20. Equivalent: 0.06 g = 60 mg

Formula Method	Proportion Expressed as Two Ratios	Proportion Expressed as Two Fractions
$\dfrac{\overset{4}{\cancel{60}} \text{ mg}}{\underset{1}{\cancel{15}} \text{ mg}} \times 5 \text{ mL} = 20 \text{ mL}$	5 mL : 15 mg : : x : 60 mg	$\dfrac{5 \text{ mL}}{15 \text{ mg}} \diagtimes \dfrac{x}{60 \text{ mg}}$

$$5 \times 60 = 15x$$

$$\frac{300}{15} = x$$

$$20 \text{ mL} = x$$

Self Test 3 Mental Drill: Oral Solids

1.	2 tablets	**6.**	½ tablet	**11.**	2 tablets
2.	½ tablet	**7.**	1 tablet	**12.**	½ tablet
3.	2 tablets	**8.**	1 tablet	**13.**	2 tablets
4.	2 tablets	**9.**	½ tablet		
5.	2 tablets	**10.**	2 tablets		

Self Test 4 Mental Drill: Oral Liquids

1.	10 mL	**3.**	10 mL	**5.**	15 mL	**7.**	15 mL	**9.**	6 mL
2.	25 mL	**4.**	5 mL	**6.**	20 mL	**8.**	5 mL	**10.**	2.5 mL

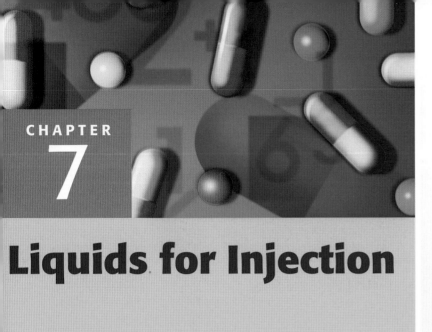

LEARNING OBJECTIVES

1. Solving injection-from-liquid problems

2. Syringes and marking

3. Preparing medications from 1 vial, glass ampoule, and from 2 vials.

4. Insulin injections

5. Mixing insulins

6. Sliding-scale insulin calculations

7. Principles for reconstituting drugs from powder form
   Reading and understanding drug manufacturer's label and package insert directions
   Storing reconstituted drugs safely
   Labelling reconstituted drugs

Liquid drugs for injection are prepared by pharmaceutical companies as sterile solutions, powders, or suspensions. Aseptic techniques are used to prepare and administer them. As with oral medications, the nurse may have to calculate the correct dosage. The nurse must also follow correct administration techniques and special considerations (e.g., correct dilution, injection site, size of needle, speed of IV injection).

RULE   **CALCULATING LIQUID INJECTIONS**

To solve liquid injection problems, use the same rule as for oral solids and liquids.

Formula Method	*Proportion Expressed as Two Ratios*	*Proportion Expressed as Two Fractions*
$\dfrac{\text{Desire}}{\text{Have}} \times \text{Supply} = \text{Amount}$	$\text{Supply} : \text{Have} :: x : \text{Desire}$	$\dfrac{\text{Supply}}{\text{Have}} = \dfrac{x}{\text{Desire}}$

Example   Order: Midazolam 1.5 mg IM q6h prn

Supply: Read the label

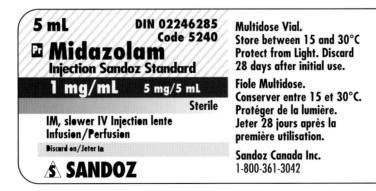

Desire: the amount ordered, 1.5 mg

Have: strength of the drug supplied, here, 1 mg

Supply: the unit form of the drug, here, 1 mL (For liquid calculations, the supply is usually 1 mL.)

Amount or *Answer:* how much liquid to give by injection in mL. "x" is used in all 3 methods.

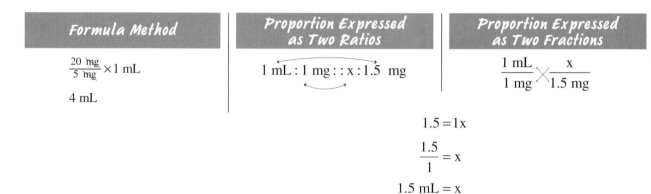

Formula Method	**Proportion Expressed as Two Ratios**	**Proportion Expressed as Two Fractions**
$\dfrac{20 \text{ mg}}{5 \text{ mg}} \times 1 \text{ mL}$ 4 mL	$1 \text{ mL} : 1 \text{ mg} :: x : 1.5 \text{ mg}$	$\dfrac{1 \text{ mL}}{1 \text{ mg}} \times \dfrac{x}{1.5 \text{ mg}}$

$$1.5 = 1x$$

$$\frac{1.5}{1} = x$$

$$1.5 \text{ mL} = x$$

Calculating Injection Problems

Syringes

When you're calculating injection answers, the degree of accuracy depends on the syringe you use.

3-mL Syringe

Figure 7-1 shows a 3-mL syringe marked in millilitres to the nearest tenth. *To calculate millilitre answers for this 3-mL syringe, carry out the arithmetic to the hundredth place and then round off the answer to the nearest tenth (follow standard rounding rules).*

   1.25 mL becomes 1.3 mL

1-mL Precision Syringe

Figure 7-2 shows a 1-mL precision syringe marked in millilitres to the nearest hundredth. *To calculate millilitres when the 1-mL syringe is used, carry out the arithmetic to the thousandth place and then round off the answer to the nearest hundredth (follow standard rounding rules).*

   0.978 mL becomes 0.98 mL

   Each of the following examples provides a syringe. Calculate millilitres to the degree of accuracy required by the syringe markings. Draw a line on the syringe to indicate your answer for millilitres.

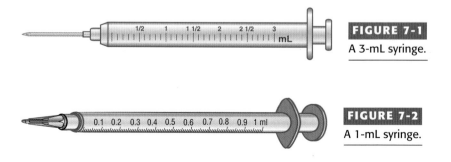

FIGURE 7-1
A 3-mL syringe.

FIGURE 7-2
A 1-mL syringe.

Example   Order: Demerol (meperidine HCl) 75 mg IM q4h prn

Supply: Read the label.

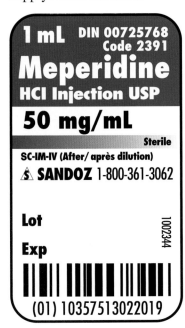

© Copyright of Sandoz Canada Inc. All rights reserved.

Formula Method	Proportion Expressed as Two Ratios	Proportion Expressed as Two Fractions
$\dfrac{\overset{3}{\cancel{75}} \text{ mg}}{\underset{2}{\cancel{50}} \text{ mg}} \times 1 \text{ mL} = \dfrac{3}{2} = 1.5 \text{ mL}$	$1 \text{ mL} : 50 \text{ mg} :: x : 75 \text{ mg}$	$\dfrac{1 \text{ mL}}{50 \text{ mg}} = \dfrac{x}{75 \text{ mg}}$

$$\frac{75}{50} = x$$

$$1.5 \text{ or } 1\frac{1}{2} \text{ mL} = x$$

Give 1.5 mL IM.

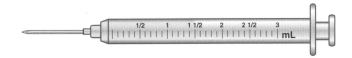

Example Order: heparin sodium 1500 units subcutaneous bid
Supply: Read the label.

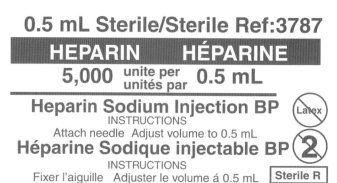

0.5 mL Sterile/Sterile Ref:3787
HEPARIN   HÉPARINE
5,000 unite per / unités par **0.5 mL**

Heparin Sodium Injection BP (Latex)
INSTRUCTIONS
Attach needle Adjust volume to 0.5 mL
Héparine Sodique injectable BP (2)
INSTRUCTIONS
Fixer l'aiguille   Adjuster le volume á 0.5 mL [Sterile R]

[Lot] 7531   Exp:2009 AL

MedXL Inc. Montreal, Canda (514) 695-7474   Used with permission of MedXL Inc.

Formula Method	*Proportion Expressed as Two Ratios*	*Proportion Expressed as Two Fractions*
$\frac{\overset{3}{\cancel{1500}}\ \text{units}}{\underset{10}{\cancel{5000}}\ \text{units}} \times 0.5\ \text{mL} = \frac{3}{10} = 0.3\ \text{mL}$ $0.3\ \text{mL} \times 0.5 = 0.15\ \text{mL}$	$0.5\ \text{mL} : 5000\ \text{units} :: \text{x} : 1500\ \text{units}$	$\frac{0.5\ \text{mL}}{5000\ \text{units}} \times \frac{\text{x}}{1500\ \text{units}}$ $\frac{750}{5000} = \text{x}$ $0.15\ \text{mL} = \text{x}$

Give 0.15 mL.

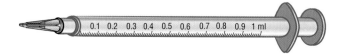

Heparin can also be administered intravenously—this will be covered in Chapter 9.

Preparing the Dose

To prevent incompatibility of drugs, ordinarily you draw up only one medication in a syringe. If you are giving two drugs in one syringe, first determine that the drugs are compatible and then follow the procedure for mixing.

Drugs That Are Liquids in Vials

1. Clean the top of the vial with an alcohol pad.

2. Draw up into the syringe an amount of air equivalent to the desired amount of solution.

3. Insert the syringe needle (or needleless device) through the rubber diaphragm into the vial.

4. Inject the air from the syringe into the vial (Fig 7-3A). This increases the pressure in the vial and makes it easier to withdraw the medication.

5. Invert the vial, hold it at eye level, and draw up the desired amount into the syringe (see Fig. 7-3B). While the needle remains in the vial, tap the needle gently to cause any air bubbles to rise to the top of

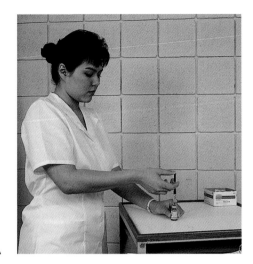 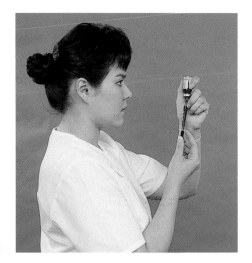

A B

FIGURE 7-3

(**A**) Injecting air into the vial. (**B**) Invert the vial and draw up the desired amount of medication into the syringe.

the needle where they can be injected back into the vial. Ensure there are no bubbles as this will alter the amount of medication.

6. Withdraw the needle (or needleless device) quickly from the vial.

7. If needle is to be used for a parenteral injection (IM, subcutaneous, or ID), change the needle to one of the correct length and gauge to maximize patient comfort during the injection.

Drugs in Glass Ampoules

1. Tap the top of the ampoule with your finger to clear out any trapped drug (this may need to be repeated until all the medication is cleared).

2. Place an unopened alcohol pad around the neck of the ampoule to protect your fingers and thumb while opening the ampoule.

3. Hold the base of the ampoule in your nondominant hand between your thumb and fingers.

4. Grasp the top of the ampoule with your dominant hand, thumb in front, fingers behind so you can "snap" the ampoule at the scored neck. (Both thumbs will be in front of ampoule.)

5. Break off the top of the ampoule with a sharp snapping motion away from yourself. Discard the top into a sharps container.

6. Invert the ampoule, hold it at eye level, insert the syringe needle with a filter (to ensure no microscopic glass shards are withdrawn), and withdraw the dose (Fig. 7-4).

   IMPORTANT: Do not add air before removing the dose, because if you do, medication will leak from the ampoule. Also, keep the needle below the upper level of the fluid so the vacuum seal is not broken, which would also cause medication to leak from the ampoule.

7. You should remove slightly more liquid from the ampoule than the required amount as there will be air bubbles in the syringe. Remove needle from ampoule.

8. Tap the syringe with your finger to cause the bubbles to rise to the top and then gently pull back on the plunger and slowly expel the air. Ensure that you pull back slightly after each "tap" to clear the needle/hub of fluid or this fluid will spray out when you expel the excess air.

9. Ensure that the correct dosage/volume of medication is in the syringe.

10. Discard the ampoule in a sharps container.

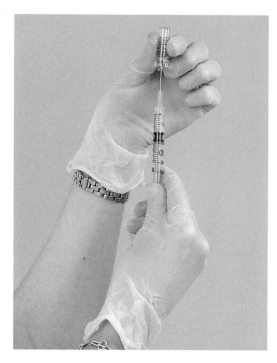

Drugs in Unit-Dose Cartidge and Holder Systems

1. Insert the cartridge into the metal or plastic holder, and screw it into place.

2. Move the plunger forward until it engages the shaft of the cartridge, then twist the plunger until it is locked into the cartridge

3. The holder is reusable, but the cartridge is not.

4. Place the cartridge in a sharps container after use.

Drugs in Unit-Dose Prefilled Syringes

1. The medication is already in the syringe. Some prefilled syringes are simple and require no action other than removing the needle cover; others are packaged for compactness and include directions for preparing the syringe for use.

2. These prefilled syringes are disposable.

Mixing Two Medications in One Syringe

GENERAL PRINCIPLES

- Consult a standard reference to determine that the drugs are compatible.

- When in doubt about compatibility, prepare medications separately and administer them into different injection sites.

- When medications are in both a vial and an ampoule, draw up the medication from the vial first; and then add the medication from the ampoule following the steps listed above.

- When preparing two types of insulin in one syringe, first draw into the syringe the vial containing regular insulin. (Regular insulin has not been adulterated with protein as have other insulins used as protamine zinc insulin.)

METHOD FOR TWO VIALS

1. Clean both vials with an alcohol pad.

2. Choose one vial as the primary. Example: with vials of a narcotic and a nonnarcotic, the narcotic is the primary. With two insulins, regular insulin is the primary.

3. Draw up and inject air into the second vial, in an amount equaling the medication to be withdrawn. Do not let the needle touch the medication. Remove needle from vial.

4. Draw up and inject air into the primary vial, in an amount equaling the medication to be withdrawn, and then withdraw the mediation in the usual way. Make sure there are NO air bubbles.

5. Insert the needle (or needleless device) into the second vial. Do not touch the plunger, because if you do you might push the primary medication into the second vial.

6. Slowly withdraw the *exact* amount of drug needed from the second vial. The two medications are now combined.

7. Remove the needle or needleless device from the second vial and carefully recap it, using a one-handed technique.

IV Medications

IV push (IVP) medications must be diluted and administered either according to directions in a nursing drug book or according to hospital policy. First, calculate the correct dose.

Example Order: Lanoxin (digoxin) 120 mcg IV every day. Use a 1-mL precision syringe.

Supply: Read the label.

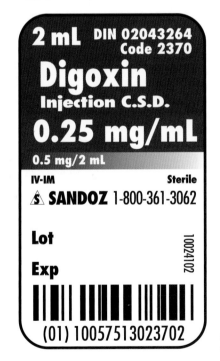

Formula Method	Proportion Expressed as Two Ratios	Proportion Expressed as Two Fractions
$\frac{120 \text{ mcg}}{250 \text{ mcg}} \times 1 \text{ mL} = \frac{0.48}{25 \overline{)12.00}}$ $\frac{100}{200}$ $\frac{200}{}$	$1 \text{ mL} : 250 \text{ mcg} :: x : 120 \text{ mcg}$	$\frac{1 \text{ mL}}{250 \text{ mcg}} \times \frac{x}{120 \text{ mcg}}$

$$\frac{120}{250} = x$$

$$0.48 \text{ mL} = x$$

Give 0.48 mL IV.

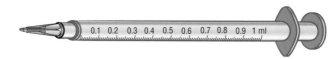

Digoxin IVP is given either undiluted or diluted in 4 mL sterile water and administered over 5 minutes.

Example   Order: Lasix (furosemide) 20 mg IV q12h

Supply: Read the label.

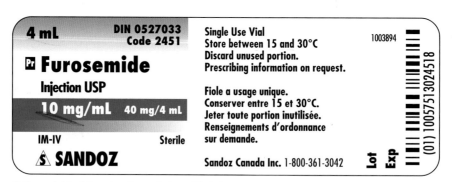

Formula Method	Proportion Expressed as Two Ratios	Proportion Expressed as Two Fractions
$\frac{20 \text{ mg}}{10 \text{ mg}} \times 1 \text{ mL}$	$1 \text{ mL} : 10 \text{ mg} :: x : 20 \text{ mg}$	$\frac{1 \text{ mL}}{10 \text{ mg}} \times \frac{x}{20 \text{ mg}}$

$$20 = 10x$$

$$\frac{20}{10} = x$$

$$2 \text{ mL} = x$$

Give 2 mL IV.

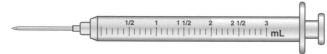

Lasix IVP is given undiluted at a rate of 20 mg over 1 minute.

Example Order: Promethazine 12.5 mg IV q4–6h prn

Supply: Read the label.

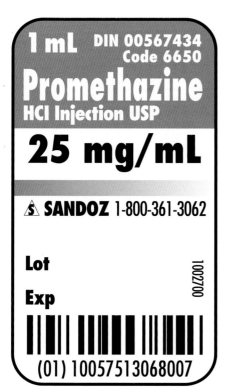

1 mL DIN 00567434
Code 6650
Promethazine
HCl Injection USP
25 mg/mL

⚠ **SANDOZ** 1-800-361-3062

Lot

Exp

10027.00

(01) 10057513068007

Formula Method	Proportion Expressed as Two Ratios	Proportion Expressed as Two Fractions
$\dfrac{12.5 \text{ mg}}{25 \text{ mg}} \times 1 \text{ mL} = x$	$1 \text{ mL} : 25 \text{ mg} :: x : 12.5 \text{ mg}$	$\dfrac{1 \text{ mL}}{25 \text{ mg}} \diagdown \dfrac{x}{12.5 \text{ mg}}$
$0.5 \text{ mL} = x$		

$$12.5 \text{ mg} = 25x$$

$$\frac{12.5}{25} = x$$

$$0.5 \text{ mL} = x$$

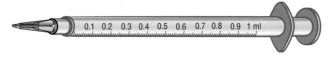

Promethazine IVP is given undiluted if less than 25 mg. Give each 25 mg over 1 minute.

SELF TEST 1   Calculation of Liquids for Injection

Practice calculations of injections from a liquid. Report your answer in millilitres; mark the syringe in millilitres. Answers appear at the end of the chapter.

1. Order: Clindamycin (cleocin) 0.3 g IM q6h
Supply: liquid in a vial labelled 300 mg/2 mL

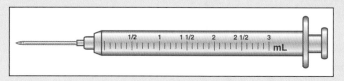

2. Order: morphine 12 mg IV stat
Supply: vial of liquid labelled 15 mg/mL

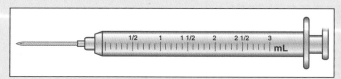

3. Order: vitamin B$_{12}$ 1 mg IM every day
Supply: vial of liquid labelled 1000 mcg/mL

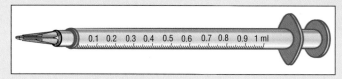

4. Order: gentamicin 9 mg IM q8h
Supply: pediatric ampule labelled 20 mg/2 mL

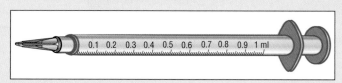

5. Order: Lanoxin (digoxin) 0.5 mg IV q6h × 3 doses
Supply: vial labelled 0.25 mg/mL

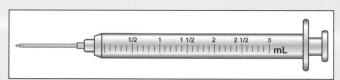

6. Order: gentamicin 50 mg IM q8h
Supply: vial labelled 40 mg/mL

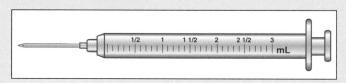

(continued)

7. Order: phenobarbital 100 mg IM stat
   Supply: ampoule labelled 130 mg/mL

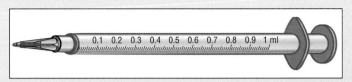

8. Order: Lanoxin (digoxin) 0.25 mg IV stat
   Supply: ampoule labelled 0.5 mg/2 mL

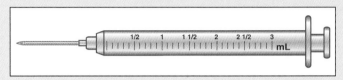

9. Order: heparin 6000 units subcutaneous q4h
   Supply: vial labelled 10,000 units/mL

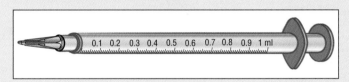

10. Order: Terbutaline (brethine) 0.25 mg subcutaneous for preterm contractions
    Supply: ampoule labelled 1 mg/1 mL

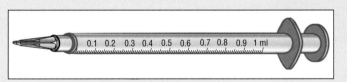
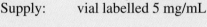

11. Order: Normadyne (labetolol) 20 mg IV stat
    Supply: vial labelled 5 mg/mL

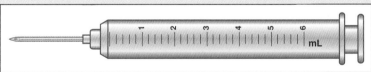

12. Order: Haldol (haloperidol) 2.5 mg IM q4–8h
    Supply: vial labelled 5 mg/mL

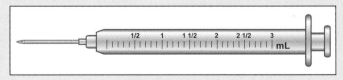

(continued)

13. Order: Methadone 3 mg subcutaneous now
      Supply: vial labelled 10 mg per mL

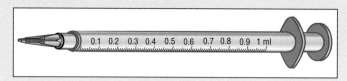

14. Order: Endep (amitriptyline) 0.025 g IM tid
      Supply: vial labelled 10 mg/mL

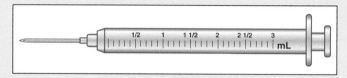

15. Order: Thorazine (chlorpromazine) 50 mg IM now
      Supply: vial labelled 25 mg/mL

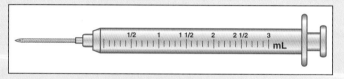

16. Order: Fragmin (dalteparin) 2500 units subcutaneous every day
      Supply: syringe labelled 5000 units in 0.2 mL

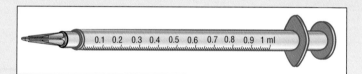

Special Types of Problems in Injections from a Liquid

When Supply Is a Ratio

Labels may state the strength of a drug as a ratio.

Example   Adrenalin 1:1000

Ratios are always interpreted in the metric system as grams per millilitres. In the example given, 1:1000 means 1 g in 1000 mL. Ratios may be stated in three ways:

    1 g per 1000 mL

    1 g = 1000 mL

    1 g/1000 mL

SELF TEST 2   Ratios

Write the following ratios in three ways. Answers appear at the end of the chapter.

RATIO	? g per ? mL	? g = ? mL	? g/? mL
1:20			
2:15			
1:500			
2:2000			
1:4			
2:25			
4:50			
1:100			
3:75			
5:1000			

The label below shows epinephrine that is a 1:1000 solution. 1:1000 means 1 g in 1000 mL. 1 g is equivalent to 1000 mg. Therefore, you can interpret the solution as 1000 mg = 1000 mL. If 1000 mL contains 1000 mg, then 1 mL contains 1 mg.

$$\frac{\cancel{1000}\ \text{mg}}{\cancel{1000}\ \text{mL}} = \frac{1\ \text{mg}}{1\ \text{mL}}$$

When reading and writing milligram (mg) and millilitre (mL), remember that milligram is the solid measure; millilitre is the liquid measure.

Example

Order: epinephrine 1 mg subcutaneous stat

Supply: ampoule labelled 1:1000

Equivalent: 1:1000 means

    1 g in 1000 mL

    1 g = 1000 mg

Therefore, 1000 mL contains 1000 mg.

Epinephrine Injection USP
Épinéphrine injectable USP

1:1000 (1 mg/mL)

SYMPATHOMIMETIC
Each mL contains: Epinephrine 1 mg, sodium metabisulfite 0.90 mg as an antioxidant, sodium chloride for tonicity, and hydrochloric acid for pH adjustment.
Dosage: Varies with routes of administration: intramuscular, intravenous, intracardiac, endotracheal, or subcutaneous (preferred), and indications.
For allergic manifestations - Adults: 0.2 to 1 mg (0.2 to 1 mL) s.c.   **Children:** 0.01 mL/kg (maximum 0.5 mL) s.c.; may be repeated every 4 hours.
WARNINGS: CONTAINS SODIUM METABISULFITE: USE WITH CAUTION. MAY CAUSE ALLERGIC-TYPE REACTIONS, INCLUDING ANAPHYLACTIC SYMPTOMS OR LIFE THREATENING OR LESS SEVERE ASTHMATIC EPISODES IN CERTAIN SUSCEPTIBLE PERSONS.
See insert for details.
Storage: 15 - 25°C. **Protect from light.** Do not use the solution if its colour is pinkish or darker than slightly yellow, or if it contains a precipitate. Discard unused portion.

SYMPATHOMIMÉTIQUE
Composition de 1 mL: Épinéphrine 1 mg, métabisulfite de sodium 0,90 mg (comme antioxydant), chlorure de sodium pour la tonicité et acide chlorhydrique pour ajuster le pH.
Posologie: Varie selon la voie d'administration, soit intramusculaire, intraveineuse, intracardiaque, endotrachéale ou sous-cutanée (de préférence), et selon les indications.
Dans les cas de manifestations allergiques - Adultes: De 0,2 à 1 mg (de 0,2 à 1 mL) s.-c.   **Enfants:** 0,01 mL/kg (maximum 0,5 mL) s.-c.; peut être répétée aux 4 heures.
MISE EN GARDE: RENFERME DU MÉTABISULFITE DE SODIUM: EMPLOYER AVEC PRUDENCE. PEUT CAUSER DES RÉACTIONS DE TYPE ALLERGIQUE, Y COMPRIS, CHEZ CERTAINES PERSONNES SENSIBLES, DES SYMPTÔMES ANAPHYLACTIQUES OU DES CRISES D'ASTHME POUVANT ALLER JUSQU'À METTRE LA VIE DU PATIENT EN DANGER.
Pour plus de détails, voir le dépliant.
Entreposage: 15 - 25°C. **Craint la lumière.** N'utiliser que si la solution est incolore ou jaune pâle et exempte de précipité.
Jetez tout reste.

Hospira Healthcare Corporation
Corporation de Soins de la Santé Hospira
Montréal, Qc H4P 1A5   K183437H

Hospira

8 82135 72411 8

Courtesy of Hospira.

Formula Method	**Proportion Expressed as Two Ratios**	**Proportion Expressed as Two Fractions**
$\dfrac{1\text{mg}}{1000\ \text{mg}} \times 1000\ \text{mL} = 1\ \text{mL}$	1000 mL : 1000 mg : : x : 1 mg	$\dfrac{1000\ \text{mL}}{1000\ \text{mg}} \times \dfrac{\text{x}}{1\ \text{mg}}$

$$\frac{1000}{1000} = x$$

$$1\ \text{mL} = x$$

Give 1 mL subcutaneously.

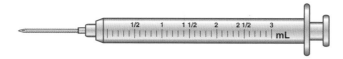

Example   Order: Isuprel (isoproterenol) HCl 0.2 mg IM stat

Supply: ampoule labelled 1:5000

Equivalents: 1:5000 means

    1 g in 5000 mL

    1 g = 1000 mg

Therefore, 5000 mL contains 1000 mg.

Formula Method	**Proportion Expressed as Two Ratios**	**Proportion Expressed as Two Fractions**
$\dfrac{0.2\ \text{mg}}{1000\ \text{mg}} \times \overset{5}{5000}\ \text{mL} = \dfrac{\overset{5}{\times}\ 0.2}{1.0\ \text{mL}}$	5000 mL : 1000 mg : : x : 0.2 mg	$\dfrac{5000\ \text{mL}}{1000\ \text{mg}} \times \dfrac{\text{x}}{0.2\ \text{mg}}$

$$\frac{1000}{1000} = x$$

$$1\ \text{mL} = x$$

Give 1 mL IM.

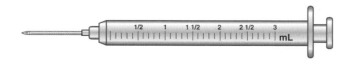

SELF TEST 3 Using Ratios with Liquids for Injection

Solve these problems involving ratios. Answers appear at the end of the chapter.

1. Order: neostigmine 0.5 mg subcutaneous
   Supply: ampoule labelled 1:2000

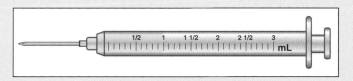

2. Order: Isuprel (isoproterenol) 1 mg: add to IV
   Supply: vial labelled 1:5000

   A 10-mL syringe is available.

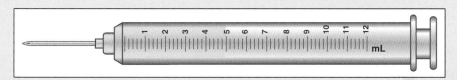

3. Order: neostigmine methylsulfate 0.75 mg subcutaneous
   Supply: ampoule labelled 1:1000

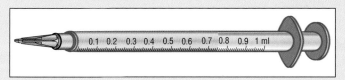

4. Order: epinephrine 0.5 mg subcutaneous stat
   Supply: ampoule labelled 1:1000

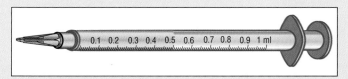

5. Order: neostigmine methylsulfate 1.5 mg IM tid
   Supply: ampoule labelled 1:2000

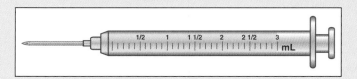

When Supply Is a Percent

Labels may state the strength of a drug as a percent. Percent means parts per hundred. *Percentages are always interpreted in the metric system as grams per 100 mL.*

Example	Lidocaine 2% = 2 g in 100 mL

Percents may be stated in three ways:

     2 g per 100 mL

     2 g = 100 mL

     2 g/100 mL

SELF TEST 4   **Percentages**

Write the following percentage in three ways. Answers appear at the end of the chapter.

PERCENTAGE	? g per 100 mL	? g = 100 mL	? g/100 mL
0.9%	_____	_____	_____
10%	_____	_____	_____
0.45%	_____	_____	_____
50%	_____	_____	_____
0.33%	_____	_____	_____
5%	_____	_____	_____
30%	_____	_____	_____
1.5%	_____	_____	_____
1%	_____	_____	_____
20%	_____	_____	_____

To solve percent problems, state the percent as the number of grams per mL.

Example	Order: lidocaine 30 mg for injection before suturing wound

Supply: Read the label.

DIN 01901950   MULTI DOSE VIAL 20 mL

℗LIDOCAINE 1% HCI (10mg/mL)

Epinephrine 1:10000 injection (100 mcg/mL)

FOR INFILTRATION / BLOCK
NOT FOR EPIDURAL OR CAUDAL USE

WARNING: CONTAINS A PRESERVATIVE

Store at room temperature (15-30°C)

DIRECTIONS FOR USE: See package insert.

EXP DEC. 2011

Equivalents: 1% means

> 1 g in 100 mL

> 1 g = 1000 mg

Supply is 1000 mg in 100 mL. Note 10 mg/mL is indicated on label.

Formula Method	Proportion Expressed as Two Ratios	Proportion Expressed as Two Fractions
$\frac{30 \text{ mg}}{10 \text{ mg}} \times 1 \text{ mL} = x$	1mL : 10 mg :: x : 30 mg	$\frac{1 \text{ mL}}{10 \text{ mg}} \times \frac{x}{30 \text{ mg}}$

Formula Method:

$$\frac{30 \text{ mg}}{2000 \text{ mg}}$$

$$\frac{1}{100} = \frac{3}{2} \quad \frac{1.5}{2)3.0}$$

$$\frac{30 \text{ mg}}{1000 \text{ mg}} \times 100$$

Proportion Expressed as Two Fractions:

$$\frac{30}{10} = x$$

$$3 = x$$

Prepare 3 mL.

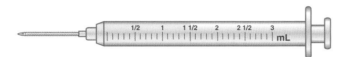

Example

Order: magnesium sulfate 1 g; add to IV stat

Supply: Read the label

DIN 00392618   10mL

℞ **Magnesium Sulphate 50%**

Injection (0.5 g/mL)

500 mg / mL

4.06 mEq/mL

For IM/IV Use

Single Dose Vial: DISCARD UNUSED PORTION

Consult package insert for complete instructions

Store between 15–30°C

EXP DEC.2012

Equivalent: 50% means 50 g in 100 mL

Formula Method	Proportion Expressed as Two Ratios	Proportion Expressed as Two Fractions
$\frac{1 \text{ g}}{50 \text{ g}} \times 100 \text{ mL} = 2 \text{ mL}$	100 mL : 50 g :: x : 1 g	$\frac{100 \text{ mL}}{50 \text{ g}} \times \frac{x}{1 \text{ g}}$

$$\frac{100}{50} = x$$

$$2 \text{ mL} = x$$

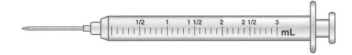

SELF TEST 5   Using Percentages with Liquids for Injection

Solve these problems involving percentages. Answers appear at the end of the chapter. Answers are in millilitres (mL).

1. Order: epinephrine 5 mg subcutaneous stat
   Supply: ampoule labelled 1%

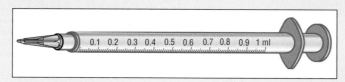

2. Order: lidocaine 15 mg subcutaneous
   Supply: ampoule labelled 1%

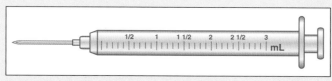

3. Order: Neo-Synephrine (phenylephrine HCl) 3 mg subcutaneous stat
   Supply: ampoule labelled 1%

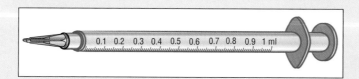

4. Order: Prepare for IV use calcium gluconate 0.3 g
   Supply: ampoule labelled 10%

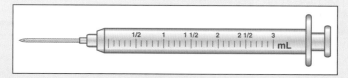

5. Order: Prepare for IV use dextrose 5 g IV
   Supply: syringe labelled 50%

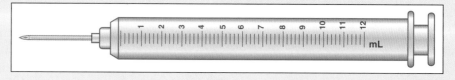

Insulin Injections

Types of Insulin

Insulin is a hormone that regulates glucose metabolism. It is measured in units and is administered by injection. Insulin is most commonly supplied in 10-mL vials containing 100 units/mL. Several types of insulin are currently available: those prepared from animal tissue, or semisynthetically, or synthetically using recombinant DNA.

Insulin cannot be given orally because enzymes in the gastrointestinal (GI) tract destroy it. Instead, insulins are administered subcutaneously—except for regular insulin, which can be given either subcutaneously or IV. An insulin nasal spray is being developed and also an insulin patch that will continuously deliver a low dose of insulin through the skin.

Insulins are classified as short, rapid, intermediate, or long acting. Because onset of action, time of peak activity, and duration of action vary, nurses must be careful to choose and calculate the correct insulin. Table 7-1 summarizes the onset, peak, and duration of various insulins.

Many hospitals and other institutions require that two licensed nurses double-check the type and amount of insulin prepared. Know the policy of your institution, and follow it.

SHORT-ACTING INSULINS. These begin acting within 30 minutes and peak in 2 to 3 hours; actions may last 6 to 7 hours. Insulins are administered subcutaneously except for regular insulin, which can also be given IV.

A large "R" on the label immediately tells you that this is **regular** insulin. Most insulin used clinically is human insulin, Humulin, which is synthesized in the laboratory using recombinant DNA technology.

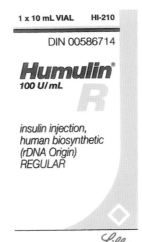

Used with permission of Eli Lilly Canada, Inc.

TABLE 7-1 Types of Insulin Approved for Use in Canada

Type	Brand Names	Onset	Peak	Duration
Rapid-acting analogue	Humalog[R] NovaRapid[R] Apidra[R]	10–15 min	60–90 min	3–5 hr
Short-acting	Humulin[R]-R Novolin[R] ge Toronto	30 min	2–3 hr	6.5 hr
Intermediate-acting	Humulin[R]-N Novolin[R] ge NPH	1–3 hr	5–8 hr	Up to 18 hr
Long-acting analogue	Lantus[R] Levemir[R]	90 min	None	• Up to 24 hr • 16–24 hr
Pre-mixed: a single vial or cartridge contains a fixed ratio of insulin	Premixed regular insulin—NPH • Humulin[R] (30/70) • Novolin[R] ge (30/70, 40/60, 50/50) Premixed Insulin analogues • Humalog[R] Mix 25 and Mix 50 • NovoMix 30	Depends on the combination		

Source: The Canadian Diabetic Association, http://www.diabetes.ca/

HUMALOG—A UNIQUE, RAPID-ACTING INSULIN. Humalog (lispro) insulin is the newest human insulin product made by recombinant DNA technology. Like regular insulin, it lowers blood sugar, but much more rapidly. Humalog starts acting 10 to 15 minutes after injection, peaks in 1 hour, and lasts 3 to 5 hours. Owing to the rapid onset, a food source must be readily available when administering.

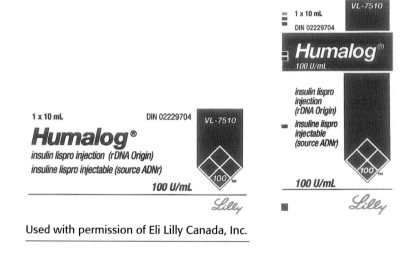

Used with permission of Eli Lilly Canada, Inc.

INTERMEDIATE-ACTING INSULINS (ISOPHANE) These begin action in 1 to 3 hours, peak around 5 to 8 hours, and may last up to 18 hours. On the label, the letter "N" indicates that regular insulin has been modified, through the addition of zinc and protamine (a basic protein), to delay absorption and prolong the time of action. The label may also show the letters "NPH", which denote intermediate action: N, means the solution is neutral pH; P, indicates the protamine content; H, stands for Hagedorn, the laboratory that first prepared this type of insulin.

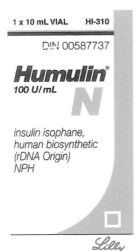

1 x 10 mL VIAL   HI-310

DIN 00587737

Humulin®
100 U/mL
N

insulin isophane,
human biosynthetic
(rDNA Origin)
NPH

Lilly   Used with permission of Eli Lilly Canada, Inc.

LONG-ACTING INSULINS. Lantus (insulin glargine) and Levemir (insulin detemir) are given subcutaneously and must not be mixed with other insulins. Onset is 90 minutes, there is no peak, and duration is up to 24 hours (Levemir lasts 16–24 hours). This long duration makes them similar to the normal insulin secretion in the human body.

Indication: LANTUS [insulin glargine injection (rDNA origin)] is a novel recombinant human insulin analog indicated for once-daily subcutaneous administration in the treatment of patients over 17 years of age with Type 1 or Type 2 diabetes mellitus who require basal (long-acting) insulin for the control of hyperglycemia. LANTUS is also indicated in the treatment of pediatric patients with Type 1 diabetes mellitus who require basal (long-acting) insulin for the control of hyperglycemia. **Dosage:** The desired blood glucose levels as well as the doses and timing of antidiabetic medications must be determined and adjusted individually. Blood glucose monitoring is recommended for all patients with diabetes. See the package insert for adequate directions for use. **Preservative:** 2.7 mg m-cresol. Product Monograph available to health professionals upon request. **Warning: Keep out of reach of children.**

EXPORT PROHIBITED
Unopened Vial: Unopened LANTUS® vials should be stored in a refrigerator, between 2°C - 8°C. LANTUS should not be stored in the freezer and it should not be allowed to freeze. If refrigeration is not possible, unopened LANTUS can be kept unrefrigerated (15 - 30°C) for up to 28 days away from direct heat and light, as long as the temperature is not greater than 30°C. If LANTUS freezes or overheats, discard it.

Opened (In Use) Vial: Opened LANTUS vials whether or not refrigerated, must be discarded after 28 days even if they contain insulin. The opened vial can also be kept unrefrigerated (15 - 30°C) for up to 28 days away from direct heat and light, as long as the temperature is not greater than 30°C.
Opened LANTUS vials should not be stored in the freezer and should not be allowed to freeze. If a vial freezes or overheats, discard it.
Do not use a vial of LANTUS after the expiration date stamped on the label or if it is cloudy or if you see particles.

DIN 02245689

Lantus®

Insulin Glargine Injection
(rDNA origin) /
*Insuline glargine injectable
(ADN recombiné)*

100 U/mL

Sterile Solution /
Solution stérile

Subcutaneous Injection /
Pour injection sous-cutanée

Antidiabetic Agent /
Antidiabétique

One 10 mL vial /
1 fiole de **10 mL**

sanofi aventis

EXPORTATION INTERDITE
Fioles intactes : Les fioles LANTUS® qui n'ont pas été conservées au réfrigérateur, à une température se situant entre 2 et 8 °C. LANTUS ne doit pas être gardé au congélateur ni exposé au gel. Si on ne peut pas réfrigérer le produit, les contenants intacts de LANTUS se conservent jusqu'à 28 jours à une température se situant entre 15 et 30 °C, pourvu qu'ils soient gardés à l'abri de la chaleur et de la lumière directes, et que la température ne dépasse pas 30 °C. Si le produit gèle ou qu'il est exposé à une chaleur excessive, il doit être jeté.

Fioles ouvertes (en cours d'utilisation) : Les fioles LANTUS qui ont été ouvertes, qu'elles aient été réfrigérées ou non, doivent être jetées au bout de 28 jours, même si elles contiennent de l'insuline. Les fioles LANTUS ouvertes peuvent aussi se conserver non réfrigérées jusqu'à 28 jours à une température se situant entre 15 et 30 °C, pourvu qu'elles soient gardées à l'abri de la chaleur et de la lumière directes, et que la température ne dépasse pas 30 °C.
Les fioles LANTUS qui ont été ouvertes ne doivent pas être gardées au congélateur ni exposées au gel. Si les fioles gèlent ou qu'elles sont exposées à une chaleur excessive, elles doivent être jetées.
N'utilisez pas une fiole de LANTUS dont la date de péremption indiquée sur l'étiquette est dépassée ou si la solution qu'elle contient est trouble ou présente des particules.

Indication : LANTUS [insuline glargine injectable [ADN recombiné]] est un nouvel analogue de l'insuline humaine obtenu par recombinaison génétique pour administration uniquotidienne par voie sous-cutanée, indiqué dans le traitement des patients de plus de 17 ans atteints de diabète de type 1 ou de type 2 devant prendre de l'insuline basale (à action prolongée) afin de maîtriser leur glycémie. LANTUS est aussi indiqué dans le traitement des enfants atteints de diabète de type 1 devant prendre de l'insuline basale (à action prolongée) afin de maîtriser leur glycémie. **Posologie :** Les cibles glycémiques, les doses et l'horaire d'administration des antidiabétiques doivent être déterminés et ajustés en fonction de chaque patient. La surveillance de la glycémie est recommandée chez tous les patients atteints de diabète. Voir la notice ci-incluse pour connaître les directives d'emploi du produit. **Agent de conservation :** 2,7 mg de m-crésol. Monographie du produit fournie sur demande aux professionnels de la santé. **Mise en garde : Tenir hors de la portée des enfants.**

Manufactured by sanofi-aventis Canada Inc.,
Laval, Quebec, Canada H7L 4A8
1-888-8LANTUS (1-888-852-6887)
www.sanofi-aventis.ca
B50057791-C

Fabriqué par sanofi-aventis Canada Inc.,
Laval (Québec) Canada H7L 4A8
1-888-8LANTUS (1-888-852-6887)
www.sanofi-aventis.ca

Used with permission of Sanofi-Aventis Canada, Inc.

MIXED INSULINS. A single vial or cartridge contains a fixed ratio of insulin. Mixed insulins combine rapid and intermediate insulin. They save nursing time in preparation and are also more convenient for the patient, who must learn to draw up and self-administer an injection.

The numbers refer to the percent of rapid-or short-acting insulin related to the percent of intermediate-acting insulin.

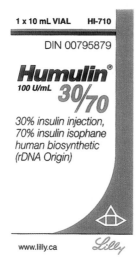

1 x 10 mL VIAL   HI-710

DIN 00795879

Humulin®
100 U/mL **30/70**

30% insulin injection,
70% insulin isophane
human biosynthetic
(rDNA Origin)

www.lilly.ca   *Lilly*   Used with permission of Eli Lilly Canada, Inc.

Regular insulin should appear clear and colourless; it is the only insulin that may be given IV. Other insulins appear cloudy. Gently rotate (don't shake) cloudy insulin vials between your hands to resuspend the particles.

Types of Insulin Syringes

Only an insulin syringe should be used to administer insulin doses. Insulin syringes have unit markings that decrease the possibility of errors as insulin in Canada is supplied as 100 units/mL. All insulin orders must be in units. Insulin syringes are marked as U 100 and have small-gauge needles attached. Standard sizes are ½ mL and 1 mL (Fig. 7-6).

Preparing an Injection Using an Insulin Syringe

The physician or healthcare provider's order for insulin is written as units; the stock comes in 100 units/mL. Both syringes are calibrated (lined) for 100 units/mL.

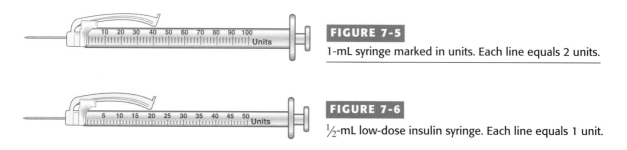

FIGURE 7-5

1-mL syringe marked in units. Each line equals 2 units.

FIGURE 7-6

½-mL low-dose insulin syringe. Each line equals 1 unit.

Example

Order: 60 units Humulin N subcutaneous every day

Supply: Read the label

Ask yourself three questions:

1. What is the order? Humulin N 60 units
2. What is the supply? Humulin N 100 units/mL
3. Is a U 100 insulin syringe available? Yes.

Using aseptic technique, draw up the amount required into the syringe.

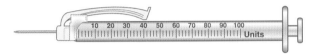

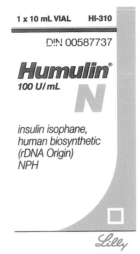

1 x 10 mL VIAL   HI-310

DIN 00587737

Humulin®
100 U/mL
N

insulin isophane,
human biosynthetic
(rDNA Origin)
NPH

Lilly

Used with permission of
Eli Lilly Canada, Inc.

Example

Order: 35 units Humulin R insulin subcutaneous stat

Supply: Read the label

Ask yourself three questions:

1. What is the order? Humulin R insulin 35 units
2. What is the supply? Humulin R 100 units/mL
3. What syringe should be used? Low-dose insulin syringe

Using aseptic technique, draw up the amount required into the syringe.

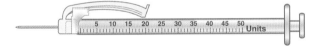

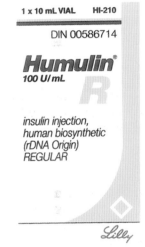

1 x 10 mL VIAL   HI-210

DIN 00586714

Humulin®
100 U/mL
R

insulin injection,
human biosynthetic
(rDNA Origin)
REGULAR

Lilly

Used with permission of
Eli Lilly Canada, Inc.

Mixing Two Insulins in One Syringe

Sometimes the physician or healthcare provider will order regular insulin to be mixed with another insulin and injected together at the same site. Remember two points:

1. Always draw up the regular insulin into the syringe first.
2. The total number of units in the syringe equals the two insulin orders added together.

Regular insulin is often ordered with NPH insulin. Since regular insulin is clear and NPH insulin is cloudy, the mnemonic "clear to cloudy" may help you to remember which insulin to draw up first.
To prepare two insulins with one syringe:

1. Inject into the NPH vial the amount of air equal to the amount of NPH insulin ordered, being careful not to let the needle touch the medication.
2. Inject into the regular vial the amount of air equal to the amount of regular insulin ordered.
3. Withdraw the correct amount of regular insulin ("clear").
4. Withdraw the correct amount of NPH insulin ("cloudy").
5. The total number of units will be the regular insulin amount plus the NPH insulin amount.

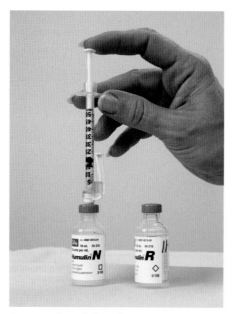

Step 1. Inject air into the NPH (Humulin N) vial.

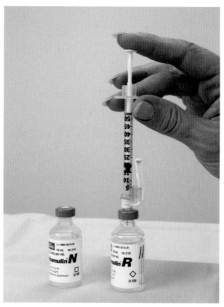

Step 2. Inject air into the regular (Humulin R) vial.

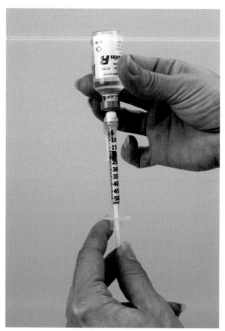

Step 3. Withdraw the correct amount of regular (Humulin R) insulin.

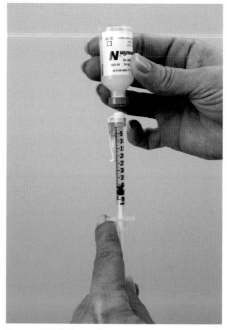

Step 4. Withdraw the correct amount of NPH (Humulin R) insulin.

(Used with permission from Evans-Smith, P. [2005]. *Taylor's clinical nursing skills.* Philadelphia: Lippincott Williams & Wilkins, pp. 128–129.)

Example Order: Humulin R insulin 15 units ⎱ every morning, at breakfast, subcutaneously
Humulin N insulin 10 units ⎰

Supply: Humulin R insulin 100 units/mL
Humulin N insulin 100 units/mL

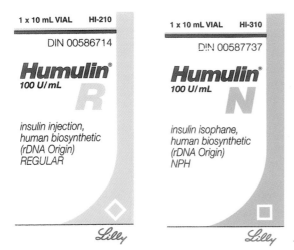

Used with permission of Eli Lilly Canada, Inc.

1. What are the orders? Humulin R 15 units; Humulin N 10 units

2. What is the supply? Humulin R 100 units/mL; Humulin N 100 units/mL

3. Is there an insulin syringe? Yes

4. What will be the total units in the syringe? 25 units

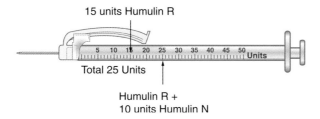

Sliding-Scale Regular Insulin Dosages

Sliding-scale insulin orders refer to a method of insulin administration that is based on the blood glucose (BG) result. The BG result often comes from a finger-stick and uses some type of glucometer such as an Accucheck monitor. The order will read something like this:

Accuchecks every 4 hours. Give Humulin R as per sliding scale below:

- For blood sugar < 4.0 mmol/L: Call physician

- For blood sugar 4.1–8.0 mmol/L: Give 0 units Humulin R

- For blood sugar 8.1–11.4 mmol/L: Give 2 units Humulin R

- For blood sugar 11.5–14.0 mmol/L: Give 4 units Humulin R

- For blood sugar 14.1–17.0 mmol/L: Give 6 units Humulin R

- For blood sugar 17.1–20.0 mmol/L: Give 8 units Humulin R

- If blood sugar > 20.1 mmol/L: Call physician

In this example, the nurse assesses the BG using a glucometer and, according to the results, gives the ordered amount of insulin. Most hospitals still require that another licensed nurse double-check both the physician's order and the amount of insulin drawn into the syringe.

Insulin Pens and Prefilled Insulin Devices

Insulin pens and prefilled insulin devices contain insulin in a cartridge. The dosage is calculated in the same manner: a needle is attached to the pen or prefilled insulin device, and then the number of units is set with a small dial on the insulin pen or prefilled insulin device (Fig. 7-7). The injection is given subcutaneously and held in place for 6 to 10 seconds. Then the needle is removed from the pen or prefilled insulin device and discarded safely. The insulin pen or prefilled insulin device can be used until the insulin cartridge is empty. Usually the insulin pen or prefilled insulin device is primed with 1 to 2 units before giving the actual dose. There are several advantages, including portability and ease of measuring an accurate dose. However, not all insulins can be supplied, and there is no way to mix insulins with an insulin pen or prefilled insulin device. In a hospital setting, the insulin pen or prefilled insulin device is supplied for only one patient and usually doses must be verified by two licensed nurses.

An insulin pump can administer insulin continuously by the subcutaneous route. A pump is placed near the abdominal area of the patient. The pump is preset at a certain rate to deliver the insulin via tubing through a needle inserted in the subcutaneous tissue. Settings can be adjusted to the patient's insulin needs. The site and tubing are usually changed every 2 to 3 days or as needed (Fig. 7-8).

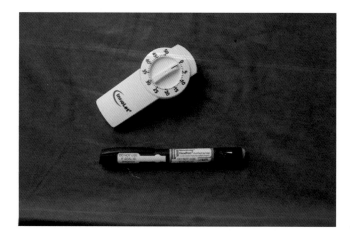

FIGURE 7-7

Insulin pen. (Copyright © 2008 Lacey-Bordeaux Photography.)

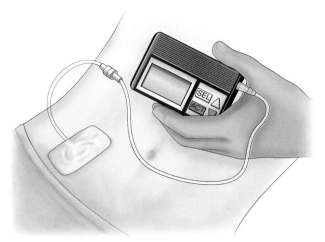

FIGURE 7-8

Insulin pump. (With permission from Taylor, C. [2008]. *Fundamentals of nursing*. Philadelphia: Lippincott Williams and Wilkins, p. 797.)

SELF TEST 6 | Insulin Calculations

Solve these insulin problems. Draw a line on the syringe to indicate the dose you would prepare. Answers appear at the end of the chapter.

1. Order: NPH insulin 56 units subcutaneous every day
     Supply: vial of NPH insulin 100 units/mL

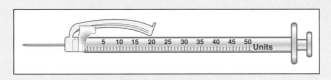

2. Order: 7 units regular insulin and 20 units NPH insulin subcutaneous every day at 0700h
     Supply: vial of regular insulin 100 units/mL and NPH 100 units/mL

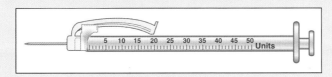

3. Order: Humulin R insulin 4 units subcutaneous stat
     Supply: vial Humulin R insulin 100 units/mL

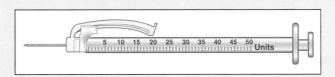

4. Order: Lantus 28 units subcutaneous
     Supply: Lantus insulin zinc suspension 100 units/mL

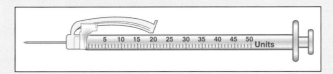

5. Order: 20 units of NPH subcutaneous every day
     Supply: vial of NPH 100 units/mL

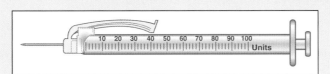

6. Order: regular insulin 16 units with NPH insulin 64 units subcutaneous every day
     Supply: vial of regular insulin 100 units/mL and vial of NPH 100 units/mL

(continued)

Use the following sliding scale to calculate the insulin dosages. Draw a line on the syringe to indicate the dose you would prepare.

Accuchecks q4h.

For BG >18.1 mmol/L call physician.

For BG 14.1–18.0 mmol/L give 5 units of regular insulin subcutaneous.

For BG 11.5–14.0 mmol/L give 3 units of regular insulin subcutaneous.

For BG 8.1–11.4 mmol/L give 2 units of regular insulin subcutaneous.

For BG 4.1–8.0 mmol/L give 0 units of regular insulin subcutaneous.

For BG < 4.0 mmol/L give 1 ampoule of D50 and call physician.

7. Accucheck 10.6 mmol/L

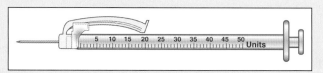

8. Accucheck 13.8 mmol/L

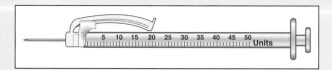

9. Accucheck 19.1 mmol/L

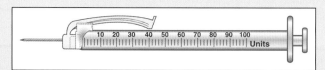

10. Accucheck 3.6 mmol/L

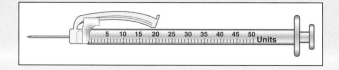

Injections from Powders

Some medications are prepared in a dry form, powder, or crystal. As liquids, they are unstable and lose potency over time. The drug must be reconstituted according to the manufacturer's directions, which will give the type and amount of diluent to use.

In some hospitals and other healthcare settings, the pharmacy is responsible for reconstituting medications. Sometimes, however, this task becomes the nurses' responsibility; that's why this book includes these kinds of dosage calculations. Some drugs are reconstituted using a special reconstitution device within an IV bag. (See Chapter 8 for more information.) Others use traditional needle (or needleless) device and syringe.

To solve injection-from-powder problems, you use the same rule as for oral medications and for injection from a liquid. This is because once the powder is dissolved, the powdered drug takes liquid form.

Preparing the Dose

Drugs That Are Powders in Vials

1. Clean the top of the vial with an alcohol pad.

2. Draw up the amount of calculated diluent from a vial of sterile water or normal saline for injection. If a different diluent is indicated, follow pharmaceutical directions.

3. Add the diluent to the powder and roll the vial between your hands to cause the powder to dissolve completely

4. Label the vial with the concentration made, your initials, and the date and time of reconstitution.

5. Clean the top of the vial with an alcohol pad.

6. Draw up into the syringe an amount of air equivalent to the amount of solution desired.

7. Insert the syringe needle (or needleless device) through the rubber diaphragm into the vial.

8. Inject the air from the syringe into the vial. This increases the pressure in the vial and makes it easier to withdraw the medication.

9. Invert the vial, hold it at eye level, and draw up the desired amount into the syringe (see Fig. 7-1B). Ensure there are no bubbles as this will alter the amount of medication.

10. Withdraw the needle (or needleless device) quickly from the vial.

11. If needle is to be used for a parenteral injection (IM, subcutaneously, or ID) change the needle to one of the correct length and gauge to maximize patient comfort during the injection.

12. Check the directions for storing any remaining drug.

Application of the Rule for Injections from Powders

RULE

Formula Method	Proportion Expressed as Two Ratios	Proportion Expressed as Two Fractions
$\dfrac{\text{Desire}}{\text{Have}} \times \text{Supply} = \text{Amount}$	Supply : Desire :: x : Have	$\dfrac{x}{\text{Desire}} = \dfrac{\text{Supply}}{\text{Have}}$

Example   Order: cefonicid sodium 0.65 g IM every day.

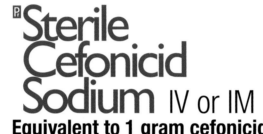

DIN 11223456

℞ Sterile Cefonicid Sodium IV or IM
Equivalent to 1 gram cefonicid

Before reconstitution, protect from light and refrigerate (2–8°C)

For IM or IV Direct Injections: Add 2.5 mL Sterile Water for injection. Shake well. Provides an approximate volume of 3.1 mL

325 mg/mL usual Adult Dose: 1 gram every 24 hrs. as a single dose.

DATE / TIME:
INITIALS:

Storage: After reconstitution:
24 h at room temperature
72 h if refrigerated (5°C)

Label directions: Add 2.5 mL sterile water for injection. Shake well. Provides an approximate volume of 3.1 mL (325 mg/mL). Stable 24 hours at room temperature or 72 hours if refrigerated (5°C).

Desire: The order in the example is 0.65 g.

Have: The strength of the drug supplied. The example is 1 g as a dry powder; when reconstituted, it is 325 mg/mL. Remember that the manufacturer gives the strength of the solution; the nurse does not have to determine it.

Supply: The fluid portion of the solution made. In this example, it is 1 mL = 325 mg.

Answer: How much liquid to give, stated as mL.

Equivalent: 0.65 g = 650 mg

Formula Method	Proportion Expressed as Two Ratios	Proportion Expressed as Two Fractions
$\frac{D}{H} \times S = x \frac{\overset{2}{\cancel{650}} \text{ mg}}{\underset{1}{\cancel{325}} \text{ mg}} \times 1 \text{ mL} = 2 \text{ mL}$	$1 \text{ mL} : 325 \text{ mg} :: x \text{ mL} : 650 \text{ mg}$	$\frac{x \text{ mL}}{650 \text{ mg}} \times \frac{1 \text{ mL}}{325 \text{ mg}}$

$$650 = 325x$$

$$2 \text{ mL} = x$$

Give 2 mL. Store the remaining solution in the refrigerator. Label the vial with the date, the time, the solution made (325 mg/mL), the expiration date (year/month/day) + time, and the initials of the nurse who dissolved the powder.

> *325 mg/mL*
>
> *10/Oct/24 1600 h*
>
> *BP*
>
> *Expires 10/Oct/27 1600h*

Distinctive Features of Injections from Powders

Aseptic technique is used to prepare and administer the medication, which is given parenterally (usually IM, IV, or IVPB). The dry drug is supplied in vials of powder or crystals and may come in different strengths. Because powders deteriorate in solution, choose the strength closest to the amount ordered.

The powder is usually diluted with one of the following:

- Sterile water for injection
- Bacteriostatic water for injection with a preservative added
- Normal saline for injection (0.9% sodium chloride)

Directions will state which fluids may be used. Read this information carefully because some fluids may be incompatible (i.e., unsuitable) as diluents. When the powder goes into solution, *displacement* occurs. This means that as the powder dissolves, it increases the volume added to the vial. There is no uniformity in the way powders go into solution.

Refer to the label for Cefonicid again. The manufacturer tells the nurse to add 2.5 mL sterile water to provide an approximate volume of 3.1 mL. In this example, 0.6 mL is the displacement volume. *Injections-from-powder problems are solved by using the solution made, not the displacement volume.* The manufacturer will give the solution.

Example   The package insert information concerning the dilution of Cefobid (cefoperazone) injection is reproduced in Figure 7-9. Examine the directions with the intention of solving the following problem, then read the explanation:

Order: Cefobid (cefoperazone) 0.5 g IM q12h

Supply: 1-g vial of powder

Search the directions for three pieces of information to dissolve your supply, which is 1 g:

1. Type of fluid needed to dissolve the powder
2. Amount of fluid to add
3. Solution made

Explanation

1. Figure 7-9 gives *Solutions for Initial Reconstitution:* sterile water for injection, bacteriostatic water for injection, and 0.9% sodium chloride injection. Choose one.

2. The heading *Preparation for Intramuscular Injection* states that when a concentration of 250 mg or more is to be administered, a 2% lidocaine solution should be used together with sterile water for injection in a two-step dilution.

3. Two tables are given. The upper table has the two-step dilution; the lower one does not. Because the order requires two steps, use the directions in the top table.

4. Two strengths of powder are listed in the upper table. Look at the extreme left. They are for a 1-g vial and a 2-g vial. Our supply is a 1-g vial. Follow directions for 1 g.

5. The next heading is *Final Cefoperazone Concentration.* Two possibilities are given for the dilution: 333 mg/mL and 250 mg/mL. Because the order calls for 0.5 g, choose 250 mg/mL. 0.5 g = 500 mg so you will need 2 mL of solution.

6. To make the solution of 250 mg/mL, add the following: 2.8 mL sterile water and 1.0 mL 2% lidocaine.

7. The last column on the right, headed *Withdrawable Volume,* lists 4 mL. Ignore this column; it does not affect the answer: When you add 2.8 mL and 1.0 mL, you expect to have 3.8 mL. The package insert states you will end up with 4 mL. The manufacturer is giving the displacement.

RECONSTITUTION

The following solutions may be used for the initial reconstitution of CEFOBID sterile powder:

Table 1. Solutions for Initial Reconstitution

5% Dextrose Injection (USP)	0.9% Sodium Chloride Injection (USP)
5% Dextrose and 0.9% Sodium Chloride Injection (USP)	Normosol® M and Dextrose Injection
5% Dextrose and 0.2% Sodium Chloride Injection (USP)	Normosol® R
10% Dextrose Injection (USP)	Sterile Water for Injection*
Bacteriostatic Water for Injection [Benzyl Alcohol or Parabens] (USP)*†	

* Not to be used as a vehicle for intravenous infusion.
† Preparation containing Benzyl Alcohol should not be used in neonates.

Preparation for Intramuscular Injection

Any suitable solution listed above may be used to prepare CEFOBID sterile powder for intramuscular injection. When concentrations of 250 mg/ml or more are to be administered, a lidocaine solution should be used. These solutions should be prepared using a combination of Sterile Water for Injection and 2% Lidocaine Hydrochloride Injection (USP) that approximates a 0.5% Lidocaine Hydrochloride Solution. A two-step dilution process as follows is recommended: First, add the required amount of Sterile Water for Injection and agitate until CEFOBID powder is completely dissolved. Second, add the required amount of 2% lidocaine and mix.

	Final Cefoperazone Concentration	Step 1 Volume of Sterile Water	Step 2 Volume of 2% Lidocaine	Withdrawable Volume*†
1 g vial	333 mg/ml	2.0 ml	0.6 ml	3 ml
	250 mg/ml	2.8 ml	1.0 ml	4 ml
2 g vial	333 mg/ml	3.8 ml	1.2 ml	6 ml
	250 mg/ml	5.4 ml	1.8 ml	8 ml

When a diluent other than Lidocaine HCl Injection (USP) is used reconstitute as follows:

	Cefoperazone Concentration	Volume of Diluent to be Added	Withdrawable Volume*
1 g vial	333 mg/ml	2.6 ml	3 ml
	250 mg/ml	3.8 ml	4 ml
2 g vial	333 mg/ml	5.0 ml	6 ml
	250 mg/ml	7.2 ml	8 ml

* There is sufficient excess present to allow for withdrawal of the stated volume.
† Final lidocaine concentration will approximate that obtained if a 0.5% Lidocaine Hydrochloride Solution is used as diluent.

STORAGE AND STABILITY

CEFOBID sterile powder is to be stored at or below 25°C (77°F) and protected from light prior to reconstitution. After reconstitution, protection from light is not necessary.

The following parenteral diluents and approximate concentrations of CEFOBID provide stable solutions under the following conditions for the indicated time periods. (After the indicated time periods, unused portions of solutions should be discarded.)

Controlled Room Temperature (15°–25°C/59°–77°F)

24 Hours   Approximate

Bacteriostatic Water for Injection [Benzyl Alcohol or Parabens] (USP)	300 mg/ml
5% Dextrose Injection (USP)	2 mg to 50 mg/ml
5% Dextrose and Lactated Ringer's Injection	2 mg to 50 mg/ml
5% Dextrose and 0.9% Sodium Chloride Injection (USP)	2 mg to 50 mg/ml
5% Dextrose and 0.2% Sodium Chloride Injection (USP)	2 mg to 50 mg/ml
10% Dextrose Injection (USP)	2 mg to 50 mg/ml
Lactated Ringer's Injection (USP)	2 mg/ml
0.5% Lidocaine Hydrochloride Injection (USP)	300 mg/ml
0.9% Sodium Chloride Injection (USP)	2 mg to 300 mg/ml
Normosol® M and 5% Dextrose Injection	2 mg to 50 mg/ml
Normosol® R	2 mg to 50 mg/ml
Sterile Water for Injection	300 mg/ml

Reconstituted CEFOBID solutions may be stored in glass or plastic syringes, or in glass or flexible plastic parenteral solution containers.

Refrigerator Temperature (2°–8°C/36°–46°F)

5 Days   Approximate Concentrations

Bacteriostatic Water for Injection [Benzyl Alcohol or Parabens] (USP)	300 mg/ml
5% Dextrose Injection (USP)	2 mg to 50 mg/ml
5% Dextrose and 0.9% Sodium Chloride Injection (USP)	2 mg to 50 mg/ml
5% Dextrose and 0.2% Sodium Chloride Injection (USP)	2 mg to 50 mg/ml
Lactated Ringer's Injection (USP)	2 mg/ml
0.5% Lidocaine Hydrochloride Injection (USP)	300 mg/ml
0.9% Sodium Chloride Injection (USP)	2 mg to 300 mg/ml
Normosol® M and 5% Dextrose Injection	2 mg to 50 mg/ml
Normosol® R	2 mg to 50 mg/ml
Sterile Water for Injection	300 mg/ml

Reconstituted CEFOBID solutions may be stored in glass or plastic syringes, or in glass or flexible plastic parenteral solution containers.

FIGURE 7-9

Reconstitution directions for Cefobid (cefoperazone sodium). (Courtesy of Pfizer Laboratories.)

8. You now have all the information needed to prepare the dose ordered. Your solution is 250 mg/mL. Equivalent: 0.5 g = 500 mg.

Formula Method	Proportion Expressed as Two Ratios	Proportion Expressed as Two Fractions
$\dfrac{\overset{2}{\cancel{500}} \text{ mg}}{\underset{1}{\cancel{250}} \text{ mg}} \times 1 \text{ mL} = 2 \text{ mL}$	$1 \text{ mL} : 250 \text{ mg} :: x : 500 \text{ mg}$	$\dfrac{1 \text{ mL}}{250 \text{ mg}} \times \dfrac{x}{500 \text{ mg}}$

$$\frac{500}{250} = x$$

$$2 \text{ mL} = x$$

Give 2 mL IM.

9. Write on the label the solution you made, the date, time, expiration date, and your initials.

10. Note the storage directions and stability expiration.

Where to Find Information about Reconstitution of Powders

Information about reconstitution of powders may be found from

- The label on the vial of powder
- The package insert that comes with the vial of powder
- Nursing drug handbooks
- Other references such as the *Physician's Desk Reference (PDR)*

STEPS FOR RECONSTITUTING POWDERS WITH DIRECTIONS

1. Read the order.
2. Identify the supply.
3. Dilute the fluid.
4. Identify the solution and new supply.
5. Apply the rule and arithmetic.
6. Obtain the amount to give.
7. Write on the label the solution made, date, time, expiration date, and your initials.
8. Store according to directions.

Example   Order: Ancef (cefazolin sodium) 0.3 g IM (Fig. 7-10)

Supply: 500 mg powder

Diluting fluid: 2 mL sterile water for injection

Solution and new supply: 225 mg/mL

RECONSTITUTION
Preparation of Parenteral Solution
Parenteral drug products should be SHAKEN WELL when reconstituted, and inspected visually for particulate matter prior to administration. If particulate matter is evident in reconstituted fluids, the drug solutions should be discarded. When reconstituted or diluted according to the instructions below, Ancef (sterile cefazolin sodium, SK&F) is stable for 24 hours at room temperature or for 96 hours if stored under refrigeration. Reconstituted solutions may range in color from pale yellow to yellow without a change in potency.
Single-Dose Vials
For I.M. injection, I.V. direct (bolus) injection, or I.V. infusion, reconstitute with Sterile Water for Injection according to the following table. SHAKE WELL.

Vial Size	Amount of Diluent	Approximate Concentration	Approximate Available Volume
250 mg.	2.0 ml.	125 mg./ml.	2.0 ml.
500 mg.	2.0 ml.	225 mg./ml.	2.2 ml.
1 gram	2.5 ml.	330 mg./ml.	3.0 ml.

FIGURE 7-10

Reconstitution directions for Ancef (cefazolin sodium). (Courtesy of GlaxoSmithKline.)

Formula Method	Proportion Expressed as Two Ratios	Proportion Expressed as Two Fractions

Equivalent: 0.3 g = 300 mg

$$1 \text{ mL} : 225 \text{ mg} :: x \text{ mL} : 300 \text{ mg}$$

$$\frac{1 \text{ mL}}{225 \text{ mg}} \times \frac{x \text{ mL}}{300 \text{ mg}}$$

$$\frac{300}{225} = x$$

1.33 or 1.3 mL = x

$$\frac{\cancel{300}^{4} \text{ mg}}{\cancel{225}_{3} \text{ mg}} \times 1 \text{ mL} = \frac{4}{3} \overline{)4.00}\,^{1.33}$$

Give 1.3 mL IM.

Write on label: 225 mg/mL, date, time, expiration date, initials.

Storage: Refrigerate; stable for 96 hours.

Example Order: penicillin G potassium 1 million units IM q6h (Fig. 7-11)

Supply powder: 5 million-unit vial

Diluting fluid and number of millilitres: Use sterile water for injection. Write out the directions for the 5 million-unit vial (supply).

23 mL will provide 200,000 units/mL.

18 mL will provide 250,000 units/mL.

8 mL will provide 500,000 units/mL.

3 mL will provide 1 million units/mL.

Choose 3 mL to dilute the powder.

Solution and new supply: 1 million units/mL.

PENICILLIN G POTASSIUM for injection
Preparation of Solutions
Use sterile water for injection
  RECONSTITUTION

1,000,000 u vial	
Diluent	Desired Concentration
9.6 mL	100,000 u/mL
4.6 mL	200,000 u/mL
3.6 mL	250,000 u/mL
5,000,000 u vial	
Diluent	Desired Concentration
23 mL	200,000 u/mL
18 mL	250,000 u/mL
8 mL	500,000 u/mL
3 mL	1,000,000 u/mL

Storage
Prepared solutions may be kept in the refrigerator one week.

FIGURE 7-11
Preparation of solution for the 1 million-unit and the 5 million-unit vials of penicillin G potassium.

Formula Method	Proportion Expressed as Two Ratios	Proportion Expressed as Two Fractions
$\dfrac{1 \text{ million units}}{1 \text{ million units}} \times 1 \text{ mL} = 1 \text{ mL}$	1 mL : 1 million units : : x mL : 1 million units	$\dfrac{1 \text{ mL}}{1 \text{ million units}} \times \dfrac{x}{1 \text{ million units}}$

$$\frac{1 \text{ million units}}{1 \text{ million units}} = x$$

$$1 \text{ mL} = x$$

Give 1 mL IM.

Write on label: 1 million units/mL, date, time, expiration date, initials

Storage: Refrigerate; stable for 1 week

Note: This solution (1 million units/mL) may be so concentrated that it is painful when injected. To make a less painful solution, you can dilute the powder with 8 mL to make 500,000 units/mL and give 2 mL to the patient.

Here are a few tips before you begin Self Test 7.

- When reading the directions for reconstitution, look first at the solutions you can make. Think the problem through mentally and choose one dilution, so that you will have a focus as you read.

- If your answer is more than 3 mL for an IM injection, consider using two syringes and injecting in two different sites.

- Experience in administering injections will guide you in choosing the solution's concentration. Stronger concentrations, although smaller in volume, may be more painful; a more dilute solution may be more suitable despite its larger volume.

- Each powder problem is unique. Carefully read the directions.

- Choose one diluting fluid for injection: generally sterile water or 0.9% sodium chloride. You do not need to list all of the fluids in your answer.

- For the following practice problems and self tests, assume that the doses ordered and the order are correct. Chapter 12 discusses the nurse's responsibilities in drug knowledge. Dosages for infants and children are discussed in Chapter 10.

Solve the following problems in injections from powders and write your answers using the steps. Answers appear at the end of the chapter.

1. Order: Ceftazidime 1 g IM q6h
   Supply: 1 g powder

   a. Diluting fluid and number of millilitres:
   b. Solution and new supply:
   c. Rule and arithmetic:
   d. Answer:
   e. Write on label:
   f. Storage:

<table>
<tr><td colspan="4" align="center">**CEFTAZIDIME INJECTION**</td></tr>
<tr><td colspan="4">Reconstitution</td></tr>
<tr><td colspan="4">Single dose vials: Reconstitute with sterile water. Shake well.</td></tr>
<tr><td>**Vial Size**</td><td>**Diluent**</td><td>**Approx. Avail. Volume**</td><td>**Approx. Avg. Concentration**</td></tr>
<tr><td>IM or IV bolus injection</td><td></td><td></td><td></td></tr>
<tr><td>1 g</td><td>3.0 mL</td><td>3.6 mL</td><td>280 mg/mL</td></tr>
<tr><td>IV infusion</td><td></td><td></td><td></td></tr>
<tr><td>1 g</td><td>10 mL</td><td>10.6 mL</td><td>95 mg/mL</td></tr>
<tr><td>2 g</td><td>10 mL</td><td>11.2 mL</td><td>180 mg/mL</td></tr>
<tr><td colspan="4">Stable for 18 hours at room temperature or 7 days if refrigerated.</td></tr>
</table>

Label and reconstitution directions for ceftazidime.

2. Order: ampicillin 250 mg IM q6h
   Supply: 500-mg vial of powder

   a. Diluting fluid and number of millilitres:
   b. Solution and new supply:
   c. Rule and arithmetic:
   d. Answer:
   e. Write on label:
   f. Storage:

AMPICILLIN
Reconstitution
Dissolve contents of a vial with the amount of Sterile Water or Bacteriostatic Water.

Amount Ordered	Recommended Amount of Diluent	Withdraw Volume	Concentration in mg/ml
500 mg	1.8 mL	2.0 mL	250 mg
1.0 g	3.4 mL	4.0 mL	250 mg
2.0 g	6.8 mL	8.0 mL	250 mg

Storage
Use within 1 hour of reconstitution.

Reconstitution directions for ampicillin for IM or IV injection.

(continued)

3. Order: Ancef (cefazolin sodium) 225 mg IM q6h

     Supply: On the shelf, there are three vial sizes of powder: 250 mg, 500 mg, 1 g

    a. Supply chosen:

    b. Diluting fluid and number of millilitres:

    c. Solution and new supply:

    d. Rule and arithmetic:

    e. Answer:

    f. Write on label:

    g. Storage:

RECONSTITUTION

Preparation of Parenteral Solution

Parenteral drug products should be SHAKEN WELL when reconstituted, and inspected visually for particulate matter prior to administration. If particulate matter is evident in reconstituted fluids, the drug solutions should be discarded. When reconstituted or diluted according to the instructions below, Ancef (sterile cefazolin sodium, SK&F) is stable for 24 hours at room temperature or for 96 hours if stored under refrigeration. Reconstituted solutions may range in color from pale yellow to yellow without a change in potency.

Single-Dose Vials

For I.M. injection, I.V. direct (bolus) injection, or I.V. infusion, reconstitute with Sterile Water for Injection according to the following table. SHAKE WELL.

Vial Size	Amount of Diluent	Approximate Concentration	Approximate Available Volume
250 mg.	2.0 ml.	125 mg./ml.	2.0 ml.
500 mg.	2.0 ml.	225 mg./ml.	2.2 ml.
1 gram	2.5 ml.	330 mg./ml.	3.0 ml.

Reconstitution directions for Ancef (cefazolin sodium). (Courtesy of GlaxoSmithKline.)

---

4. Order: Cefazolin 500 mg IM q6h

     Supply: 1 g powder

    a. Diluting fluid and number of millilitres:

    b. Solution:

    c. Rule and arithmetic:

    d. Answer:

    e. Write on label:

    f. Storage:

Sterile   **DIN 02108127**

           10 x 1 g vials

℞ CEFAZOLIN for Injection, USP

1 g

Cefazolin per vial

ANTIBIOTIC

Intramuscular or intravenous use only

For intramuscular use, add 2.5 mL Sterile Water for Injection for a 334 mg/mL solution.

For direct intravenous (bolus) use, further dilute reconstituted solution to a minimum of 10 mL with Sterile Water for Injection. **SHAKE WELL.**

For intermittent intravenous infusion, further dilute in 50 to 100 mL of one of the recommended intravenous solutions. Use reconstituted solution within 24 hours when stored at controlled room temperature not exceeding 25°C, or within 72 hours if refrigerated (2°C to 8 °C), protected from light. Consult package insert for dosage and prescribing information.

Product Monograph available upon request.

Store powder between 15°C and 25°C. Protect from light.

®-Reg'd Trademark of Novopharm Limited, Toronto, Canada M1B 2K9

69397CT-0110   Rev. 03

LOT 360226
EXP 05.2011

Used with permission of Novopharm.

(continued)

5. Order: Mefoxin (cefoxitin sodium) 200 mg IM q4h
   Supply: vial of powder labelled 1 g

   a. Diluting fluid and number of millilitres:
   b. Solution made and new supply:
   c. Rule and arithmetic:
   d. Answer:
   e. Write on label:
   f. Storage:

Table 3 — Preparation of Solution			
Strength	Amount of Diluent to be Added (mL) + +	Approximate Withdrawable Volume (mL)	Approximate Average Concentration (mg/mL)
1 gram Vial	2 (Intramuscular)	2.5	400
2 gram Vial	4 (Intramuscular)	5	400
1 gram Vial	10 (IV)	10.5	95
2 gram Vial	10 or 20 (IV)	11.1 or 21.0	180 or 95
1 gram Infusion Bottle	50 or 100 (IV)	50 or 100	20 or 10
2 gram Infusion Bottle	50 or 100 (IV)	50 or 100	40 or 20
10 gram Bulk	43 or 93 (IV)	49 or 98.5	200 or 100

+ + Shake to dissolve and let stand until clear.

Intramuscular
   MEFOXIN, as constituted with Sterile Water for Injection, Bacteriostatic Water for Injection, or 0.5 percent or 1 percent lidocaine hydrochloride solution (without epinephrine), maintains satisfactory potency for 24 hours at room temperature, for one week under refrigeration (below 5°C), and for at least 30 weeks in the frozen state.

Directions to reconstitute Mefoxin (cefoxitin sodium). (Courtesy of Merck Co. Inc.)

For the next set of problems, you must choose the direction you need to give the ordered dose. Directions for these problems are located throughout Chapter 7. For each problem, provide the answer for

a. Diluting fluid and number of millilitres
b. Solution made and new supply
c. Answer
d. Label

6. Order: Ceptaz (ceftazidime sodium) 90 mg IM q12h (Refer to label for problem 1.)
   Supply: vial of powder labelled Ceptaz 1 g

   Refer to label for problem 1.

7. Order: Ancef (cefazolin sodium) 0.45 g IM q12h
   Supply: vial of powder labelled cefazolin sodium 500 mg (Refer to label for problem 3.)

8. Order: ampicillin sodium 400 mg IM q6h (Refer to label for problem 2.)
   Supply: 500 mg

9. Order: Cefazolin 0.5 g IM q6h (Refer to label for problem 4.)
   Supply: 1 g

10. Order: Mefoxin (cefoxitin sodium) 0.5 g IM q12h
   Supply: vial of powder labelled Mefoxin 1 g (Refer to label for problem 5.)

CRITICAL THINKING: TEST YOUR CLINICAL SAVVY

You are a nursing student about to graduate from one of the most prestigious nursing schools in Canada. On your last day of clinical, you are to give insulin to the last patient in your nursing school career. The patient has been insulin dependent for 15 years. The ordered dose is 30 units of NPH insulin and 20 units of regular insulin. Unfortunately, the nursing unit has run out of insulin syringes.

1. Could you use a 1-mL syringe to draw up insulin? If so, how would this be done and what would be the precautions?
2. What would be the danger in using a 1-mL syringe?

You are working in a medical-surgical unit of a large city hospital. A patient is to receive 500,000 units of penicillin G potassium, IV, q12h. Normally a vial containing 1 million units is considered stock drug (reconstituted: 250,000 units = 1 mL). Because of a nationwide shortage, a vial with 5 million units of penicillin G potassium is supplied (reconstituted 1,000,000 units = 1 mL).

1. What should you do to ensure no mistakes are made for the initial dosing and for subsequent dosing of penicillin?
2. What is the danger in administering too much of any drug?
3. What is the danger in administering too much penicillin and/or potassium?

Putting It Together

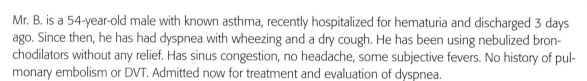

Mr. B. is a 54-year-old male with known asthma, recently hospitalized for hematuria and discharged 3 days ago. Since then, he has had dyspnea with wheezing and a dry cough. He has been using nebulized bronchodilators without any relief. Has sinus congestion, no headache, some subjective fevers. No history of pulmonary embolism or DVT. Admitted now for treatment and evaluation of dyspnea.

Past Medical History: renal cell carcinoma, hypertension, asthma, type 2 diabetes, hypercholesterolemia. Previous surgeries: hemorrhoidectomy, hiatal hernia repair, nephrectomy. Obstructive sleep apnea. Social history: life-long smoker, no alcohol. Lives with his son.

Allergies: Keflex causing rash. Augmentin causing rash. Phenergan causing leg spasm.

Current Vital Signs: Pulse is 96, BP 170/100, RR of 18, sat 96% afebrile.

Medication Orders

Lasix (furosemide) *diuretic* 40 mg IV q12h

Epogen (epoetin) *erythropoietin* 8000 units subcutaneous Tuesday/Thursday/Saturday

Heparin *anticoagulant* 2500 units subcutaneous q8h

Theodur (theophylline) *bronchodilator* 300 mg po q12h

Flovent (fluticasone) *corticosteroid* 1 puff bid

Norvasc (amlodipine) *antihypertensive* 10 mg po daily

Mevacor (lovastatin) *antihyperlipidemic* 50 mg po daily

Putting It Together

Solu-Medrol (methylprednisolone) *corticosteroid, glucocorticoid* 100 mg IVP daily

Phenergan (promethazine) *antiemetic* 12.5 mg IV q6h prn nausea.

Vancocin (vancomycin) *antiinfective* 1 g IV q12h

Vasotec (enalapril) *antihypertensive* 0.625 mg IV q6h over 5 minutes prn SBP >160

Accuchecks ac and hs. For BG >11.4 mmol/L Sliding scale: Give 7.5 units Humulin R subcutaneous

Calculations

1. Calculate how many mL of Lasix to administer. Available supply is 10 mg/mL.

2. Calculate how many mL of heparin to administer. Available supply is 5000 units/mL.

3. Calculate how many mL of Epogen to administer. Available supply is 20,000 units/mL.

4. Calculate how much (if any) insulin to give for BG of 12.1 mmol/L.

5. Calculate how many mL of Solu-Medrol to administer. Available supply is 125 mg in 2 mL.

6. Calculate how many mL to administer of Pherergan to administer. Available supply is 25 mg/mL.

7. What prn medication should be given (if any) for the patient's blood pressure? Calculate how many mL if available supply is 1.25 mg/mL.

8. Calculate the amount of vancomycin to add to an IVPB for infusion. Available supply is 500 mg/mL after reconstitution.

Critical Thinking Questions

1. What are precautions that need to be taken with IVP drugs?

2. What are precautions that need to be taken with insulin calculations and administration?

3. What are common mistakes that could happen with insulin dosages?

4. What are common mistakes that could happen with heparin dosages?

5. Why would this patient be on insulin coverage if the patient has type 2 diabetes?

6. What medications should be held and why?

Answers in Appendix B.

PROFICIENCY TEST 1 Calculations of Liquid Injections

Name: _____

Solve these injection problems. Draw a line on the syringe indicating the amount you would prepare in millilitres. See Appendix A for answers.

1. Order: sodium amytal 0.1 g IM at 0700h
   Supply: ampoule of liquid labelled 200 mg/3 mL

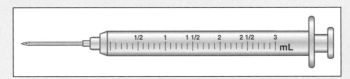

2. Order: morphine sulfate 5 mg IV stat
   Supply: vial of liquid labelled 15 mg/mL

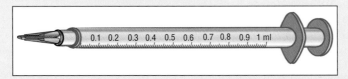

3. Order: Benadryl (diphenhydramine) 25 mg IM q4h prn
   Supply: ampoule of liquid labelled 50 mg (2-mL size)

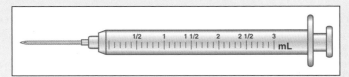

4. Order: NPH insulin 15 units and Humulin R insulin 5 units subcutaneous every day at 0700h
   Supply: vials of NPH insulin 100 units/mL and Humulin R insulin 100 units/mL

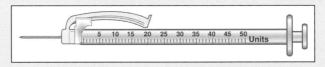

5. Order: add 20 mEq potassium chloride to IV stat
   Supply: vial of liquid labelled 40 mEq (3 g) per 20 mL

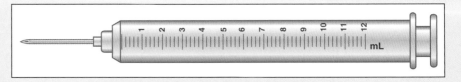

(continued)

6. Order: scopolamine 0.6 mg subcutaneous stat
Supply: vial labelled 0.4 mg/mL

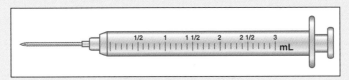

7. Order: atropine sulfate 0.8 mg IV at 0700h
Supply: vial labelled 0.4 mg/mL

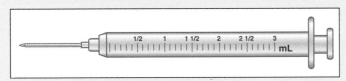

8. Order: add 0.5 g dextrose 25% to IV stat
Supply: vial of liquid labelled infant 25% dextrose injection 250 mg/mL

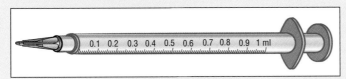

9. Order: Vitamin C (ascorbic acid) 200 mg IM bid
Supply: ampoule labelled 500 mg/2 mL

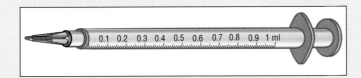

10. Order: epinephrine 7.5 mg SC stat
Supply: ampoule labelled 1:100

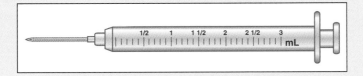

11. Order: Valium (diazepam) 10 mg IV now
Supply: vial labelled 5 mg/mL

(continued)

12. Order: Librium (chlordiazepoxide) 25 mg IM bid
Supply: vial labelled 100 mg per 2 mL

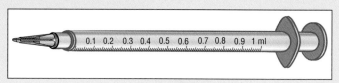

13. Order: Vistaril (hydroxyzine) 50 mg IM bid
Supply: vial labelled 25 mg/mL

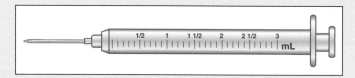

14. Order: Ativan (lorazepam) 0.5 mg IV q4h
Supply: vial labelled 2 mg/mL

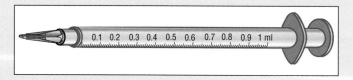

15. Order: Dilantin (phenytoin) 0.2 g IM stat
Supply: vial labelled 200 mg/2 mL

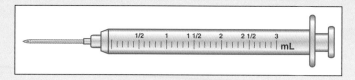

PROFICIENCY TEST 2 Calculations of Liquid Injections

Name: _____

Solve these problems for injections from a liquid. Draw a line on the syringe indicating the amount you would prepare in millilitres. See Appendix A for answers.

1. Order: morphine sulfate 10 mg IV stat
   Supply: vial labelled 15 mg/mL

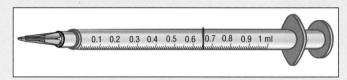

2. Order: Demerol (meperidine) 25 mg IM stat
   Supply: vial of liquid labelled 100 mg in 1 mL

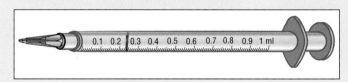

3. Order: phenobarbital 0.1 g IM q6h
   Supply: ampoule of liquid labelled 200 mg/3 mL

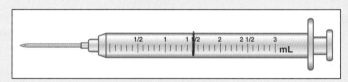

4. Order: vitamin B$_{12}$ 1000 mcg IM every day
   Supply: vial labelled 5000 mcg/mL

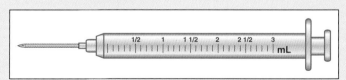

5. Order: prepare 25 mg lidocaine
   Supply: vial of liquid labelled 1%

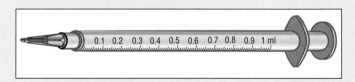

(continued)

6. Order: scopolamine 0.5 mg subcutaneous stat
Supply: vial labelled 0.4 mg/mL

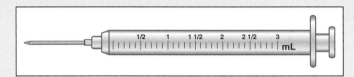

7. Order: NPH insulin 10 units and Humulin R insulin 3 units subcutaneous every day at 0700h
Supply: vials of NPH insulin 100 units/mL and Humulin R insulin 100 units/mL

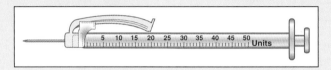

8. Order: add sodium bicarbonate 1.2 mEq to IV stat
Supply: vial labelled infant 4.2% sodium bicarbonate 5 mEq (0.5 mEq/mL)

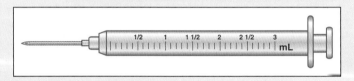

9. Order: Masteron (dromostanolone proprionate) 75 mg IM three times a week
Supply: vial labelled 50 mg/mL

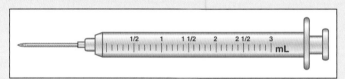

10. Order: epinephrine 500 mcg subcutaneous stat
Supply: ampoule of liquid labelled 1:1000

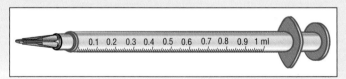

PROFICIENCY TEST 3 Calculations of Liquid Injections

Name: _____

Aim for 90% or better on this test. Assume you have only a 3-mL syringe. See Appendix A for answers.

1. Order: Lanoxin (digoxin) 0.25 mg IM every day
   Supply: ampoule labelled 0.5 mg/2 mL

2. Order: Benadryl (diphenhydramine hydrochloride) 40 mg IM stat
   Supply: ampoule labelled 50 mg (2-mL size)

3. Order: morphine sulfate 8 mg IV q4h prn
   Supply: vial labelled 15 mg/mL

4. Order: Demerol (meperidine) 25 mg IM q4h prn
   Supply: vial labelled 100 mg/mL

5. Order: Vitamin C (ascorbic acid) 200 mg IM every day
   Supply: ampoule labelled 500 mg/2 mL

6. Order: vitamin B_{12} 1500 mcg every day IM
   Supply: vial labelled 5000 mcg/mL

7. Order: atropine sulfate 0.6 mg IV at 0730h
   Supply: vial labelled 0.4 mg/mL

8. Order: sodium amytal 0.1 g IM stat
   Supply: ampoule 200 mg/3 mL

9. Order: Dilaudid (hydromorphone HCl) 1.5 mg IM q4h prn
   Supply: vial labelled 2 mg/mL

10. Order: penicillin G procaine 600,000 units IM q12h
    Supply: vial labelled 500,000 USP units/mL

11. Order: add nitroglycerin 200 mcg to IV stat
    Supply: vial labelled 0.8 mg/mL

12. Order: neostigmine methylsulfate 500 mcg subcutaneous
    Supply: ampoule labelled 1:4000

13. Order: Levo-Dromoran (levorphanol tartrate) 3 mg subcutaneous
    Supply: vial labelled 2 mg/mL

14. Order: epinephrine 0.4 mg subcutaneous stat
    Supply: ampoule labelled 1:1000 (2-mL size)

15. Order: magnesium sulfate 500 mg IM
    Supply: ampoule labelled 50% (2-mL size)

(continued)

16. Order: Numorphan (oxymorphone HCl) 0.75 mg subcutaneous
     Supply: vial labelled 1.5 mg/mL

17. Order: add lidocaine 100 mg to IV stat
     Supply: ampoule labelled 20%

18. Order: Lanoxin (digoxin) 0.125 mg IV at 1000h
     Supply: ampoule labelled 0.25 mg/2 mL

19. Order: Nubain (nalbuphine HCl) 12 mg IM
     Supply: vial 10 mg/mL

20. Order: add 10 mEq KCl to IV
     Supply: vial 40 mEq/20 mL

PROFICIENCY TEST 4   Mental Drill in Liquids-for-Injection Problems

Name: _____

As you develop proficiency in solving problems, you will be able to calculate many answers without written work. This drill combines your knowledge of equivalents and dosages. Solve these problems mentally and write only the amount to give. See Appendix A for answers.

Order	Supply	Give
1. 0.5 g IM	250 mg/mL	_____
2. 10 mEq IV	40 mEq/20 mL	_____
3. 0.5 mg IM	0.25 mg/mL	_____
4. 100 mg IM	0.2 g/2 mL	_____
5. 50 mg IM	100 mg/1 mL	_____
6. 0.25 mg IM	0.5 mg/2 mL	_____
7. 0.3 mg subcutaneous	0.4 mg/mL	_____
8. 1 mg subcutaneous	1:1000 solution	_____
9. 1 g IV	5% solution	_____
10. 0.1 g IM	200 mg/5 mL	_____
11. 400,000 units IM	500,000 units/mL	_____
12. 0.5 mg IM	0.5 mg/2 mL	_____
13. 1 g IV	50% solution	_____
14. 75 mg IM	100 mg/2 mL	_____
15. 15 mg IM	1:100 solution	_____
16. 35 mg IM	100 mg/mL	_____
17. 0.6 mg subcutaneous	0.4 mg per mL	_____
18. 0.15 g IM	0.2 g/2 mL	_____

Name: _____

Solve the problems. See Appendix A for answers.

1. Order: Cefazolin 250 mg IM q8h
    Supply: vial of powder labelled 1-g powder (refer to Figure on p. 169)

    a. Diluting fluid and number of millilitres:
    b. Solution and new supply:
    c. Rule and arithmetic:
    d. Amount to give:
    e. Write on label:
    f. Storage:

2. Order: Ticar (ticarcillin disodium) 1 g IM
    Supply: vial of powder labelled Ticar 1 g

    a. Diluting fluid and number of millilitres:
    b. Solution and new stock:
    c. Rule and arithmetic:
    d. Amount to give:
    e. Write on label:
    f. Storage:

> **DIRECTIONS FOR USE**
> **—1 Gm, 3 Gm and 6 Gm Standard Vials—**
> **INTRAMUSCULAR USE:** (Concentration of approximately 385 mg/ml).
> For initial reconstitution use Sterile Water for Injection, USP, Sodium Chloride Injection, USP or 1% Lidocaine Hydrochloride solution* (without epinephrine).
> Each gram of Ticarcillin should be reconstituted with 2 ml of Sterile Water for Injection, U.S.P., Sodium Chloride Injection, U.S.P. or 1% Lidocaine Hydrochloride solution* (without epinephrine) and **used promptly.** Each 2.6 ml of the resulting solution will then contain 1 Gm of Ticarcillin.
> *[For full product information, refer to manufacturer's package insert for Lidocaine Hydrochloride.]
> As with all intramuscular preparations, TICAR (Ticarcillin Disodium) should be injected well within the body of a relatively large muscle, using usual techniques and precautions.

Directions for use of ticarcillin disodium (Ticar).
(Courtesy of GlaxoSmithKline.)

3. Order: ampicillin sodium 300 mg IM q8h
    Supply: vial of 500 mg powder (refer to Figure on p. 182)

    a. Diluting fluid and number of millilitres:
    b. Solution and new supply:
    c. Rule and arithmetic:
    d. Amount to give:
    e. Write on label:
    f. Storage:

Intramuscular Use: 125 mg vial: Add 1 ml Sterile Water for Injection, USP, or Bacteriostatic Water for Injection, USP (TUBEX® Sterile Cartridge-Needle Unit) to give a final concentration of 125 mg per ml. For fractional doses, withdraw the ampicillin sodium solution as follows:

Dose	Withdraw
25 mg	0.2 ml
50 mg	0.4 ml
75 mg	0.6 ml
100 mg	0.8 ml
125 mg	1 ml

250 mg vial: Add 0.9 ml Sterile Water for Injection, USP, or Bacteriostatic Water for Injection, USP (TUBEX) to give a final concentration of 250 mg/ml. For fractional doses, withdraw the ampicillin sodium solution as follows:

Dose	Withdraw
125 mg	0.5 ml
150 mg	0.6 ml
175 mg	0.7 ml
200 mg	0.8 ml
225 mg	0.9 ml
250 mg	1 ml

For dilution of 500-mg, 1-gram, and 2-gram vials, dissolve contents of a vial with the amount of Sterile water for Injection, USP, or Bacteriostatic Water for Injection, USP, listed in the table below:

Label Claim	Recommended Amount of Diluent	Withdrawable Volume	Concentration in mg/ml
500 mg	1.8 ml	2.0 ml	250 mg
1.0 gram	3.4 ml	4.0 ml	250 mg
2.0 gram	6.8 ml	8.0 ml	250 mg

While the 1-gram and 2-gram vials are primarily for intravenous use, they may be administered intramuscularly when the 250-mg or 500-mg vials are unavailable. In such instances, dissolve in 3.4 or 6.8 ml Sterile Water for Injection, USP, or Bacteriostatic Water for Injection, USP, to give a final concentration of 250 mg/ml
The above solutions must be used within one hour after reconstitution.

Reconstitution directions for ampicillin sodium for IM or IV injection.

(continued)

4. Order: Mefoxin 300 mg IM q4h
   Supply: vial of powder 1 g

   a. Diluting fluid and number of millilitres:
   b. Solution and new supply:
   c. Rule and arithmetic:
   d. Amount to give:
   e. Write on label:
   f. Storage:

	— Preparation of Solution		
Strength	Amount of Diluent to be Added (mL) + +	Approximate Withdrawable Volume (mL)	Approximate Average Concentration (mg/mL)
1 gram Vial	2 (Intramuscular)	2.5	400
2 gram Vial	4 (Intramuscular)	5	400
1 gram Vial	10 (IV)	10.5	95
2 gram Vial	10 or 20 (IV)	11.1 or 21.0	180 or 95
1 gram Infusion Bottle	50 or 100 (IV)	50 or 100	20 or 10
2 gram Infusion Bottle	50 or 100 (IV)	50 or 100	40 or 20
10 gram Bulk	43 or 93 (IV)	49 or 98.5	200 or 100

+ +Shake to dissolve and let stand until clear.

Intramuscular
MEFOXIN, as constituted with Sterile Water for Injection, Bacteriostatic Water for Injection, or 0.5 percent or 1 percent lidocaine hydrochloride solution (without epinephrine), maintains satisfactory potency for 24 hours at room temperature, for one week under refrigeration (below 5°C), and for at least 30 weeks in the frozen state.

Directions to reconstitute Mefoxin (cefoxitin sodium). (Courtesy of Merck Co. Inc.)

5. Order: Ancef (cefazolin sodium) 0.33 g IM q8h
   Supply: vial of powder labelled 1 g (see label on p. 168)

   a. Diluting fluid and number of millilitres:
   b. Solution and new supply:
   c. Rule and arithmetic:
   d. Amount to give:
   e. Write on label:
   f. Storage:

Answers to Self Tests

Self Test 1 Calculation of Liquids for Injection

1. Equivalent: 0.3 g = 300 mg

Formula Method	*Proportion Expressed as Two Ratios*	*Proportion Expressed as Two Fractions*
$\dfrac{\overset{1}{\cancel{300}} \text{ mg}}{\underset{1}{\cancel{300}} \text{ mg}} \times 2 \text{ mL} = 2 \text{ mL}$	2 mL : 300 mg : : x : 300 mg	$\dfrac{2 \text{ mL}}{300 \text{ mg}} \times \dfrac{\text{x}}{300 \text{ mg}}$

$$\frac{600}{300} = \text{x}$$

$$2 \text{ mL} = \text{x}$$

Give 2 mL IM.

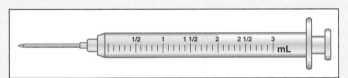

2.

Formula Method	*Proportion Expressed as Two Ratios*	*Proportion Expressed as Two Fractions*
$\dfrac{\overset{4}{\cancel{12}} \text{ mg}}{\underset{5}{\cancel{15}} \text{ mg}} \times 1 \text{ mL} = \dfrac{4}{5} \overline{)\dfrac{0.8}{4.0}}$	1 mL : 15 mg : : x : 12 mg	$\dfrac{1 \text{ mL}}{15 \text{ mg}} \times \dfrac{\text{x}}{12 \text{ mg}}$

$$\frac{12}{15} = \text{x}$$

$$0.8 \text{ mL} = \text{x}$$

Give 0.8 mL IV. Follow directions for dilution and rate of administration.

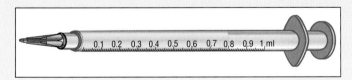

3. Equivalent: 1 mg = 1000 mcg

Formula Method	Proportion Expressed as Two Ratios	Proportion Expressed as Two Fractions
$\dfrac{\overset{1}{\cancel{1000}}\ \cancel{mcg}}{\underset{1}{\cancel{1000}}\ \cancel{mcg}} \times 1\ \text{mL} = 1\ \text{mL}$	1 mL : 1000 mcg :: x : 1000 mcg	$\dfrac{1\ \text{mL}}{1000\ \text{mcg}} \bowtie \dfrac{\text{x}}{1000\ \text{mcg}}$

$$\frac{1000}{1000} = x$$

$$1\ \text{mL} = x$$

Give 1 mL IM.

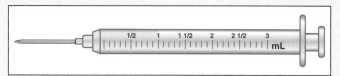

4.

Formula Method	Proportion Expressed as Two Ratios	Proportion Expressed as Two Fractions
$\dfrac{9\ \cancel{mg}}{20\ \cancel{mg}} \times 2\ \text{mL} = \dfrac{18}{20} \overset{0.9}{\left)\overline{\begin{matrix}18.0\\ \underline{18.0}\end{matrix}}\right.}$	2 mL : 20 mg :: x : 9 mg	$\dfrac{2\ \text{mL}}{20\ \text{mg}} \bowtie \dfrac{\text{x}}{9\ \text{mg}}$

$$\frac{18}{20} = x$$

$$0.9\ \text{mL} = x$$

Give 0.9 mL IM using a 1-mL precision syringe.

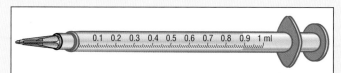

5.

Formula Method	Proportion Expressed as Two Ratios	Proportion Expressed as Two Fractions
$\dfrac{\overset{2}{\cancel{0.50}}\ \cancel{mg}}{\underset{1}{\cancel{0.25}}\ \cancel{mg}} \times 1\ \text{mL} = 2\ \text{mL}$	1 mL : 0.25 mg :: x : 0.5 mg	$\dfrac{1\ \text{mL}}{0.25\ \text{mg}} \bowtie \dfrac{\text{x}}{0.5\ \text{mg}}$

$$\frac{0.5}{0.25} = x$$

$$2\ \text{mL} = x$$

Give 2 mL IV. Follow dilution and administration guidelines.

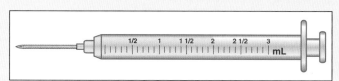

6.

Formula Method	Proportion Expressed as Two Ratios	Proportion Expressed as Two Fractions

$$\frac{50 \text{ mg}}{40 \text{ mg}} \times 1 \text{ mL} = \frac{5}{4} \overline{)5.00}^{1.25}$$
$$\underline{4}$$
$$1\ 0$$
$$\underline{8}$$
$$2\ 0$$
$$\underline{2\ 0}$$

$$1 \text{ mL} : 40 \text{ mg} :: x : 50 \text{ mg}$$

$$\frac{1 \text{ mL}}{40 \text{ mg}} \times \frac{x}{50 \text{ mg}}$$

$$\frac{50}{40} = x$$

$$1.25 \text{ mL} = x$$

Give 1.3 mL IM.

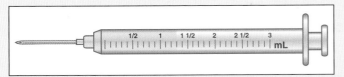

7.

Formula Method	Proportion Expressed as Two Ratios	Proportion Expressed as Two Fractions

$$\frac{100 \text{ mg}}{130 \text{ mg}} \times 1 \text{ mL} = \frac{10}{13} \overline{)10.000}^{0.769}$$
$$\underline{9\ 1}$$
$$9\ 0$$
$$\underline{7\ 8}$$
$$1\ 20$$
$$\underline{1\ 17}$$
$$3$$

$$1 \text{ mL} : 130 \text{ mg} :: x : 100 \text{ mg}$$

$$\frac{1 \text{ mL}}{130 \text{ mg}} \times \frac{x}{100 \text{ mg}}$$

$$\frac{100}{130} = x$$

$$0.769 \text{ or } 0.77 \text{ mL} = x$$

Give 0.77 mL IM using a 1-mL precision syringe (millilitres to the nearest hundredth).

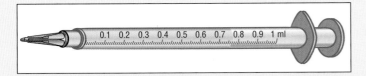

8.

Formula Method	Proportion Expressed as Two Ratios	Proportion Expressed as Two Fractions

$$\frac{\overset{1}{0.25} \text{ mg}}{\underset{2}{0.50} \text{ mg}} \times \overset{1}{2} \text{ mL} = 1 \text{ mL}$$

$$2 \text{ mL} : 0.5 \text{ mg} :: x : 0.25 \text{ mg}$$

$$\frac{2 \text{ mL}}{0.5 \text{ mg}} \times \frac{x}{0.25 \text{ mg}}$$

$$\frac{0.5}{0.5} = x$$

$$1 \text{ mL} = x$$

Give 1 mL IV. Follow directions for dilution and rate of medication administration.

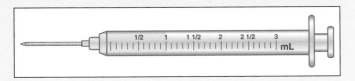

9.

Formula Method	Proportion Expressed as Two Ratios	Proportion Expressed as Two Fractions
$\dfrac{6000 \text{ units}}{10\,000 \text{ units}} \times 1 \text{ mL} = \dfrac{6}{10} = 0.6$	1 mL : 10000 units : : x : 6000 units	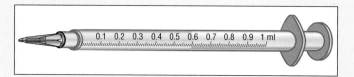

$$\frac{6000}{10000} = x$$

$$0.6 \text{ mL} = x$$

Give 0.6 mL subcutaneous.

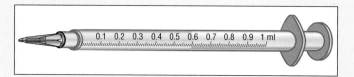

10.

Formula Method	Proportion Expressed as Two Ratios	Proportion Expressed as Two Fractions
$\dfrac{0.25 \text{ mg}}{1 \text{ mg}} \times 1 \text{ mL}$ 0.25 mL	1 mL : 1 mg : : x : 0.25 mg	$\dfrac{1 \text{ mL}}{1 \text{ mg}} \times \dfrac{x}{0.25 \text{ mg}}$

$$0.25 \text{ mL} = x$$

Give 0.25 mL subcutaneous.

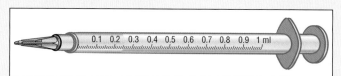

11.

Formula Method	Proportion Expressed as Two Ratios	Proportion Expressed as Two Fractions
$\dfrac{20 \text{ mg}}{5 \text{ mg}} \times 1 \text{ mL}$ 4 mL	1 mL : 5 mg : : x : 20 mg	$\dfrac{1 \text{ mL}}{5 \text{ mg}} \times \dfrac{x}{20 \text{ mg}}$

$$20 = 5x$$

$$\frac{20}{5} = x$$

$$4 \text{ mL} = x$$

Give 4 mL IV. Follow directions for dilution and rate of administration.

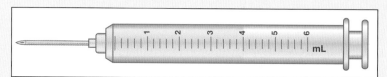

12.

Formula Method	Proportion Expressed as Two Ratios	Proportion Expressed as Two Fractions
$\dfrac{2.5 \text{ mg}}{5 \text{ mg}} \times 1 \text{ mL}$ 0.5 or ½ mL	1 mL : 5 mg :: x : 2.5 mg	$\dfrac{1 \text{ mL}}{5 \text{ mg}} \times \dfrac{x}{2.5 \text{ mg}}$ $2.5 = 5x$ 0.5 or ½ mL = x

Give 0.5 mL 1M.

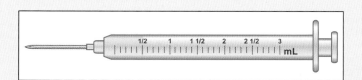

13.

Formula Method	Proportion Expressed as Two Ratios	Proportion Expressed as Two Fractions
$\dfrac{3 \text{ mg}}{10 \text{ mg}} \times 1 \text{ mL} = x$ 0.3 mL	1 mL : 10 mg :: x : 3 mg	$\dfrac{1 \text{ mL}}{10 \text{ mg}} \times \dfrac{x}{3 \text{ mg}}$ $3 = 10 \, x$ $\dfrac{3}{10} = x$ $0.3 = x$

Give 0.3 mL subcutaneous.

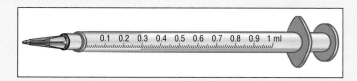

14. 0.025 g = 25 mg

Formula Method	Proportion Expressed as Two Ratios	Proportion Expressed as Two Fractions
$\dfrac{25 \text{ mg}}{10 \text{ mg}} \times 1 \text{ mL} = x$ 2.5 mL = x	1 mL : 10 mg :: x : 25 mg	$\dfrac{1 \text{ mL}}{25 \text{ mg}} \times \dfrac{x}{10 \text{ mg}}$ $25 = 10 \, x$ $\dfrac{25}{10} = x$ 2.5 mL = x

Give 2.5 mL IM.

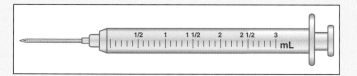

15.

Formula Method	Proportion Expressed as Two Ratios	Proportion Expressed as Two Fractions
$\dfrac{50 \ \text{mg}}{25 \ \text{mg}} \times 1 \ \text{mL} = x$ $2 \ \text{mL} = x$	$1 \ \text{mL} : 25 \ \text{mg} : : x : 50 \ \text{mg}$	$\dfrac{1 \ \text{mL}}{25 \ \text{mg}} \diagdown \dfrac{x}{50 \ \text{mg}}$ $50 = 25 \ x$ $2 \ \text{mL} = x$

Give 2 mL IM.

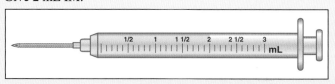

16.

Formula Method	Proportion Expressed as Two Ratios	Proportion Expressed as Two Fractions
$\dfrac{2500 \ \text{units}}{5000 \ \text{units}} \times 0.2 \ \text{mL} = x$ $0.5 \times 0.2 = x$ $0.1 \ \text{mL}$	$0.2 \ \text{mL} : 5000 \ \text{units} : : x : 2500 \ \text{units}$	$\dfrac{0.2 \ \text{mL}}{5000 \ \text{units}} \diagdown \dfrac{x}{2500 \ \text{units}}$ $0.2 \times 2500 = 5000 \ x$ $500 = 5000 \ x$ $0.1 = x$

Give 0.1 mL subcutaneous.

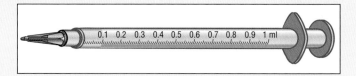

Self Test 2 Ratios

RATIO	? g per ? mL	? g = ? mL	? g/? mL
1:20	1 g per 20 mL	1 g = 20 mL	1 g/20 mL
2:15	2 g per 15 mL	2 g = 15 mL	2 g/15 mL
1:500	1 g per 500 mL	1 g = 500 mL	1 g/500 mL
2:2000	2 g per 2000 mL	2 g = 2000 mL	2 g/2000 mL
1:4	1 g per 4 mL	1 g = 4 mL	1 g/4 mL
2:25	2 g per 25 mL	2 g = 25 mL	2 g/25 mL
4:50	4 g per 50 mL	4 g = 50 mL	4 g/50 mL
1:100	1 g per 100 mL	1 g = 100 mL	1 g/100 mL
3:75	3 g per 75 mL	3 g = 75 mL	3 g/75 mL
5:1000	5 g per 1000 mL	5 g = 1000 mL	5 g/1000 mL

Self Test 3 Using Ratios with Liquids for Injection

1. Equivalent: 1:2000 means

            1 g in 2000 mL

            1 g = 1000 mg

Hence, the solution is 1000 mg/2000 mL.

Formula Method	Proportion Expressed as Two Ratios	Proportion Expressed as Two Fractions
$\dfrac{0.5 \text{ mg}}{1000 \text{ mg}} \times \overset{2}{2000} \text{ mL} = 0.5$ $\times\ 2$ $\overline{1.0}$	$2000 \text{ mL} : 1000 \text{ mg} :: x : 0.5 \text{ mg}$	$\dfrac{2000 \text{ mL}}{1000 \text{ mg}} \times \dfrac{x}{0.5 \text{ mg}}$

$$\dfrac{1000}{1000} = x$$

$$1 \text{ mL} = x$$

Give 1 mL subcutaneous.

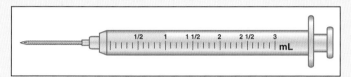

2. Equivalent: 1:5000 means
   1 g in 5000 mL
   1 g = 1000 mg
Hence, the solution is 1000 mg/5000 mL.

Formula Method	Proportion Expressed as Two Ratios	Proportion Expressed as Two Fractions
$\dfrac{1 \text{ mg}}{1000 \text{ mg}} \times \overset{5}{5000} \text{ mL} = 5 \text{ mL}$	$5000 \text{ mL} : 1000 \text{ mg} :: x : 1 \text{ mg}$	$\dfrac{5000 \text{ mL}}{1000 \text{ mg}} \times \dfrac{x}{1 \text{ mg}}$

$$\dfrac{5000}{1000} = x$$

$$5 \text{ mL} = x$$

Add 5 mL to IV. (This is correct because route is IV not IM.)

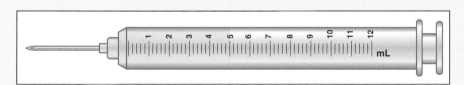

3. Equivalent: 1:1000 means
   1 g in 1000 mL
   1 g = 1000 mg
Hence, the solution is 1000 mg/1000 mL or 1 mg/mL.

Formula Method	Proportion Expressed as Two Ratios	Proportion Expressed as Two Fractions
$\dfrac{0.75 \text{ mg}}{1 \text{ mg}} \times 1 \text{ mL} = 0.75 \text{ mL}$	$1 \text{ mL} : 1 \text{ mg} :: x : 0.75 \text{ mg}$	$\dfrac{1 \text{ mL}}{1 \text{ mg}} \times \dfrac{x}{0.75 \text{ mg}}$

You have a 1-mL syringe marked in hundredths. Draw up 0.75 mL. Do not round.

$$\dfrac{0.75}{1} = x$$

$$0.75 \text{ mL} = x$$

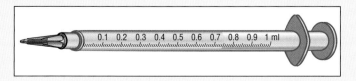

4. Equivalent: 1:1000 means

　　　　　　1 g in 1000 mL

　　　　　　1 g = 1000 mg

Hence, the solution is 1000 mg/1000 mL.

Formula Method	Proportion Expressed as Two Ratios	Proportion Expressed as Two Fractions
$\dfrac{0.5 \text{ mg}}{1000 \text{ mg}} \times 1000 \text{ mL}$ 0.5 mL	$1000 \text{ mL} : 1000 \text{ mg} :: \text{x} : 0.5 \text{ mg}$	$\dfrac{1000 \text{ mL}}{1000 \text{ mg}} \times \dfrac{\text{x}}{0.5 \text{ mg}}$ $\dfrac{500}{1000} = \text{x}$ $0.5 \text{ mL} = \text{x}$

Give 0.5 mL subcutaneous.

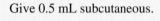

5. Equivalent: 1:2000 means

　　　　　　1000 mg in 2000 mL

　　　　　　1 mg per 2 mL

Formula Method	Proportion Expressed as Two Ratios	Proportion Expressed as Two Fractions
$\dfrac{1.5 \text{ mg}}{1 \text{ mg}} \times 2 \text{ mL} = 1.5$ $\dfrac{\times 2}{3.0} \text{ mL}$	$2 \text{ mL} : 1 \text{ mg} :: \text{x} : 1.5 \text{ mg}$	$\dfrac{2 \text{ mL}}{1 \text{ mg}} \times \dfrac{\text{x}}{1.5 \text{ mg}}$ $\dfrac{3}{1} = \text{x}$ $3 \text{ mL} = \text{x}$

Give 3 mL IM. May use 2 syringes of 1.5 mL each.

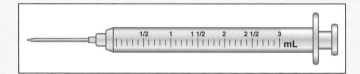

Self Test 4 Percentages

PERCENTAGE	? g per 100 mL	? g = 100 mL	? g/100 mL
0.9%	0.9 g per 100 mL	0.9 g = 100 mL	0.9 g/100 mL
10%	10 g per 100 mL	10 g = 100 mL	10 g/100 mL
0.45%	0.45 g per 100 mL	0.45 g = 100 mL	0.45 g/100 mL
50%	50 g per 100 mL	50 g = 100 mL	50 g/100 mL
0.33%	0.33 g per 100 mL	0.33 g = 100 mL	0.33 g/100 mL
5%	5 g per 100 mL	5 g = 100 mL	5 g/100 mL
30%	30 g per 100 mL	30 g = 100 mL	30 g/100 mL
1.5%	1.5 g per 100 mL	1.5 g = 100 mL	1.5 g/100 mL
1%	1 g per 100 mL	1 g = 100 mL	1 g/100 mL
20%	20 g per 100 mL	20 g = 100 mL	20 g/100 mL

Self Test 5 Using Percentages with Liquids for Injection

1. Equivalent: 1% 1 g in 100 mL

   1 g = 1000 mg

Hence, the solution is 1000 mg/100 mL.

Formula Method	Proportion Expressed as Two Ratios	Proportion Expressed as Two Fractions
$\dfrac{\overset{1}{\cancel{5}}\ mg}{\underset{2}{\cancel{1000}}\ mg} \times \overset{1}{\cancel{100}}\ mL = \frac{1}{2}\ mL$ or 0.5 mL	$\overset{\longleftrightarrow}{100\ mL : 1000\ mg :: x : 5\ mg}$	$\dfrac{100\ mL}{1000\ mg} \times \dfrac{x}{5\ mg}$ $\dfrac{500}{1000} = x$ 0.5 mL = x

Give 0.5 mL subcutaneous.

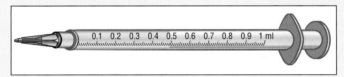

2. Equivalent: 1% 1 g in 100 mL

   1 g = 1000 mg

Hence, the solution is 1000 mg/100 mL.

Formula Method	Proportion Expressed as Two Ratios	Proportion Expressed as Two Fractions
$\dfrac{15\ mg}{\underset{10}{\cancel{1000}}\ mg} \times \overset{}{\cancel{100}}\ mL$ $\dfrac{15}{10} = 1.5\ mL$ or $1\frac{1}{2}$ mL	$\overset{\longleftrightarrow}{100\ mL : 1000\ mg :: x : 15\ mg}$	$\dfrac{100\ mL}{1000\ mg} \times \dfrac{x}{15\ mg}$ $\dfrac{1500}{1000} = x$ 1.5 or $1\frac{1}{2}$ mL = x

Give 1.5 mL subcutaneous.

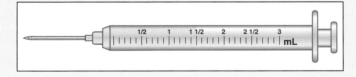

3. Equivalent:　1%　1 g in 100 mL

$$1 \text{ g} = 1000 \text{ mg}$$

Hence, the solution is 1000 mg/100 mL.

Formula Method	Proportion Expressed as Two Ratios	Proportion Expressed as Two Fractions
$\dfrac{3 \text{ mg}}{1000 \text{ mg}} \times 100 \text{ mL} = \dfrac{3}{10} = 0.3 \text{ mL}$	$100 \text{ mL} : 1000 \text{ mg} :: \text{x} : 3 \text{ mg}$	$\dfrac{100 \text{ mL}}{1000 \text{ mg}} \times \dfrac{\text{x}}{3 \text{ mg}}$

$$\frac{300}{1000} = \text{x}$$

$$0.3 \text{ mL} = \text{x}$$

Give 0.3 mL subcutaneous.

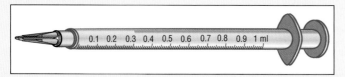

4. Equivalent:　10% means 10 g in 100 mL or 1 g in 10 mL

Formula Method	Proportion Expressed as Two Ratios	Proportion Expressed as Two Fractions
$\dfrac{0.3 \text{ g}}{1 \text{ g}} \times 10 \text{ mL} \quad \begin{array}{r} 10 \\ \times 0.3 \\ \hline 3.0 \text{ mL} \end{array}$	$10 \text{ mL} : 1 \text{ g} :: \text{x} : 0.3 \text{ g}$	$\dfrac{10 \text{ mL}}{1 \text{ g}} \times \dfrac{\text{x}}{0.3 \text{ g}}$

$$\frac{3}{1} = \text{x}$$

$$3 \text{ mL} = \text{x}$$

Prepare the syringe with 3 mL for IV use.

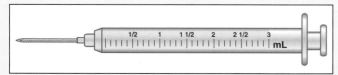

5. Equivalent:　50% means 50 g in 100 mL

Formula Method	Proportion Expressed as Two Ratios	Proportion Expressed as Two Fractions
$\dfrac{5 \text{ g}}{50 \text{ g}} \times 100 \text{ mL}$ 10 mL	$100 \text{ mL} : 50 \text{ g} :: \text{x} : 5 \text{ g}$	$\dfrac{100 \text{ mL}}{50 \text{ g}} \times \dfrac{\text{x}}{5 \text{ g}}$

$$\frac{500}{50} = \text{x}$$

$$10 \text{ mL} = \text{x}$$

Prepare the syringe with 10 mL for IV use.

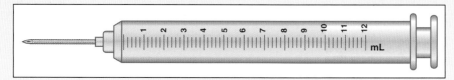

Self Test 6 Insulin Calculations

1.

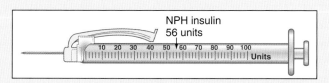

NPH insulin
56 units

2.

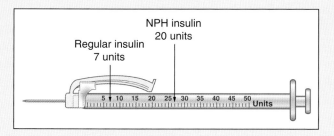

NPH insulin
20 units

Regular insulin
7 units

3.

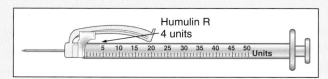

Humulin R
4 units

4.

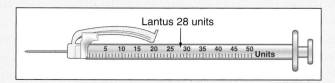

Lantus 28 units

5.

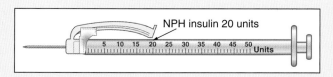

NPH insulin 20 units

6.

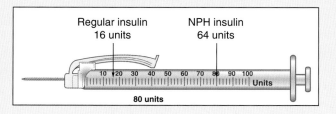

Regular insulin
16 units

NPH insulin
64 units

80 units

7.

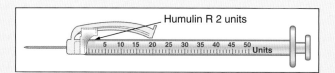

8.

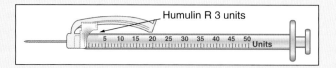

9. Call physician. No insulin given

10. Give 1 ampoule D50 and call physician.

Self Test 7 Injections from Powders

1. You want 1 g. The supply is 1 g. When you dilute the powder, you will give the whole amount of fluid, *whatever the amount is*. The manufacturer states it will be 1g in 3.6 mL. If you solve the arithmetic, you have

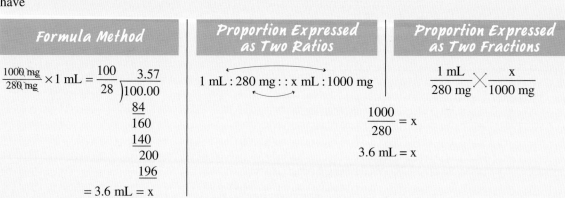

Formula Method	Proportion Expressed as Two Ratios	Proportion Expressed as Two Fractions

$$\frac{1000 \text{ mg}}{280 \text{ mg}} \times 1 \text{ mL} = \frac{100}{28} \overline{)\begin{array}{l} 3.57 \\ 100.00 \\ \underline{84} \\ 160 \\ \underline{140} \\ 200 \\ \underline{196} \end{array}}$$

$$= 3.6 \text{ mL} = x$$

1 mL : 280 mg : : x mL : 1000 mg

$$\frac{1 \text{ mL}}{280 \text{ mg}} \times \frac{x}{1000 \text{ mg}}$$

$$\frac{1000}{280} = x$$

$$3.6 \text{ mL} = x$$

a. 3 mL sterile water for injection

b. 1 g in 3.6 mL; 280 mg/mL

c. Not necessary

d. Give 3.6 mL in two syringes.

e. Discard the vial; it is empty.

f. Discard the vial in appropriate receptacle.

2. a. 1.8 mL sterile water for injection

   b. 250 mg/mL

Formula Method	Proportion Expressed as Two Ratios	Proportion Expressed as Two Fractions
c. $\dfrac{250 \text{ mg}}{250 \text{ mg}} \times 1 = 1 \text{ mL}$	1 mL : 250 mg : : x mL : 250 mg	$\dfrac{1 \text{ mL}}{250 \text{ mg}} \times \dfrac{x}{250 \text{ mg}}$

$$\frac{250}{250} = x$$

$$1 \text{ mL} = x$$

   d. Give 1 mL IM.

   e. "The above solutions must be used within 1 hour after reconstitution." You must discard the remaining fluid.

   f. None

3. a. Choose 500 mg powder. (Can you see why?)

   b. Add 2 mL sterile water for injection.

   c. 225 mg/mL

   d. Not necessary: You want 225 mg; you made 225 mg/mL.

   e. Give 1 mL IM.

   f. 225 mg/mL, date, time, expiration date: 96 hours after reconstitution, initials

   g. Refrigerate; stable for 96 hours

4. a. 2.5 mL sterile water for injection

   b. 334 mg/mL

Formula Method	Proportion Expressed as Two Ratios	Proportion Expressed as Two Fractions
c. $\dfrac{500 \text{ mg}}{334 \text{ mg}} \times 1 \text{ mL} = \dfrac{500}{334}$ $334 \overline{)500.00} = 1.49$ $\underline{334}$ 1660 $\underline{1336}$ 3240 $\underline{3006}$ 234 $= 1.5 \text{ mL} = x$	1 mL : 334 mg : : x mL : 500 mg	$\dfrac{1 \text{ mL}}{334 \text{ mg}} \times \dfrac{x}{500 \text{ mg}}$

$$\frac{500}{334} = x$$

$$1.49 \text{ or } 1.5 \text{ mL} = x$$

   d. Give 1.5 mL IM.

   e. 334 mg/mL, date, time, expiration date, initials

   f. Use reconstituted solution within 24 hours when stored at room temperature or within 72 hours if refrigerated

5. **a.** Add 2 mL sterile water for injection, bacteriostatic water in injection, or 0.5% lidocaine hydrochloride solution (without epinephrine).

    b. 400 mg/mL

Formula Method	Proportion Expressed as Two Ratios	Proportion Expressed as Two Fractions

c. $\dfrac{\overset{1}{\cancel{200}}\ \text{mg}}{\underset{2}{\cancel{400}}\ \text{mg}} \times 1\ \text{mL} = \frac{1}{2}\ \text{mL or 0.5 mL}$ 1 mL : 400 mg : : x mL : 200 mg $\dfrac{1\ \text{mL}}{400\ \text{mg}} \times \dfrac{x}{200\ \text{mg}}$

$$\frac{200}{400} = x$$

$$0.5\ \text{mL} = x$$

    d. Give ½ mL (0.5 mL).

    e. 400 mg/mL, date, time, expiration date: 1 week after reconstitution, initials

    f. Refrigerate; stable for 1 week

6. **a.** 3.0 mL sterile water for injection

    b. 280 mg/mL

    c. Give 0.32 mL (1-mL precision syringe).

    d. 280 mg/mL, date, time, expiration date: 1 week after reconstitution, initials

7. **a.** 2 mL sterile water for injection

    b. 225 mg/mL

    c. 2 mL IM

    d. 225 mg/mL, date, time, expiration date: 96 hours after reconstitution, initials

8. **a.** 1.8 mL sterile water for injection

    b. 250 mg/mL

    c. 1.6 mL

    d. 250 mg/mL, date, time, initials. Discard after use.

9. **a.** 3 mL sterile water for injection

    b. 280 mg/mL

    c. 1.8 mL

    d. 280 mg/mL, date, time, expiration date: 7 days after reconstitution, initials

10. **a.** 2 mL sterile water for injection

    b. 400 mg/mL

    c. 1.3 mL IM

    d. 400 mg/mL, date, time, expiration date: 1 week after reconstitution, initials

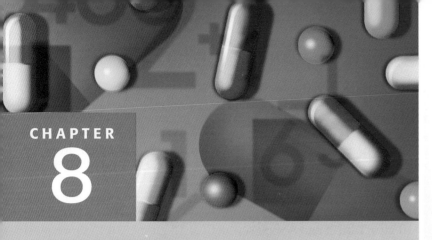

CHAPTER

8

Calculation of Basic IV Drip Rates

Administration of parenteral fluids and medications by the IV route is common medical practice and is a specialty within nursing and healthcare. Texts such as *Plumer's Principles and Practice of Intravenous Therapy* (Lippincott, 2006) present detailed and extensive information. This chapter presents basic knowledge—types of fluids, equipment, calculation of drip rates, and recording intake. Chapter 9 presents rules and calculations for special types of IV orders.

Types of Intravenous Fluids

Intravenous fluids are packaged in sterile plastic bags or glass bottles. The nurse selects the IV fluid ordered and prepares the solution. It is essential to choose the correct IV fluid to avoid serious fluid and electrolyte imbalance that may occur from infusing the wrong solution.

   If you have any doubt about the correct IV solution, always double-check with another healthcare professional.

   Common abbreviations for IV fluids are D, dextrose; W, water; and NS, normal (or isotonic) saline. An order often indicates a percent of these. For example, D5W means 5% dextrose in water; 0.9%NS means 0.9% saline in water.

Example	*Written Order*	*Supply Label*
	1000 mL D5W	1000 mL D5%W
	500 mL D5S	500 mL D5% 0.9%NS
	250 mL D5½NS	250 mL D5% 0.45%NS
	500 mL D5⅓NS	500 mL D5% 0.33%NS
	500 mL NS	500 mL 0.9%NS
	1000 mL ½NS	1000 mL 0.45%NS

Kinds of Intravenous Drip Factors

IV fluids are administered through infusion sets. These consist of plastic tubing attached at one end to the IV bag and at the other end to a needle or catheter inserted into a blood vessel. The top of the infusion set contains a chamber. Sets with a small needle in the chamber are called microdrip, because their drops are small. To deliver 1 mL fluid to the patient, 60 drops must drip in the chamber (60 gtt = 1 mL). All microdrip sets deliver 60 gtt/mL.

Infusion sets without a small needle in the chamber are called macrodrip (Fig. 8-1). Drops per millilitre differ according to the manufacturer. For example, Baxter-Travenol macrodrip sets deliver 10 gtt/mL, so 10 drops must drip in the chamber (10 gtt = 1 mL); and Abbott sets deliver 15 gtt/mL, so 15 drops must drip in the chamber (15 gtt = 1 mL). The package label states the drops per millilitre (gtt/mL). Sometimes the drop factor is also stated on the top part of the chamber. To calculate IV drip rates, you must know this information.

The tubing for these sets includes a roller clamp that you can open or close to regulate the drip rate; use a watch or a clock with a second hand to count the number of drops per minute in the chamber (Fig. 8-2).

Infusion Pumps

Electric infusion pumps also deliver IV fluid. Some are easy to operate; others are more elaborate. You must enter two pieces of information: the total number of millilitres to be infused and the number of millilitres per hour. Pumps used in specialty units also allow you to input the name of the medication, the concentration of the medication, the amount of fluid, and the patient's weight. The infusion rate can be set in mL/hr and the pump automatically calculates the dose in mg, mcg, and so forth. The pump can also calculate the dosage based on weight. Figure 8-3 shows the face of an infusion pump,

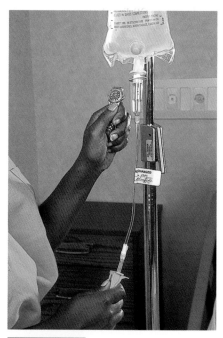

FIGURE 8-2

Timing the IV drip rate. (© B. Proud.) (With permission From Taylor, C., Lillis, C., & LeMone, P. [2004]. *Photo atlas of medication administration.* Philadelphia: Lippincott Williams & Wilkins, p. 46.)

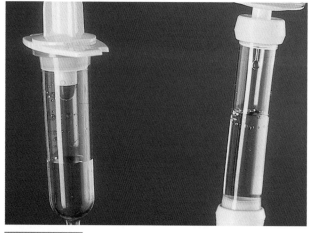

FIGURE 8-1

Drip chambers for macrodrip and microdrip IV tubing.

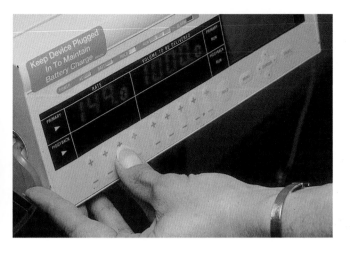

FIGURE 8-3
IV rate is programmed into the infusion pump in mL/hr.

with IV tubing connected. If an order reads "500 mL D5W IV. Run 50 mL/hr," you press the buttons on the pump that read:

- Volume for Infusion: 500 mL

- Rate for Infusion: 50 mL

- On.

The pump automatically delivers 50 mL/hr and runs over a 10-hour period.

IV pumps can also run intravenous piggybacks (IVPB). If an order reads "Ampicillin 2 g IVPB in 100 mL NS over 1 hour," you press the buttons on the pump that read:

- Secondary Volume: 100 mL

- Secondary Rate: 100 mL

- On.

The pump *interrupts* the main IV to administer the IVPB over 1 hour, then resumes the primary flow.

Labelling IVs

Every IV must be identified so that any professional can check both the fluid that is infusing and the drip rate. A typical order includes the following information:

Patient name, room, bed number, date, and time

Order: 500 mL D5W½NS. Run 50 mL/hr.

Label			
Patient	*James Latham*	Room	*1411B*
Date, Time	*09-Nov-26 1000h*	Rate	*50 gtt/min*
Order	*500 mL D5 ½NS*	Run	*50 mL/hr*
		Initials	*CB*

Note that the physician or healthcare provider ordered 50 mL/hr. Because the IV fluid amount is 500 mL, the infusion will take 10 hours to complete (500 divided by 50 = 10); the time is 1000h–2000h (10 hours). With microdrip tubing, 50 mL/hr = 50 gtt/min, the nurse sets the rate. (Instructions for calculating IV drip rates appear in the next section.) Your goal is to deliver the amount of fluid ordered, in the time ordered, and with a drip rate that is continuous and even.

Calculating Basic IV Drip Rates

Routine IV orders specify the number of millilitres of fluid and the duration of administration:

Example	250 mL D5W IV at 250 mL/hr	Fluid amount: 250 mL	Time: 1 hour
	1000 mL Ringer's lactate IV 0800h–2000h	Fluid amount: 1000 mL	Time: 12 hours
	500 mL D5½NS with 20 mEq KCl IV to run 75 mL/hr on a pump	Fluid amount: 500 mL	Time: 75 mL/hr

The equipment that you use determines the drip factor and the calculations needed. An infusion pump is set in mL/hr, so your dosage calculations are in mL/hr as well. IV tubing sets infuse at gtt/min, and the infusion rate depends on the drip rate of the tubing used. Although many institutions use only infusion pumps today, occasionally you will need to calculate and infuse IV fluid using the drip rate calculation.

RULE   **SOLVING IV CALCULATIONS WITH MICRO- AND MACRODRIP TUBING**

The terms "drop factor," "drip factor," "gtt factor," and "tubing drip factor" are all used to explain how many drops per mL the tubing delivers. In this text, we will use "tubing factor" or "TF" to mean all these terms.

Calculation:

$$\frac{\text{Number of millilitres to infuse} \times \text{TF}}{\text{Number of minutes to infuse}} = \text{drops per minute or gtt/mL.}$$

For example, the order is to infuse 120 mL of IV fluid over 60 minutes with a tubing factor of 10 gtt/mL. The calculation is:

$$\frac{120 \text{ mL} \times 10 \text{ gtt/mL}}{60 \text{ min}} = 20 \text{ gtt/min.}$$

Explanation:

TF: the tubing drip factor—either microdrip (60 gtt = 1 mL) or macrodrip

Depending on the manufacturer, macrodrip could be 10 gtt = 1 mL, 15 gtt = 1 mL, or 20 gtt = 1 mL.

min: the number of minutes, specified in every IV order. If the order reads "hour," then you convert to minutes by multiplying by 60 (60 minutes = 1 hour).

gtt/min: the drip factor, calculated to deliver an even flow of fluid over a specified time. To regulate the drip rate, use a second hand on a watch or a clock. If the drip rate is calculated to be 20 gtt/min, open the clamp and regulate the drip until you reach that amount. Usually you break this amount down into seconds, rather than counting for a full minute. For this example, 20 gtt/min becomes approximately 3 gtt every 20 seconds (divide 20 by 60, since a minute contains 60 seconds).

The problems requiring calculation in this text will supply the drip factor. When you're working in the clinical area, you must read the package label to identify the gtt/mL.

Drip rates are rounded to the nearest whole number, unless using an infusion pump that can infuse in tenths or hundredths (i.e., 8.25 mL/hr). Usually these infusion pumps are used in a specialty setting such as critical care or pediatrics.

Solving IV Calculations Using an Infusion Pump

Infusion pumps are always calculated in mL/hr. Here's how to calculate the previous example, infusing 120 mL of IV fluid over 60 minutes:

$$\frac{\text{Total number of millilitres ordered}}{\text{Number of hours to run}} = \text{mL/hr}$$

The calculation looks like this:

$$\frac{120 \text{ mL}}{1 \text{ hr}} = 120 \text{ mL/hr}$$

Note that 60 minutes was changed to 1 hour (60 minutes = 1 hour).

After calculating, connect the IV fluids to the infusion pump with the appropriate tubing, set the pump at 120 mL/hr, and start the infusion.

Explanation:

mL: The physician or healthcare provider will indicate the number of millilitres to be infused in the order.

hr: The number of hours to run depends on the way the order is written. For example, if the order is written

q8h = 8 hours at a time
1000 − 1600h = 6 hours
60 minutes = 1 hour
90 minutes = 1.5 hours (to get the number of hours, divide minutes by 60)

Applying the Rule

Example

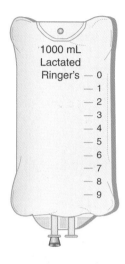

1000 mL
Lactated
Ringer's — 0
— 1
— 2
— 3
— 4
— 5
— 6
— 7
— 8
— 9

Order: 1000 mL Ringer's lactate IV 0800h—22000h

Available: an infusion pump

0800h—2000h indicates the IV will run for 12 hours. The infusion pump regulates the rate in millilitres per hour.

$$\frac{\text{number mL}}{\text{number hr}} = \text{mL/hr}$$

$$\frac{1000 \text{ mL}}{12 \text{ hr}} = \begin{array}{r} 83.3 \\ 12 \overline{\smash{)}1000.0} \\ \underline{96} \\ 40 \\ \underline{36} \\ 40 \\ \underline{36} \end{array}$$

$\frac{1000}{12}$

Label the IV.

Set the pump as follows:

Total number mL: 1000

mL/hr: 83

Example

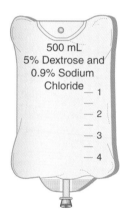

500 mL
5% Dextrose and
0.9% Sodium
Chloride — 1
— 2
— 3
— 4

Order: 500 mL D5NS IV 1200h—1600h

Available: microdrip at 60 gtt/mL; macrodrip at 20 gtt/mL

The IV will run 4 hours or 240 minutes (4 × 60 minutes). Because no pump is available, the nurse must choose the drip factor. Solve for both drip factors and choose one.

Macrodrip

$$\frac{500 \text{ mL} \times \overset{1}{\cancel{20}}}{\underset{12}{\cancel{240}}} = \begin{array}{r} 41.6 \\ 12 \overline{\smash{)}500.0} \\ \underline{48} \\ 20 \\ \underline{12} \\ 80 \end{array}$$

Macrodrip at 42 gtt/min

Microdrip

$$\frac{500 \times \overset{1}{\cancel{60}}}{\underset{4}{\cancel{240}}} = 4\overline{)500}\ \overset{125}{}$$

$$\begin{array}{r} 4 \\ \hline 10 \\ 8 \\ \hline 20 \end{array}$$

Microdrip at 125 gtt/min

Answers are macrodrip at 42 gtt/min and microdrip at 125 gtt/min. Choose one. (See the explanation for choosing the infusion set, after this discussion.)

Label the IV.

Set the drip rate.

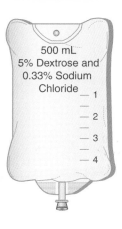

500 mL
5% Dextrose and
0.33% Sodium
Chloride

— 1
—
— 2
—
— 3
—
— 4

Example

Order: 500 mL D5⅓NS IV KVO for 24 h

Available: microdrip at 60 gtt/mL; macrodrip 10 gtt/mL

Because no pump is available, choose the IV set. The IV will run 24 hours or 1400 minutes (24 × 60 minutes). Work out the problem for micro- and macrodrip and make a nursing judgment about which tubing to use.

Macrodrip

$$\frac{500\ \text{mL} \times \overset{1}{\cancel{10}}\ \text{gtt}}{\underset{140}{\cancel{1400}}\ \text{min}} = 140\overline{)500.0}\ \overset{3.5}{}$$

$$\begin{array}{r} 420 \\ \hline 800 \\ 700 \end{array}$$

Macrodrip at 4 gtt/min

Microdrip

$$\frac{500\ \text{mL} \times 60\ \text{gtt}}{1400\ \text{min}} = \frac{3000}{140}\overline{)3000.0}\ \overset{21.4}{}$$

$$\begin{array}{r} 280 \\ \hline 200 \\ 140 \\ \hline 600 \end{array}$$

Microdrip at 21 gtt/min

A 4-gtt/min macrodrip is too slow. Choose microdrip. (See the explanation on p. 221 for choosing the infusion set.)

Label the IV.

Select a microdrip infusion set.

Set the drip rate at 21 gtt/min.

Calculate the drip factor for the following IV orders given in millilitres per hour or gtt per minute. Answers are given at the end of the chapter.

1. Order: 150 mL D5W 0.33NS IV q8h
   Available: infusion pump

2. Order: 250 mL D5W; run at 25 mL/hr
   Available: infusion pump

3. Order: 1000 mL D5NS; run 100 mL/hr
   Available: macrodrip (20 gtt/mL); microdrip (60 gtt/mL)

4. Order: 180 mL D5⅓NS 1200–1800h
   Available: macrodrip (10 gtt/mL); microdrip (60 gtt/mL)

5. Order: 1000 mL D5W 0.45NS IV 1600–2400h
   Available: macrodrip (15 gtt/mL); microdrip (60 gtt/mL)

6. Order: 250 mL D5W IV q8h
   Available: infusion pump

7. Order: 500 mL NS IV over 2 hr
   Available: infusion pump

8. Order: 1000 mL D5NS IV 0400–1600h
   Available: macrodrip (15 gtt/mL); microdrip (60 gtt/mL)

9. Order: 1000 mL D5W 0.45 NS IV; run 150 mL/hr
   Available: macrodrip (10 gtt/mL); microdrip (60 gtt/mL)

10. Order: 150 mL 0.9 NS IV; over 1 hr
    Available: macrodrip (20 gtt/mL); microdrip (60 gtt/mL)

Determining Hours an IV Will Run

Knowing how to calculate approximately how long an IV will last helps you in your work, because you can use that amount of time to prepare the next IV or note any new orders.

$$\frac{\text{number of millilitres ordered}}{\text{number of millilitres per hour}} = \text{number of hours to run}$$

Example

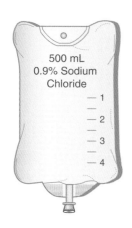

500 mL
0.9% Sodium
Chloride
— 1
— 2
— 3
— 4

Order: 500 mL NS IV; infuse at 75 mL/hr

Rule: $\frac{\text{number mL}}{\text{number mL/hr}} = \text{hr}$

$$\frac{500 \text{ mL}}{75 \text{ mL/hr}} = 75\overline{)500.00}$$

$$\begin{array}{r} 6.67 \\ \hline 450 \\ \hline 50\ 0 \\ 45\ 0 \\ \hline 5\ 00 \end{array}$$

The IV will last approximately 6.7 hours.

Example

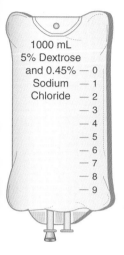

Order: 1000 mL D5½NS IV 0800–2000h

No math necessary; 0800−2000h = 12 hours

The IV will last 12 hours.

Example

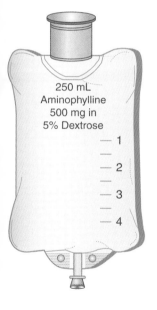

Order: aminophylline 500 mg in 250 mL D5W IV at 50 mL/hr

Rule: $\frac{\text{number mL}}{\text{number mL/hr}} = \#hr$

$\frac{250 \text{ mL}}{50 \text{ mL}} = 5 \text{ hr}$

The IV will last 5 hours.

SELF TEST 2   IV Infusions—Hours

Calculate the hours that the following IV orders will run. Answers are given at the end of this chapter.

1. Order: 250 mL D5½NS IV at 30 mL/hr
2. Order: Ringer's lactate 500 mL IV; run 60 mL/hr
3. Order: 1000 mL D5NS IV 1600h−0200h
4. Order: 1000 mL D5W IV KVO 24 hours
5. Order: 500 mL D5½NS at 70 mL/hr
6. Order: 500 mL D5W IV at 50 mL/hr
7. Order: LR 1000 mL IV 10 hours
8. Order: 250 mL NS IV at 100 mL/hr
9. Order: 1000 mL NS IV 1200h−1800h
10. Order: 500 mL NS IV over 5 hours

Choosing the Infusion Set

Experience will enable you to judge which IV tubing to use. In clinical settings, the guidelines below will help you make your choice. An electric infusion pump poses no problem, because it will deliver the amount programmed. Specialized pumps in neonatal and intensive care units can deliver 1 mL/hr and even less. Specialized syringe pumps also can deliver less than 1 mL/hr.

When an IV pump is not available, consider these guidelines:

Use Microdrip When

- the IV is to be administered over a long period
- a small amount of fluid is to be infused
- the macrodrops per minute are too few (Without an infusion pump, IV fluids flow by gravity. Blood flowing in the vein exerts a pressure. If the IV is too slow, the pressure of the blood in the vein may back up into the tubing, where it may clot and cause the IV to stop infusing.)

Use Macrodrip When

- the order specifies a large amount of fluid over a short time
- the microdrips per minute are too many and counting the drip rate becomes too difficult

Need for Continuous Observation

Many factors may interfere with the drip rate. When you are not using an infusion pump, gravity will cause the IV to vary from its starting rate; you will need to check the IV frequently. You'll need to monitor other conditions as well. As the amount of fluid decreases in the IV bag, pressure changes occur—and they, too, may affect the rate. The patient's movements can kink the tube and shut off the flow; he or she can change the position of the needle or catheter in the vein. The needle can become lodged against the side of the blood vessel, thereby altering the flow, or it may be forced out of the vessel, allowing fluid to enter the tissues (infiltration). (Signs of possible infiltration are swelling, pain, coolness, or pallor at the insertion site. If you notice any of these signs, discontinue the IV and start a new one at another insertion site.)

Infusion pumps have an alarm system that beeps to alert the nurse when the rate cannot be maintained or when the infusion is nearly finished. Be sure to check the infusion pump frequently and know how to troubleshoot the various alarms.

◉▭ Adding Medications to IVs

When a continuous IV order includes a medication, generally this medication arrives already pre-mixed in the infusion bag, or the pharmacist adds it on site. In some institutions, the nurse adds the medication to the IV and determines the rate of flow. If the task falls to you, first calculate how much of the medication to add to the IV fluids, and then calculate the drip rate.

Example   Order: 1000 mL D5W with 20 mEq KCl IV 1000h−2200h

Available: vial of KCl 40 mEq/20 mL, microdrip (60 gtt/min), macrodrip (20 gtt/min)

Formula Method	Proportion Expressed as Two Ratios	Proportion Expressed as Two Fractions
$\dfrac{\overset{1}{\cancel{20}} \text{ mEq}}{\underset{2}{\cancel{40}} \text{ mEq}} \times \overset{10}{\cancel{20}} \text{ mL} = 10 \text{ mL}$	$20 \text{ mL} : 40 \text{ mEq} :: x \text{ mL} : 20 \text{ mEq}$	$\dfrac{20 \text{ mL}}{40 \text{ mEq}} \times \dfrac{x}{20 \text{ mEq}}$

$$\frac{400}{40} = x$$

$$10 \text{ mL} = x$$

Add 10 mL KCl to the IV bag.

Choose the tubing. The IV will run 12 hours.

For macrodrip: $\dfrac{1000 \text{ mL} \times 20 \text{ gtt}}{720 \text{ min}} = 28 \text{ gtt/min}$

For microdrip: $\dfrac{1000 \text{ mL} \times 60 \text{ gtt}}{720 \text{ min}} = 83 \text{ gtt/min}$

Choose either drip rate.

Label the IV.

Example   Order: aminophylline 250 mg in 250 mL D5W IV; run at 50 mL/hr for 1 hour.

Available: ampoule of aminophylline labelled 1 g in 10 mL; Buretrol that delivers 60 gtt/mL (microdrip). See Figure 8-4.

The ampoule of aminophylline has 1 g in 10 mL. This is equivalent to 1000 mg in 10 mL. You want 250 mg.

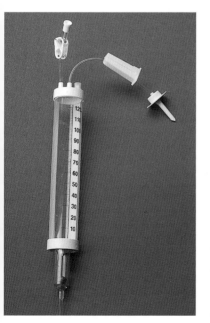

FIGURE 8-4

A Buretrol is an IV delivery system with tubing and a chamber that can hold 150 mL delivered as microdrip (1 mL = 60 drops). (This device is sometimes called a Volutrol.) The top of the Buretrol has a port so that a reservoir of fluid can be added. The Buretrol is a volume control because no more than 150 mL can be infused at one time.

Formula Method	Proportion Expressed as Two Ratios	Proportion Expressed as Two Fractions
$\dfrac{\overset{1}{\cancel{250}}}{\underset{4}{\cancel{1000}}}\times 10 = \dfrac{\cancel{10}}{4}\quad 4\overline{)10.0}\;\; 2.5\text{ mL}$	$\overleftrightarrow{10 \text{ mL} : 1000 \text{ mg}} :: \overleftrightarrow{\text{mL} : 250 \text{ mg}}$	$\dfrac{10 \text{ mL}}{1000 \text{ mg}} \times \dfrac{\text{x}}{250 \text{ mg}}$ $\dfrac{2500}{1000} = \text{x}$ $2.5 \text{ mL} = \text{x}$

Draw up 2.5 mL and inject it into 250 mL D5W. You have 250 mg aminophylline in 250 mL D5W. Label the bag.

You want 50 mL/hr, and you have a Buretrol 60 gtt/mL. Open the Buretrol device and drip in 50 mL. You will run this amount over 1 hour because that's what the order specified.

$$\frac{50 \text{ mL} \times \cancel{60} \text{ gtt}}{\cancel{60} \text{ min}} = 50 \text{ mL/hr}$$

Label the IV: Rate, 50 mL/hr

FINE POINTS

The Buretrol is microdrip. No calculation is needed.

mL/hr = gtt/min

SELF TEST 3   IV Infusion Rates

Calculate how much medication is needed (if applicable) and the infusion rate. Answers are given at the end of the chapter.

1. Order: 500 mL D5W IV with vitamin C 500 mg at 60 mL/hr
   Available: ampoule of vitamin C labelled 500 mg/2 mL; microdrip tubing at 60 gtt/mL

2. Order: 250 mg Solu Cortef (hydrocortisone sodium succinate) in 1000 mL D5W
               0800−2400h
   Available: vial of hydrocortisone sodium succinate labelled 250 mg with a 2-mL diluent; microdrip tubing

3. Order: aminophylline 250 mg in 250 mL D5W IV; run 50 mL/hr
   Available: infusion pump, vial of aminophylline labelled 500 mg/10 mL

4. Order: 250 mL D5½ NS with KCl 10 mEq IV 1200–1800h
   Available: microdrip tubing, vial of potassium chloride labelled 20 mEq/10 mL

⬤▬ Medications for Intermittent IV Administration

Some IV medications are administered not continuously but only intermittently, such as q4h, q6h, or q8h. This route is termed *intravenous piggyback* or IVPB (Fig. 8-5). The term admixture refers to the pre-mixed IVPB.

Most of these drugs are prepared in powder form. The manufacturer specifies the type and amount of diluent needed to reconstitute the drug; after reconstitution, the nurse connects the IVPB by IV tubing to the main IV line. Some IVPB medications come pre-mixed from the manufacturer. For other medications, the institutional pharmacy may reconstitute and prepare IVPB solutions in a sterile environment using a laminar flow hood. This saves nursing time. Nevertheless, the nurse still bears responsibility: You must check the diluent and volume. You must also check the dose and the expiration date of the reconstituted solution; note whether the IVPB should be refrigerated before use or whether it can remain at room temperature until hung. Finally, you must calculate the drip rate and record this information on the IVPB label before hanging the bag.

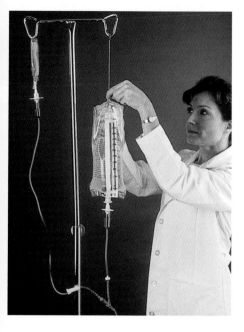

FIGURE 8-5

Photo of a primary IV line (*right*) and an IVPB (or secondary) line (*left*). Fluid flows continuously through the primary line into the patient's vein. At timed intervals, medication placed in an intravenous piggyback bag (IVPB) is attached by tubing to the primary IV for delivery to the patient. The primary fluid is lowered and the IVPB fluid flows. After the IVPB has infused, the primary fluid begins infusing again. An IV infusion pump may also be used, and medication in the IVPB is infused through the pump.

The physician or healthcare provider may write a detailed order, such as "Vancomycin 0.5 g IVPB in 100 mL D5W over 1 hr." More often, however, the physician or healthcare provider writes only the drug, route, and time interval, relying on the nurse to research the manufacturer's directions for the amount and type of diluent and the time for the infusion to run (e.g., Order: cefazolin 1 g IVPB q6h).

Explanation

To solve IVPB problems, you use a calculation much like the one you used for the IV:

$$\frac{mL \times TF}{min} = gtt/min$$

mL: The label or the package insert will state the type and amount of diluent. Nurses' drug references and the *Physicians Drug Reference* also contain this information.

TF: The tubing for IVPB is called a secondary administration set and has a macrodrip factor. It is shorter than main line IV tubing. In the clinical setting, check the label for the tubing drip factor.

min: The manufacturer may or may not indicate the number of minutes needed for the IVPB medication to be infused. When the number is not given, follow this general rule for adults: allow 30 minutes for every 50 mL solution.

Example   Order: cefazolin 1 g IVPB q6h

Supply: **package insert** IVPB dilution of cefazolin sodium. Reconstitute with 50 to 100 mL of sodium chloride injection or other solution listed under administration. Other solutions listed include D5W, D10W, D5LR, and D5NS.

Use 50 mL D5W. It is the most common IVPB diluent. No time for infusion is given in the directions for IVPB. Use 30 minutes for 50 mL.

Here's the calculation

$$\frac{mL \times TF}{min} = gtt/min$$

mL = 50 mL D5W

TF = 10 gtt/mL (For a secondary asministration, no set time for administration is given. Follow the general adult rule of 30 minutes for every 50 mL.)

min = 30

$$\frac{50 \times 10}{30} = 16.6 = 17 \text{ gtt/min}$$

Before hanging the IVPB, reconstitute the drug. You have a vial of powder labelled 1 g, and you need the whole amount. You have a 50-mL bag of D5W, and you need that whole amount as well. To mix the powder and the diluent, use a reconstitution device— (if available) a sterile implement containing two needles that connects the vial and the 50-mL bag. With this device, you can dilute the powder and place it in the IV bag without using a syringe (Fig. 8-6). Some manufacturers now enclose a reconstitution device with the IV bag. Once the powder is reconstituted, label the IV bag.

The order is q6h, and generally the administration times are 0600h, 1200h, 1800h, 2400h. The time of infusion is 30 minutes and, for this label, will run from 1200–1230h.

Rather than spending valuable time looking through package inserts for directions, check the concise information in drug references such as *Lippincott's Nursing Drug Guide*.

Medication Added		
Patient *Tom Smith*	**Room** *1503*	
Date *cefazolin 1 g*	**Flow Rate** *17 gtt/min*	
Base solution *50 mL D5W*	**Initials** *RT*	
Time to Run *1200h–1230h*	**Date** *6/14*	

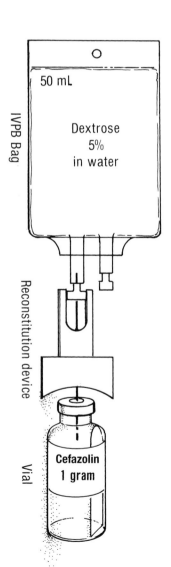

FIGURE 8-6

Reconstitution device. The IVPB bag is squeezed, forcing fluid into the vial of powder, which is then diluted. The three parts are turned to a vertical position—vial up, IVPB bag down. The IVPB bag is squeezed and released. This creates a negative pressure, allowing the diluted medication to flow into the IVPB bag.

Example	Order: Vancomycin 1 g IVPB 0700h

Supply: 500 mg powder

Package insert directions: 250 mL (1 g)/D5W

Run over 2 hours (1 g). Refrigerate for 7 days.

$$\frac{mL \times TF}{min} = gtt/min$$

$$\frac{250 \times 10}{120} = \frac{250}{12} \quad \frac{20.8}{\overline{)250.0}} = 21 \; gtt/min$$

Use a reconstitution device to add 1 g vancomycin (two vials of 500 mg) to 250 mL D5W. Label the IV. Set the rate at 21 gtt/min. The IVPB will run 2 hours.

When you're using an infusion pump for IVPB, solve the problem by setting 60 gtt as the tubing factor. Most infusion pumps have a special setting for "secondary IV administration." Choose this setting, then program the rate in mL/hr. After the IVPB has infused, the pump then either switches back to the primary IV infusion or begins beeping, letting you know that the infusion is complete.

SELF TEST 4 **IVPB Drip Factors**

Solve these drip factors for IVPB problems. Answers are given at the end of this chapter.

1. Order: Zovirax (acyclovir) 500 mg IVPB q8h
   Supply: 500 mg powder
   Package directions: 100 mL/D5W. Infuse 1 hour/once a day
   Available: macrodrip tubing at 10 gtt/mL

2. Order: Ceptaz (ceftazidime) 1 g IVPB q12h
   Supply: 1 g powder
   Package directions: 50 mL (1 g)/D5W. Infuse in 15–30 minutes/store for 7 days
                       (REFRIGERATED)
   Available: macrodrip tubing at 10 gtt/mL

3. Order: Claforan (cefotaxime) 1 g IVPB q6h
   Supply: 1 g powder
   Package directions: 50 mL (1 g)/D5W. Infuse in 15–30 minutes/store for 5 days
                       (REFRIGERATED)
   Available: macrodrip tubing at 10 gtt/mL

4. Order: Omnipen (ampicillin) 500 mg IV q6h
   Supply: 2 g in 5 mL
   Package directions: 50 mL (500 mg)/D5W. Infuse in 15–30 minutes
   Available: microdrip tubing at 60 gtt/mL

5. Order: Nebcin (tobramycin) 50 mg IV q8h
   Supply: 80 mg in 2 mL
   Package directions: 100 mL (50 mg)/D5W. Infuse in 60 minutes
   Available: macrodrip tubing at 15 gtt/mL

6. Order: Timentin (ticarcillin) 500 mg IV q6h
   Supply: 1 g in 5 mL
   Package directions: 50 mL (500 mg)/D5W. Infuse in 30 minutes
   Available: macrodrip tubing at 15 gtt/mL

Ambulatory Infusion Device

An ambulatory infusion device such as the one pictured in Figure 8-7 is used when a patient is receiving long-term antibiotic or other infusion therapy. The device is filled with the medication and a vacuum within the container infuses the medication over a specific time frame when the device is attached to the patient's IV. This is convenient for the patient, so that he or she may go home from the hospital on infusion therapy and continue in daily activities. The patient may have a peripheral IV site that has to be changed every 3–4 days, or may have a long-term indwelling IV catheter, such as a PICC (peripherally inserted central catheter) line.

Enteral Nutrition

Enteral feeding is used when a patient cannot eat or cannot eat enough. A tube is passed through the nasal or oral cavity to the stomach or duodenum (nasogastric [N/G tube] or orogastric [O/G tube]) or it is placed more permanently, as with a percutaneous endoscopic gastrostomy (PEG) tube, gastrostomy tube (G tube) or jejunostomy tube (J tube). Commercial tube feedings are used as well (Fig. 8-8); these formulas, though varied, usually carry a high caloric component. They may also include high fiber and high protein and may vary according to a patient's disease state.

Tube feedings are administered with a pump that regulates the amount of feeding. The feedings may be *intermittent*, delivering the formula at regular periods of time; *cyclic*, giving the formula over several hours of the day (over 12–16 hours); or *continuous*, infusing the formula constantly (Fig. 8–9).

Enteral feedings require careful monitoring to avoid complications and to ensure the patient's safety. Full-strength tube feeding is recommended, although diluted tube feedings are still used. Patients receiving diluted tube feedings must be carefully observed for signs of hyponatremia (water intoxication). The section below discusses common dilutions and the way to calculate the dose. For more information on enteral feedings, consult a basic nursing book such as *Fundamentals of Nursing*, by Taylor, Lillis, LeMone, and Lynn (Lippincott, 2008).

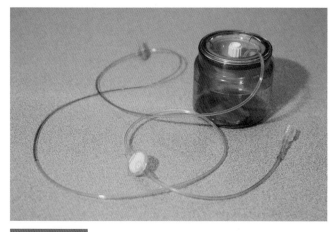

FIGURE 8-7

Ambulatory infusion device.

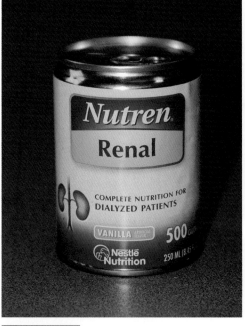

FIGURE 8-8

Commercially prepared tube feeding.

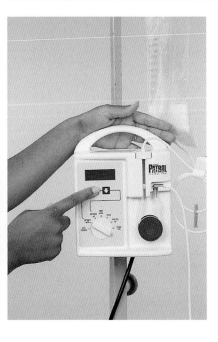

Calculation of Tube Feedings

An order for tube feedings will read:

Administer Isocal full strength at 60 mL/hr. Check for residual every 4 hours. Flush tube with 50 mL of water every 4 hours.

This order does not require calculation.

Add Isocal to a tube feeding bag, and set the tube feeding pump at 60 mL/hr.

Complete the other orders per protocol.

Follow hospital protocol for changing of tube feeding bag and tubing.

Example

Administer ½ strength Isocal at 60 mL/hr. The total volume will equal 250 mL.

For this problem, begin by taking ½ of the total volume to infuse:

½ × 250 mL = 125 mL

This number tells you how much formula to add to the tube feeding bag.

Next, subtract that number from the total volume.

250 mL − 125 mL = 125 mL

This new number tells you how much water to add to the tube feeding bag.

Now that you have diluted the formula to ½ strength, infuse it at 60 mL/hr.

> **Example**   Administer ¼ strength Isocal at 60 mL/hr. Total volume to equal 250 mL.
>
> First, take ¼ of the total volume:
>
> ¼ × 250 mL = 62.5 mL
>
> Again, this is the volume of formula to add to the tube feeding bag.
>
> Subtract this number from the total volume:
>
> 250 mL – 62.5 mL = 182.5 mL
>
> This is the volume of water to dilute.

> **Example**   Administer ¾ strength Isocal at 60 mL/hr. Total volume to equal 250 mL.
>
> Take ¾ of the total volume:
>
> ¾ × 250 mL = 182.5 mL of Isocal
>
> Subtract from the total:
>
> 250 mL – 182.5 = 62.5 mL of water to dilute.

SELF TEST 5   Calculation of Tube Feedings

Solve these problems stating how much of the feeding and how much water to add. Answers are at the end of the chapter.

1. ¾ strength Isocal must be prepared. Total volume is 275 mL. How much Isocal is to be mixed with how much water?

2. 75 mL of 75% Magnacal must be prepared. How much Magnacal is to be mixed with how much water?

3. ½ strength Osmolite must be prepared. 100 mL is the total volume. How much Osmolite is to be mixed with how much water?

4. ¼ strength Ensure must be prepared. Total volume is 85 mL. How much Ensure is to be mixed with how much water?

5. 25% Renalcal must be prepared. 400 mL is the total volume. How much Renalcal is to be mixed with how much water?

6. 50% Suplena must be prepared. 400 mL is the total volume. How much Suplena is to be mixed with how much water?

Recording Intake

Keep an accurate account of parenteral intake as well as liquids taken orally and/or enterally (e.g., tube feedings). Each institution provides a flow sheet to record fluid input over a specified period of time. Usually when an IVPB is infusing, the primary IV stops infusing. After the IVPB is completed, the primary IV flow rate begins again. (Refer to Fig. 8-5.)

SELF TEST 6   Fluid Intake

Answer the following questions regarding fluid intake. Answers are given at the end of this chapter.

1. A total of 900 mL of an IV solution is to infuse at 100 mL/hr. If it is 0900h when the infusion starts, at what time will it be completed?

2. A patient is receiving an antibiotic IVPB in 75 mL q6h to run over 1 hour plus a maintenance IV of 125 mL/hr. What is the 24-hour intake parenterally?

3. An IV of 1000 mL D5NS is infusing at 10 microdrips per minute. What is the parenteral intake for 8 hours?

4. A doctor orders 500 mL aminophylline 0.5 g to infuse at 50 mL/hr. How many mg will the patient receive each hour?

5. A total of 20,000 units of heparin is added to 500 mL D5W, and the order is to infuse IV at 30 mL/hr. How many hours will the IV run?

6. A patient is receiving an antibiotic IVPB in 50 mL q8h to run over 1 hour plus a maintenance IV of 100 mL/hr. What is the 24-hour intake parenterally?

7. A total of 500 mL of an IV solution is to infuse at 50 mL/hr. If it is 0600h when the infusion starts, at what time is it completed?

8. IV of D5W 1000 mL is infusing at 125 mL/hr. How many hours will the IV run?

9. A patient is receiving an antibiotic IVPB in 250 mL q6h. What is the 24-hour intake parenterally?

10. A physician orders 100 units regular insulin in 100 mL to infuse at 10 mL/hr. How many units will the patient receive each hour?

Solve these problems related to IV and IVPB drip rates. Answers are given at the end of the chapter.

1. Order: 1500 mL D5W 0800h–2000h $\frac{1500}{84} \times 10 = 17.8 : 18 \text{ gtt/min}$
   Available: macrodrip tubing (10 gtt/mL)
   What is the drip rate?

2. Order: 250 mL D5½ NS IV KVO (give over 12 hours)
   Available: microdrip tubing
   What is the drip rate?

3. Order: 150 mL D5⅓ NS IV; run 20 mL/hr
   Available: infusion pump

   a. What is the drip rate?
   b. How long will the IV last?

4. Order: 1000 mL D5NS with 15 mEq KCl IV; run 100 mL/hr
   Available: macrotubing (20 gtt/mL) and microdrip

   a. How many hours will this run?
   b. How many millilitres of KCl will you add to the IV if KCl comes in a vial labelled 40 mEq/20 mL?
   c. What tubing will you use?
   d. What are the gtt/min?

5. Order: aminophylline 1 g in 500 mL D5W IV at 75 mL/hr
   Available: vial of aminophylline 1 g in 10 mL; infusion pump

   a. How many mL of aminophylline should be added to the IV?
   b. How will you set the drip rate?

6. Order: Amikin (amikacin) 0.4 g IVPB q8h
   Supply: 2-mL vial labelled 250 mg/mL
   Package directions: 100 mL/D5W 30 minutes
   Available: macrodrip tubing 10 gtt/mL

   a. How many mL of amikacin should be added to the IV?
   b. What are the gtt/min?

7. Order: 500 mL D5½ NS IV q8h
   Available: microdrip tubing
   What are the gtt/min?

8. Order: 1000 mL D5W IV q24h
   Available: macrodrip tubing (15 gtt/mL)
   What is the drip rate?

9. Order: Heparin 25,000 units in 250 mL NS at 20 mL/hr
   How long will the IV last?

10. Order: 500 mL NS over 4 hr
    Available: macrodrip tubing (20 gtt/mL)
    What is the drip rate?

SELF TEST 8   IV Problems

Solve these problems related to drip rates. Answers are given at the end of this chapter.

1. Order: aqueous penicillin G 1 milliunits in 100 mL D5W IVPB q6h over 40 minutes
                  (macrodrip tubing at 10 gtt/mL) (milliunits = million units)
   Supply: vial labelled 5 million units of powder. Directions say to inject 18 mL sterile water
                  for injection to yield 20 mL solution. Reconstituted solution is stable for 1 week.

   a. How would you prepare the penicillin?
   b. What solution will you make?
   c. What amount of penicillin solution should be placed into the bag of 100 mL D5W?
   d. What is the drip factor for the IVPB?

2. A total of 1000 mL of an IV solution is to infuse at 100 mL/hr. If the infusion starts at 0800h,
   at what time will it be completed?

3. Order: gentamicin 60 mg IVPB in 50 mL D5W over 30 minutes using macrodrip
                  (20 gtt/mL)
   Supply: vial of gentamicin 40 mg/mL; 50-mL bag of D5W; order is correct

   a. How many mL of gentamicin will you add to the 50-mL bag of D5W?
   b. What is the drip factor for the IVPB?

4. Calculate the drip factor for 1500 mL D5½NS to run 12 hours by macrodrip (10 gtt/mL).

5. Intralipid, 500 mL per N/G tube q6h, is ordered for a patient together with a primary IV that is
   infusing at 80 mL/hr. Calculate the 24-hour parenteral intake. (Total will be amount of lipids
   plus primary IV amount.)

6. Order: 1000 mL D5W with 20 mEq KCl and 500 mg vitamin C at 60 mL/hr. No infusion
                  pump is available.

   a. Approximately how many hours will the IV run?
   b. Which tubing will you choose—macrodrip at 10 gtt/mL or microdrip at 60 gtt/mL?
   c. What are the drops per minute for the tubing that you choose?

Putting It Together

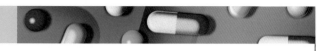

Mrs. Richardson is a 41-year-old female admitted with nausea, vomiting, and diarrhea. In the emergency room, she had a fever, leukocytosis, and potassium of 5.5.

Past Medical History: end-stage renal disease, diabetes mellitus, hypertension

Post left upper extremity graft placement.

No known drug allergies.

Current Vital Signs: BP 82/50, pulse is 111/min., respirations 20/min., oxygen saturation 86% on room air. Temp is 37°C, on admission was 38.7°C

Medication Orders

Gentamicin *anti-infective* 100 mg IV in 100 mL over 1 hour daily

Cubicin (daptomycin) *anti-infective* 500 mg in 100 mL NS every 24 hours over 30 min

Tazocin (piperacillin and tazobactam) *anti-infective* 3.375 g in 50 mL IV in NS every 6 hours

Adalat (nifedipine) XL anti-hypertensive 90 mg PO q24h

NS 1000 mL at 40 mL/hr IV

Fragmin (dalteparin) *anticoagulant* 2500 units subcutaneous qd

Reglan (metoclopramide) *anti-nausea, prokinetic agent* 20 mg IV prn q6h for nausea and vomiting. For doses over 10 mg must be IVPB

Calculations

1. Calculate the infusion rate for the Gentamicin with microdrip and macrodrip (20 gtt/mL) tubing.
2. Calculate the infusion rate for the Cubicin with microdrip and macrodrip (20 gtt/mL) tubing.
3. Calculate the infusion rate for Tazocin with microdrip and macrodrip (15 gtt/mL) tubing.
4. Calculate how many hours a 1000 mL of NS solution at 40 mL/hr will infuse. Use an infusion pump.
5. Calculate the total intake for 24 hours, including the primary IV and all antibiotics.

Critical Thinking Questions

1. What medications (PO or IV) should be held and why?
2. Why would a patient receive 3 antibiotics instead of only 1 antibiotic?
3. After 6 hours, the NS has only infused 150 mL. How much should have infused? What are some reasons that the IV solution has not infused more? Should the nurse increase the rate of the infusion in order to "catch up" on the total amount needed?
4. Is the Reglan to be infused as an IVPB? How much solution should it be mixed with and how long to infuse?

Answers in Appendix B.

Name: _____

There are 10 questions related to IV and IVPB and enteral feeding calculations. Answers are given in Appendix A.

1. Order: 1000 mL D5NS; run 150 mL/hr IV
   Supply: IV bag of 1000 mL D5NS

   a. Approximately how many hours will the IV run?
   b. Which tubing will you choose—macrodrip (10 gtt/mL) or microdrip (60 gtt/mL)?
   c. What will be the drip rate?

2. Order: 100 mL Ringer's solution 1200h−1800h IV

   a. What size tubing will you use?
   b. What are the gtt/min?

3. Order: 150 mL NS IV over 3 hours
   Supply: bag of 250 mL normal saline for IV and macrotubing, 15 gtt/mL; microtubing, 60 gtt/mL

   a. What would you do to obtain 150 mL NS?
   b. What IV tubing would you use?
   c. What are the gtt/min?

4. Order: 500 mL D5W IV KVO. Solve for 24 hours. An infusion pump is available. What should be the setting on the infusion pump?

5. Order: Vibramycin (doxycycline) 100 mg IVPB every day
   Supply: 100 mg powder
   Package directions: 250 mL/D5W to infuse over 1 hour; macrodrip tubing 10 gtt/mL

   a. State the amount and type of IV fluid you will use and the time for infusion you will use.
   b. What are the gtt/min?

6. Order: aminophylline 500 mg in 250 mL D5W to run 8 hours IV
   Available: vial of aminophylline labelled 1 g in 10 mL; microdrip tubing

   a. How much aminophylline is needed?
   b. What is the drip rate?

7. A patient is receiving a primary IV at the rate of 125 mL/hr. The doctor orders cefoxitin 1 g in 75 mL D5W q6h to run over 1 hour
   Calculate the 24-hour parenteral intake.

8. Order: 1000 mL D5½NS to run at 90 mL/hr; infusion pump available

   a. What will be the pump setting?
   b. Approximately how long will the IV run?

9. A doctor orders 500 mL aminophylline 0.5 g to infuse at 50 mL/hr. How many milligrams will the patient receive each hour?

10. Order: Bactrim (trimethoprim and sulfamethoxazole) 5 mL IVPB q6h
    Supply: vial of 5 mL; one 5-mL vial per 75 mL D5W run over 60 to 90 minutes.
    The main IV line is connected to an infusion pump. What will you do? Refer to Figure 8-4.

    a. State the type and amount of IV fluid you would use and the time for infusion.
    b. How would you program the infusion pump?

(continued)

11. ¾ strength Isocal must be prepared. 150 mL is the total volume. How much Isocal is to be mixed with how much water?

12. ½ strength Vivonex must be prepared. 500 mL is the total volume. How much Vivonex is to be mixed with how much water?

13. 25% strength Osmolite must be prepared. 400 mL is the total volume. How much Osmolite is to be mixed with how much water?

14. Full strength Isocal must be prepared. 500 mL is the total volume. How much Isocal is to be mixed with how much water?

Answers to Self Tests

Self Test 1 Calculation of Drip Factors

1. This is a continuous IV of 150 mL every 8 hours. There is a pump available. Minutes = 8 × 60 = 480.

$$\frac{150 \text{ mL}}{8\text{h}} \quad 8\overline{)150.0}^{\,18.7}$$
$$\begin{array}{r} 8 \\ \hline 70 \\ 64 \\ \hline 60 \end{array}$$

Label the IV. Set the pump: total number mL = 150; mL/hr = 19.

2. This is a continuous IV. A pump is available. The order states mL/hr. There is no calculation needed. Label the IV. Set the pump as follows: total number mL = 250; mL/hr = 25.

3. mL/hr = The order gives 100 mL/hr; mL/hr = gtt/min microdrip, so you know the microdrip is 100 gtt/min. Work out the macrodrip factor and choose the tubing.

Macrodrip

$$\frac{\text{mL/hr} \times \text{TF}}{\text{number min}} = \text{gtt/min}$$

$$\frac{100 \times \overset{1}{\cancel{20}}}{\underset{3}{\cancel{60}} \text{ min}} = \frac{100}{3} = 33.3$$

Macrodrip at 33 gtt/min

Microdrip at 100 gtt/min (mL/hr = gtt/min)

Either drip rate could be used. Label the IV.

4. This is a small volume over several hours; use microdrip. Macrodrip would be too slow (5 gtt/min). Minutes = 6 hours × 60 = 360.

$$\frac{\text{mL/hr} \times \text{TF}}{\text{min}} = \text{gtt/min}$$

$$\frac{180 \text{ mL} \times \overset{1}{\cancel{60}} \text{ gtt}}{\underset{6}{\cancel{360}} \text{ min}} = \frac{180}{6} \quad 6\overline{)180}^{\,30}$$
$$\begin{array}{r} 18 \\ \hline 0 \end{array}$$

Microdrip is 30 gtt/min because mL/hr = gtt/min.

5. This is a large volume over several hours. Solve using two steps and decide.

Microdrip

$$\frac{\text{mL/hr} \times \text{TF}}{\text{min}} = \text{gtt/min}$$

$$\frac{1000 \text{ mL} \times \overset{1}{\cancel{60}} \text{ gtt}}{\underset{8}{\cancel{480}} \text{ min}} = \frac{1000}{8} \quad 8\overline{)1000.0}^{\,125.}$$
$$\begin{array}{r} 8 \\ \hline 20 \\ 16 \\ \hline 40 \end{array}$$

microdrip will be 125 gtt/min because mL/hr = gtt/min.

Macrodrip

$$\frac{125 \times \overset{1}{\cancel{15}}}{\underset{4}{\cancel{60}} \text{ min}} = \frac{\cancel{125}}{4} \quad 4\overline{)125.0}^{\,31.2}$$
$$\begin{array}{r} 12 \\ \hline 5 \\ 4 \\ \hline 10 \\ 8 \end{array}$$

Macrodrip at 31 gtt/min

Microdrip at 125 gtt/min

Use macrodrip.

Label the IV.

6. This is a continuous IV of 250 mL every 8 hours. There is a pump available. It will run 8 hours. Minutes = 8 × 60 = 480 minutes.

$$\frac{\cancel{250} \text{ mL}}{8\text{h}} \quad 8\overline{)250.0}^{\,31.2 \text{ mL/hr}}$$
$$\begin{array}{r} 24 \\ \hline 10 \\ 8 \\ \hline 2.0 \end{array}$$

Label the IV. Set the pump: total number mL = 250; mL/hr = 31.

7. This is a continuous IV of 500 mL over 2 hours. There is a pump available.

It will run 2 hours. Minutes = $2 \times 60 = 120$.

$$
\frac{500\ \text{mL}}{2\text{h}}\overset{250.0\ \text{mL/hr}}{)\overline{500.0}}
$$

$$
\begin{array}{r}
250.0\ \text{mL/hr} \\
2\text{h}\,)\overline{500.0} \\
\underline{4} \\
10 \\
\underline{10} \\
0
\end{array}
$$

Label the IV. Set the pump: total number mL = 500; mL/hr = 250.

8. This is a large volume over several hours; macrodrip. Solve using two steps.

$$\frac{\text{mL/hr} \times \text{TF}}{\text{min}} = \text{gtt/min}$$

Macrodrip

$$
\frac{1000 \times \overset{1}{\cancel{15}}}{\underset{48}{\cancel{720}}\ \text{min}} = 48\,\overset{20.8}{)\overline{1000.0}}
$$

$$
\begin{array}{r}
20.8 \\
48\,)\overline{1000.0} \\
\underline{96} \\
400 \\
\underline{384} \\
6
\end{array}
$$

Microdrip

$$
\frac{1000 \times \overset{1}{\cancel{60}}}{\underset{12}{\cancel{720}}\ \text{min}} = 12\,\overset{83}{)\overline{1000}}
$$

$$
\begin{array}{r}
83 \\
12\,)\overline{1000} \\
\underline{96} \\
40 \\
\underline{36} \\
4
\end{array}
$$

Macrodrip at 21 gtt/min, microdrip at 83 gtt/min
Use macrodrip.
Label the IV.

9. This is a large volume at a fast rate. Use macrodrip. Solve using step 2 only.

$$\frac{\text{mL/hr} \times \text{TF}}{\text{min}} = \text{gtt/min}$$

$$
\frac{150 \times \overset{1}{\cancel{10}}}{\underset{6}{\cancel{60}}\ \text{min}} = \frac{150}{6}\overset{25.0\ \text{gtt/min}}{)\overline{150.0}}
$$

$$
\begin{array}{r}
25.0\ \text{gtt/min} \\
6\,)\overline{150.0} \\
\underline{12} \\
30 \\
\underline{30} \\
0
\end{array}
$$

Macrodrip at 25 gtt/min, microdrip at 150 gtt/min
Use macrodrip.
Label the IV.

10. This is a large volume over a short time. Use macrodrip tubing. The rate is 150 mL/hr (150 mL over 1 hour). Use step 2 only.

$$\frac{\text{mL/hr} \times \text{TF}}{\text{min}} = \text{gtt/min}$$

$$
\frac{150 \times \overset{1}{\cancel{20}}}{\underset{3}{\cancel{60}}\ \text{min}} = \frac{150}{3}\overset{50\ \text{gtt/min}}{)\overline{150.0}}
$$

$$
\begin{array}{r}
50\ \text{gtt/min} \\
3\,)\overline{150.0} \\
\underline{15} \\
0
\end{array}
$$

Macrodrip at 50 gtt/min, microdrip at 150 gtt/min
Use macrodrip.
Label the IV.

Self Test 2 IV Infusions—Hours

1. 8.3 hours approximately $\left(\frac{250}{30} = 8.3\right)$

2. 8.3 hours approximately $\left(\frac{500}{60} = 8.3\right)$

3. 10 hours (no math)

4. 24 hours (no math)

5. 7.1 hours approximately $\left(\frac{500}{70} = 7.1\right)$

6. 10 hours $\left(\frac{500}{50} = 10\right)$

7. 10 hours (no math)

8. 2.5 hours $\left(\frac{250}{100} = 2.5\right)$

9. 6 hours (no math)

10. 5 hours (no math)

Self Test 3 IV Infusion Rates

1. You want vitamin C 500 mg and the supply is 500 mg in 2 mL. Use a syringe to add the 2 mL to 500 mL D5W. You have microdrip available. The IV is to run at 60 mL/hr. Remember mL/hr = gtt/min for microdrip. No math necessary. Set the microdrip at 60 gtt/min. Label the IV.

$$\frac{60 \text{ mL} \times \cancel{60} \text{ gtt}}{\cancel{60} \text{ min}} = 60 \text{ mL/hr}$$

2. You want 250 mg hydrocortisone sodium succinate, and it comes 250 mg with a 2-mL diluent. Use a syringe to reconstitute the hydrocortisone with 2 mL diluent and add it to the IV. 8000–2400h is 16 hours.

mL/hr = gtt/min for microdrip. No math for microdrip. Microdrip = 63 gtt/min. Label the IV. Minutes = 60 × 16 = 960.

$$\frac{1000 \text{ mL} \times \overset{1}{\cancel{60}} \text{ gtt}}{\underset{16}{\cancel{960}} \text{ min}} = 16\overline{)1000.0}^{\;62.5}$$

$$\begin{array}{r} \underline{96} \\ 40 \\ \underline{32} \\ 80 \\ 80 \end{array}$$

3. You want 250 mg aminophylline. Supply is 500 mg/10 mL.

Formula Method	Proportion Expressed as Two Ratios	Proportion Expressed as Two Fractions
$\dfrac{250 \text{ mg}}{500 \text{ mg}} \times 10 \text{ mL} = 5 \text{ mL}$	10 mL : 500 mg :: x mL : 250 mg	$\dfrac{10 \text{ mL}}{500 \text{ mg}} \times \dfrac{x}{250 \text{ mg}}$

$$\frac{2500}{500} = x$$

$$5 = x$$

Add 5 mL aminophylline to 250 mL D5W. Order is 50 mL/hr. You have an infusion pump. No math. Set the pump as follows: total number mL = 250; mL/hr = 50.

4. You want KCl 10 mEq. Supply is 20 mEq/10 mL.

Formula Method	Proportion Expressed as Two Ratios	Proportion Expressed as Two Fractions
$\dfrac{10 \text{ mEq}}{20 \text{ mEq}} \times 10 \text{ mL} = 5 \text{ mL}$	10 mL : 10 mEq :: x mL : 20 mEq	$\dfrac{10 \text{ mL}}{20 \text{ mEq}} \times \dfrac{x}{10 \text{ mEq}}$

$$\frac{100}{20} = x$$

$$5 \text{ mL} = x$$

Add 5 mL KCl to 250 mL D5W½NS. 1200–1800h is 6 hours. 6 hours = 6 × 60 = 360 minutes.

$$\frac{250 \text{ mL} \times \overset{1}{\cancel{60}} \text{ gtt}}{\underset{6}{\cancel{360}} \text{ min}} = \frac{\cancel{250}}{6} \quad 6\overline{)250.0}^{\;41.6} = 42 \text{ mL/hr}$$

$$\begin{array}{r} \underline{24} \\ 10 \\ \underline{6} \\ 4\ 0 \\ \underline{3\ 6} \end{array}$$

mL/hr = gtt/min microdrip

Set the microdrip at 42 gtt/min.

Label the IV.

Self Test 4 IVPB Drip Factors

1. Zovirax (acyclovir) comes in 500 mg powder. Use a reconstitution device to add the powder to 100 mL D5W; min = 60; TF = 10 gtt/mL for IVPB.

   Rule: $\frac{mL \times TF}{min} = gtt/min$

   $$\frac{100 \times 10}{60 \ min} = \frac{100}{6} \overline{)100.0}^{\ 16.6} = 17 \ gtt/min$$

   Label the IVPB.

   Set the rate at 17 gtt/min.

2. Ceptaz (ceftazidime) comes in a 1-g powder

   Use a reconstitution device to add the powder to 50 mL D5W; min, 30; TF, 10 gtt/mL for IVPB

   Rule: $\frac{mL \times TF}{min} = gtt/min$

   $$\frac{50 \times 10}{30 \ min} = \frac{50}{3} = 16.6 = 17 \ gtt/min$$

   Label the IVPB.

   Set the rate at 17 gtt/min.

3. Claforan (cefotaxime) comes as a 1-g powder

   Use a reconstitution device to add the powder to 50 mL D5W; min, 30; TF, 10 gtt/mL for IVPB

   $\frac{mL \times TF}{min} = gtt/min$

   $$\frac{50 \times 10}{30 \ min} = 16.6 = 17 gtt/min$$

   Label the IVPB

   Set the rate at 17 gtt/min.

4. Omnipen (ampicillin) comes as a 2-g powder.

   Reconstitute in 4.5 mL diluent = total volume 5 mL (2 g = 5 mL, 2000 mg = 5 mL)

Formula Method	Proportion Expressed as Two Ratios	Proportion Expressed as Two Fractions
$\frac{500 \ mg}{2000 \ mg} \times 5 \ mL = 1.25 \ mL$	5 mL : 2000 mg : : x mL : 500 mg	$\frac{5 \ mL}{2000 \ mg} \times \frac{x}{500 \ mg}$

$$\frac{2500}{2000} = x$$

$$1.25 \ mL = x$$

Add 1.25 mL to 50 mL D5W. Total min = 30; TF = 60 gtt/mL.

$\frac{mL \times TF}{min} = gtt/min$

$$\frac{50 \times \overset{2}{60}}{\underset{1}{30} \ min} = 100 \ gtt/min$$

Label the IVPB.

Set the rate at 100 gtt/min.

5. Nebcin (tobramycin) comes as 80-mg. Reconstitute in 2 mL diluent = 2 mL (80 mg = 2 mL)

Formula Method	Proportion Expressed as Two Ratios	Proportion Expressed as Two Fractions
$\dfrac{50 \text{ mg}}{80 \text{ mg}} \times 2 \text{ mL} = 1.25 \text{ mL}$	2 mL : 80 mg : : x mL : 50 mg	$\dfrac{2 \text{ mL}}{80 \text{ mg}} \times \dfrac{x}{50 \text{ mg}}$

$$\frac{100}{80} = x$$

$$1.25 \text{ mL} = x$$

Add 1.25 mL to 100 mL D5W.

Total min = 60; TF = 15 gtt/mL

$$\frac{mL \times TF}{min} = gtt/min$$

$$\frac{100 \times \overset{1}{\cancel{15}}}{\underset{4}{\cancel{60} \text{ min}}} = 25 \text{ gtt/min}$$

Label the IVPB.

Set the rate at 25 gtt/min.

6. Timentin (ticarcillin) comes as a 1-g powder. Reconstitute in 4.5 mL of diluent = 5 mL (1 g or 1000 mg = 5 mL)

Formula Method	Proportion Expressed as Two Ratios	Proportion Expressed as Two Fractions
$\dfrac{500 \text{ mg}}{1000 \text{ mg}} \times 5 \text{ mL} = 2.5 \text{ mL}$	5 mL : 1000 mg : : x mL : 500 mg	$\dfrac{5 \text{ mL}}{1000 \text{ mg}} \times \dfrac{x}{500 \text{ mg}}$

$$\frac{2500}{1000} = x$$

$$2.5 \text{ mL} = x$$

Add 2.5 mL to 50 mL D5W.

Total min, 30; TF, 15 gtt/mL

$$\frac{mL \times TF}{min} = gtt/min$$

$$\frac{50 \times \overset{1}{\cancel{15}}}{\underset{2}{\cancel{30} \text{ min}}} = 25 \text{ gtt/min}$$

Set the rate at 25 gtt/min.

Self Test 5 Calculation of Tube Feedings

1. 206.25 mL of Isocal. 68.75 mL water.

2. 56.25 mL Magnacal. 18.75 mL water.

3. 50 mL Osmolite. 50 mL water.

4. 21.25 mL Ensure. 63.75 mL water.

5. 100 mL Renalcal. 300 mL water.

6. 200 mL Suplena. 200 mL water.

Self Test 6 Fluid Intake

1. 900 mL at 100 mL/hr = 9 hours to run. If the IV starts at 0900h, + 9 hours = 1800h.

2. IVPB is 75 mL q6h or four times in 24 hours

$$
\begin{array}{r}
75 \\
\times\ 4 \\
\hline
300\ \text{mL}
\end{array}
$$

   The patient is receiving 125 mL for 20 hours (24 hours − 4 hours that the IVPB is running).

$$
\begin{array}{r}
125 \\
\times\ 20 \\
\hline
000 \\
250 \\
\hline
2500\ \text{mL}
\end{array}
$$

$$
\begin{array}{r}
2500\ \text{mL} \\
+\ 300\ \text{mL} \\
\hline
2800\ \text{mL in 24 hours}
\end{array}
$$

3. IV is infusing at 10 microdrips/min. It takes 60 microdrips to make 1 mL., so 1 mL in 6 min, 10 mL in 60 min.

   10 mL in 60 min (1 hr)

$$
\begin{array}{r}
\times\ 8\ \text{hr} \\
\hline
80\ \text{mL in 8 hr}
\end{array}
$$

4. The IV is 0.5 g or 500 mg in 500 mL. This is equal to 1 mg/mL. The patient receives 50 mL/hr, so the patient receives 50 mg each hour.

5. The IV is infusing at 30 mL/hr and the solution is 500 mL.

$$
\frac{500\ \text{mL}}{30\ \text{mL/hr}} = \frac{50}{3} = 16.6\ \text{hours (approximately)}
$$

6. IVPB 50 mL q8h or three times in 24 hours

$$
\begin{array}{r}
50 \\
\times\ 3 \\
\hline
150\ \text{mL}
\end{array}
$$

   The patient is receiving 100 mL for 21 hours (24 hours − 3 hours that the IVPB is running).

$$
\begin{array}{r}
100 \\
\times\ 21 \\
\hline
100 \\
+\ 200 \\
\hline
2100\ \text{mL}
\end{array}
$$

$$
\begin{array}{r}
2100\ \text{mL} \\
+\ 150\ \text{mL} \\
\hline
2250\ \text{mL in 24 hours}
\end{array}
$$

7. 500 mL at 50 mL/hr = 10 hours to run. If the IV starts at 0600h + 10 hours = 1600h.

8. The IV is infusing at 125 mL/hr and the solution is 1000 mL.

$$
\frac{1000\ \text{mL}}{125\ \text{mL/hr}} = 8\ \text{hours}
$$

9. IVPB is 250 mL q6h or four times in 24 hours

$$
\begin{array}{r}
250 \\
\times\ 4 \\
\hline
1000\ \text{mL in 24 hours}
\end{array}
$$

10. The IV is 100 units in 100 mL or 1 unit/mL. The patient receives 10 mL/hr so the patient receives 10 units/hr.

Self Test 7 IV Drip Rates

1. Macrodrip $\qquad$ $12 \times 60 = 720$ min

$$\frac{mL/hr \times TF}{min} = gtt/min \qquad \frac{1500\ mL \times \overset{1}{\cancel{10}}\ gtt}{\underset{72}{\cancel{720}}\ min} = 72\overline{\smash{\big)}\begin{array}{r} 20.8 \\ 1500.0 \end{array}}$$
$$\underline{144}$$
$$600$$
$$\underline{570}$$

$= 21$ gtt/min

2. $\dfrac{250\ mL \times \overset{1}{\cancel{60}}\ gtt}{\underset{12}{\cancel{720}}\ min} = \dfrac{\cancel{250}}{12} \quad 12\overline{\smash{\big)}\begin{array}{r} 20.8 \\ 250.0 \end{array}} = 21$ ml/hr
$$\underline{24}$$
$$100$$
$$\underline{96}$$

You could also say mL/hr = gtt/min microdrip, so 21 mL/hr = 21 gtt/min.

3. $\dfrac{150\ mL}{20\ mL/hr} = \dfrac{\overset{15}{\cancel{15}}}{2} \quad 2\overline{\smash{\big)}\begin{array}{r} 7.5\ hr \\ 15.0\ hr \end{array}}$

    a. The drip rate is 20 mL/hr. No math is necessary. Set the infusion pump.

    b. The IV will last approximately 7½ hours.

4. a. $\dfrac{\overset{10}{\cancel{1000}}\ mL}{\underset{}{\cancel{100}}\ mL/hr} = 10$ hr

    b.

Formula Method	Proportion Expressed as Two Ratios	Proportion Expressed as Two Fractions
$\dfrac{D}{H} \times S = x$	$20\ mL : 40\ mEq :: x\ mL : 15\ mEq$	$\dfrac{20\ mL}{40\ mEq} \diagdown \dfrac{x}{15\ mEq}$
$\dfrac{15\ mEq}{\underset{2}{\cancel{40}}\ mEq} \times \overset{1}{\cancel{20}}\ mL = \dfrac{15}{2} = 7.5\ mL$		

$$\frac{300}{40} = 7.5\ mL$$

    c. Microdrip

$$\frac{100\ ml \times \overset{}{\cancel{60}}\ gtt}{\underset{}{\cancel{60}}\ min} = 100$$

Order states to run at 100 mL/hr. mL/hr = gtt/min microdrip, so microdrip at 100 gtt/min.

Macrodrip

$$\frac{100 \times \overset{1}{\cancel{20}}}{\underset{3}{\cancel{60}}} = \frac{100}{3} = 33\ gtt/min$$

Choose either tubing.

    d. 33 gtt/min macrodrip: 100 gtt/min microdrip

5. a. You desire 1 g. Aminophylline comes 1 g in 10 mL. Add 10 mL to the IV of 500 mL D5W and label.

    b. You have an infusion pump; there is no math.

       Set the pump:

       total # mL = 500; mL/hr = 75

6. 0.4 g = 400 mg

a.

Formula Method	Proportion Expressed as Two Ratios	Proportion Expressed as Two Fractions
$\dfrac{\overset{8}{\cancel{400}}\ \text{mg}}{\underset{5}{\cancel{250}}\ \text{mg}} \times 1\ \text{mL}$	$1\ \text{mL} : 250\ \text{mg} :: x\ \text{mL} : 400\ \text{mg}$	$\dfrac{1\ \text{mL}}{250\ \text{mg}} \times \dfrac{x}{400\ \text{mg}}$

$\dfrac{\cancel{8}}{5}\,\overset{1.6\ \text{mL}}{\big)8.0}$

$\dfrac{400}{250} = x$

$1.6\ \text{mL} = x$

b. Add 1.6 mL Amikin (amikacin) to 100 mL D5W.

TF = 10 gtt/mL for IVPB. Total min, 30

$\dfrac{\text{mL} \times \text{TF}}{\text{min}} = \text{gtt}/\text{min}$

$\dfrac{100\ \text{mL} \times \cancel{10}}{\cancel{30}} = \dfrac{100}{3} = 33.3$

$= 33\ \text{gtt/min}$

Label the IV.

Set the rate at 33 gtt/min.

7. $\dfrac{500\ \text{mL} \times \overset{1}{\cancel{60}}\ \text{gtt}}{\underset{8}{\cancel{480}}\ \text{minutes}} = \dfrac{500}{8}\ \overset{62.5}{\big)500.0} = 63\ \text{mL/hr}$

$\dfrac{48}{20}$
$\dfrac{16}{4\,0}$
$\dfrac{4\,0}{}$

You are using microdrip tubing, so mL/hr = gtt/min. Set the rate at 63 gtt/min.

8. 24 hours × 60 minutes = 1440 minutes.

$\dfrac{1000\ \text{mL} \times \overset{1}{\cancel{15}}\ \text{gtt}}{\underset{96}{\cancel{1440}}\ \text{minutes}} = 96\ \overset{10.4}{\big)1000.0}$

$\dfrac{96}{40}$
$\dfrac{0}{400}$

$\dfrac{\text{mL}/\text{hr} \times \text{TF}}{\text{min}} = \text{gtt}/\text{min}\qquad 10\ \text{gtt/min}$

9. $\dfrac{250\ \text{mL}}{20\ \text{mL/hr}} = \dfrac{250}{20}\ \overset{12.5}{\big)250.0}$

$\dfrac{20}{50}$
$\dfrac{40}{10\,0}$

The IV will last 12.5 hours.

10. $\dfrac{500 \text{ mL} \times \overset{1}{\cancel{20}} \text{ gtt}}{\underset{12}{\cancel{240} \text{ min}}} = 12\overline{)500.0} \begin{array}{r} 41.6 \\ \hline \end{array}$

$$\begin{array}{r} \underline{48} \\ 20 \\ \underline{12} \\ 80 \end{array}$$

$$\dfrac{\text{mL/hr} \times \text{TF}}{\text{min}} = \text{gtt/min} \qquad = 42 \text{ gtt/min}$$

Self Test 8 IV Problems

1. a. Add 18 mL sterile water for injection to the vial of 5 million units.

  b. Solution is 5 milliunits/20 mL. (milliunits = million units)

  c. You want 1 milliunit.

Formula Method	Proportion Expressed as Two Ratios	Proportion Expressed as Two Fractions
$\dfrac{1 \text{ milliunit}}{\cancel{5} \text{ milliunit}} \times \overset{4}{\cancel{20}} \text{ mL} = 4 \text{ mL}$	$20 \text{ mL} : 5 \text{ milliunits} :: x \text{ mL} : 1 \text{ milliunit}$	$\dfrac{20 \text{ mL}}{5 \text{ milliunits}} \times \dfrac{x}{1}$

$$\dfrac{20}{5} = 4 \text{ mL}$$

  d. $\dfrac{\text{mL} \times \text{TF}}{\text{min}} = \text{gtt/min} \qquad \dfrac{\overset{25}{\cancel{100}} \text{ mL} \times \overset{1}{\cancel{10}}}{\underset{1}{\cancel{40}}} = 25 \text{ gtt/min}$

2. 1000 mL is infusing at 100 mL/hr, so the IV will take

$$\dfrac{\overset{10}{\cancel{1000}}}{\underset{1}{\cancel{100}}} = 10 \text{ hours to complete.}$$

If it starts at 0800h, it should finish 10 hours later at 1800h.

3. a.

Formula Method	Proportion Expressed as Two Ratios	Proportion Expressed as Two Fractions
$\dfrac{\overset{3}{\cancel{60}} \text{ mg}}{\underset{2}{\cancel{40}} \text{ mg}} \times 1 \text{ mL}$ $\dfrac{3}{2} = 1.5 \text{ mL}$	$1 \text{ mL} : 40 \text{ mg} :: x \text{ mL} : 60 \text{ mg}$	$\dfrac{1 \text{ mL}}{40 \text{ mg}} \times \dfrac{x \text{ mL}}{60 \text{ mg}}$

$$\dfrac{60}{40} = x$$

$$1.5 \text{ mL} = x$$

Add 1.5 mL gentamicin.

  b. $\dfrac{\text{mL} \times \text{TF}}{\text{min}} = \text{gtt/min}$

$$\dfrac{50 \text{ mL} \times \overset{}{\cancel{20}}}{\cancel{30} \text{ min}} = \dfrac{\overset{100}{\cancel{100}}}{3} \, \overline{)100.00} \begin{array}{r} 33.3 \\ \hline \end{array} = 33 \text{ gtt/min}$$

4. 12 hours × 60 = 720 minutes

$$\frac{1500 \text{ mL} \times \overset{1}{\cancel{10}} \text{ gtt}}{\underset{72}{\cancel{720}} \text{ min}} = 72\overline{)1500.0}$$

$$\begin{array}{r} 20.8 \\ 72\overline{)1500.0} \\ \underline{194} \\ 60\ 0 \\ \underline{57\ 6} \end{array}$$

Set the rate at 21 gtt/min.

5. Intralipid 500 mL q6h means the patient is receiving 500 mL four times every 24 hours

$$\begin{array}{r} 500 \\ \times\ \ 4 \\ \hline 2000 \text{ mL} \end{array}$$

The IV is infusing 80 mL/hr. There are 24 hours in a day, so

$$\begin{array}{r} 24 \\ \times\ 80 \\ \hline 1920 \end{array}$$

Adding these we have $\begin{array}{r} 2000 \text{ mL} \\ +1920 \text{ mL} \\ \hline 3920 \text{ mL} \end{array}$

6. **a.** You have 1000 mL running at 60 mL/hr, therefore

$$\begin{array}{r} 16.6 \\ 60\overline{)1000.0} \\ \underline{60} \\ 400 \\ \underline{360} \\ 40\ 0 \end{array} = \text{approximtely } 16\ \tfrac{1}{2} \text{ hours}$$

b. If you want 60 mL/hr and use microdrip tubing, the drip factor will be 60 gtt/min:

$$\frac{1000 \text{ mL} \times \overset{1}{\cancel{60}} \text{ gtt}}{\underset{16}{\cancel{960}} \text{ minutes}} = 16\overline{)1000} = 63 \text{ gtt/min}$$

$$\begin{array}{r} 62.5 \\ 16\overline{)1000} \\ \underline{96} \\ 40 \\ \underline{32} \\ 80 \end{array}$$

If you use macrodrip tubing you have

16 hours × 60 min = 960 minutes.

$$\frac{1000 \text{ mL} \times \overset{1}{\cancel{10}} \text{ gtt}}{\underset{96}{\cancel{960}} \text{ minutes}} = 96\overline{)1000.0}$$

$$\begin{array}{r} 10.4 \\ 96\overline{)1000.0} \\ \underline{96} \\ 400 \end{array}$$

Because the IV will run over 16 hours, choose *microdrip tubing.*

c. The drip factor will be 60 gtt/min. *Note:* It is not incorrect to choose the macrodrip at 10 gtt/min. However, because the IV will run so many hours, a good flow might help to keep the IV running.

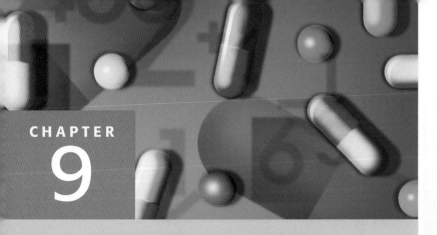

Special Types of Intravenous Calculations

LEARNING OBJECTIVES

1. Amount of drug in a solution

2. Rules and calculations for special IV orders

3. Units/hr, mg/hr, g/hr, mL/hr, mg/min, milliunits/min, mcg/min, mcg/kg/min

4. Use of the body surface nomogram

5. Calculating metres squared for IV medications

6. Special types of calculation: heparin, insulin

7. Patient-controlled analgesia

In Chapter 8, we studied calculations for microdrip and macrodrip factors, the use of the infusion pump, and IVPB orders. In this chapter, we consider calculations for orders written in units, milliunits, milligrams, and micrograms; special types of calculations in relation to continuous heparin infusion and continuous insulin infusion; methods of calculating the safety of doses based on kilograms of body weight and body surface area (BSA); and the handling of orders for patient-controlled analgesia (PCA).

This chapter's dosage calculations are for medications mixed in IV fluids and delivered as continuous infusions. Administering these medications via infusion pumps ensures a correct rate and accuracy of dose (Fig. 9-1). Many infusion pumps can deliver rates less than 1 (e.g., 0.5 mL/hr, 0.25 mL/hr), and they also can be programmed with the amount of drug, amount of solution, patient's weight, and time unit (minutes or hours). Once the pump is set at an infusion rate, the pump calculates how much drug the patient is receiving. The nurse, however, still bears the responsibility for double-checking the calculation and entering the correct information on the infusion pump.

Because many of the medications that infuse via continuous infusions are very potent, small changes in the infusion rate can greatly affect the body's physiologic response. In particular, vasopressor drugs such as dopamine, epinephrine, dobutamine, and Levophed can affect the patient's blood pressure and heart rate, even in small doses. In many hospital settings, the pharmacy prepares medications and IV solutions.

Amount of Drug in a Solution

These calculations can be complicated. One helpful technique is reduction: Start with the entire amount of drug mixed in solution, and then reduce it to the amount of the drug in only 1 mL of solution. Here's an example:

Heparin is mixed 25,000 units in 500 mL D5W.

How much heparin is in 1 mL of fluid?

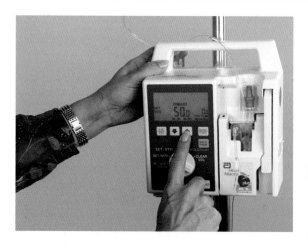

FIGURE 9-1

Infusion pump. (With permission from Evans-Smith, P. [2005]. *Taylor's clinical nursing skills.* Philadelphia: Lippincott Williams & Wilkins.)

Formula Method	Proportion Expressed as Two Ratios	Proportion Expressed as Two Fractions
$\dfrac{25000 \text{ units}}{500 \text{ mL}} \times 1 \text{ mL} = x$ 50 units	$25000 \text{ units} : 500 \text{ mL} :: x : 1 \text{ mL}$	$\dfrac{25000 \text{ units}}{500 \text{ mL}} \times \dfrac{x}{1 \text{ mL}}$ $25000 = 500x$ $\dfrac{25000}{500} = x$ $50 \text{ units} = x$

Here's a simple formula you can use to find concentration:

$$\frac{\text{Amount of Drug}}{\text{Amount of Fluid (mL)}} = \text{Amount of Drug in 1 mL}$$

Occasionally, the amount of medication to be added to an IV solution exceeds the capacity of the contained (bag/bottle) by approximately 10% or more (e.g., <10 mL in a 100-mL bag). If this occurs, an amount equal to the medication volume being added must first be removed using aseptic techniques (needle and syringe).

⬤▭ Medications Ordered in Units/hr or mg/hr

Sometimes patient medications are administered as continuous IVs. For these medications, solutions are standardized to decrease the possibility of error. Check the guidelines (institutional or drug references) to verify dose, dilution, and rate. If any doubts exist, consult with the prescribing physician or healthcare provider.

Units/hr–Rule and Calculation

The order will indicate the amount of drug to be added to the IV fluid and also the amount to administer.

Example   Order: heparin, infuse 800 units/hr

Available: heparin 40,000 units in 1000 mL D5W infusion pump

You know the solution and the amount to administer. Because you'll be using an infusion pump, the answer will be in mL/hr.

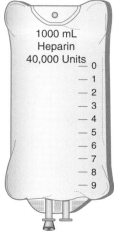

Formula Method	**Proportion Expressed as Two Ratios**	**Proportion Expressed as Two Fractions**
$\dfrac{\overset{20}{\cancel{800}\ \text{units/hr}}}{\underset{\underset{1}{40}}{\cancel{40,000}\ \text{units}}} \times \cancel{1000}\ \text{mL} =$	1000 mL : 40000 units : : x mL : 800 units	$\dfrac{\text{x mL}}{800\ \text{units}} \times \dfrac{1000\ \text{mL}}{40000\ \text{units}}$

20 mL/hr on a pump

Note that units cancel out and the answer is mL/hr.

$$40,000\text{x} = 800000$$

$$\frac{800000}{40000} = \text{x}$$

$$20\ \text{mL/hr} = \text{x}$$

How many hours will the IV run?

$$\frac{\text{Number mL}}{\text{Number mL/hr}}$$

$$\frac{1000\ \text{mL}}{20\ \text{mL/hr}} = 50\ \text{hours}$$

Note: Most hospitals require changing the IV fluids every 24 hours.

Example

Order: heparin sodium 1100 units/hr IV

Supply: infusion pump, standard solution of 25,000 units in 250 mL D5W

With an infusion pump, the answer will be in mL/hr.

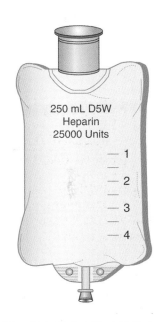

250 mL D5W
Heparin
25000 Units

— 1
— 2
— 3
— 4

Formula Method	**Proportion Expressed as Two Ratios**	**Proportion Expressed as Two Fractions**
$\dfrac{1100\ \text{units/hr}}{25,000\ \text{units}} \times 250\ \text{mL} =$	250 mL : 25000 units : : x mL : 1100 units	$\dfrac{\text{x mL}}{1100\ \text{units}} \times \dfrac{250\ \text{mL}}{25000\ \text{units}}$

$= 11\ \text{mL/hr}$

$$\frac{275000}{25000} = \text{x mL}$$

$$11\ \text{mL/hr} = \text{x}$$

How many hours will the IV run?

$$\frac{\text{Number mL}}{\text{Number mL/hr}}$$

$$\frac{250\ \text{mL}}{11\ \text{mL/hr}} = 22.75\ \text{or}\ 23\ \text{hours}$$

Example	Order: regular insulin 10 units/hr IV

Available: infusion pump, standard solution of 125 units regular insulin in 250 mL NS

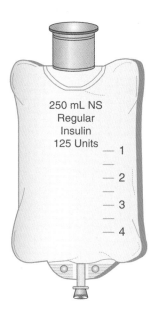

250 mL NS
Regular
Insulin
125 Units
— 1
— 2
— 3
— 4

Formula Method	Proportion Expressed as Two Ratios	Proportion Expressed as Two Fractions
$$\dfrac{10 \ \text{units}}{\underset{1}{125} \ \text{units}} \times \overset{2}{250} \ \text{mL}$$ $$= 20 \ \text{mL/hr on a pump}$$	$$250 \ \text{mL} : 125 \ \text{units} : : \ \text{x mL} : 10 \ \text{units}$$ $$\dfrac{2500}{125 \ \text{units}} = \text{x mL}$$ $$20 \ \text{mL/hr} = \text{x}$$	$$\dfrac{\text{x mL}}{10} \times \dfrac{2500}{125}$$

How many hours will the IV run?

$$\dfrac{\text{Number mL}}{\text{Number mL/hr}}$$

$$\dfrac{250 \ \text{mL}}{20 \ \text{mL/hr}} = 12.5 \text{ or approximately 13 hours}$$

mg/hr; g/hr—Rule and Calculation

The order will indicate the amount of drug added to the IV fluid and the amount to administer.

Example	Order: calcium gluconate 2 g in 100 mL D5W; run 0.25 g/hr IV via infusion pump.

Because we know the solution and the amount of drug per hour, we can solve the problem and administer the drug in mL/hr per infusion pump. Round the final answer to the nearest whole number.

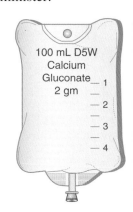

100 mL D5W
Calcium
Gluconate
2 gm — 1
— 2
— 3
— 4

Formula Method	Proportion Expressed as Two Ratios	Proportion Expressed as Two Fractions
$\dfrac{0.25\,\text{g/hr}}{\underset{1}{\cancel{2\,\text{g}}}} \times \overset{50}{\cancel{100}}\ \text{mL} = 12.5$ 13 mL/hr on a pump	100 mL : 2 g : : x mL : 0.25 g	$\dfrac{\text{x mL}}{0.25\ \text{g/hr}} \times \dfrac{100\ \text{mL}}{2\ \text{g}}$ $\dfrac{25}{2} = \text{x}$ 12.5 or 13 mL/hr = x

How many hours will the IV run?

$\dfrac{\text{Number mL}}{\text{Number mL/hr}}$

$\dfrac{100\ \text{mL}}{13\ \text{mL/hr}} = 7.6$ or approximately 8 hours

Example Order: aminophylline 250 mg in 250 mL D5W; run 65 mg/hr IV per infusion pump.

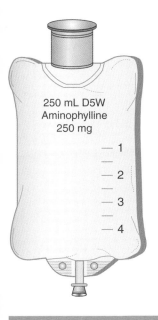

Formula Method	Proportion Expressed as Two Ratios	Proportion Expressed as Two Fractions
$\dfrac{65\ \text{mg/hr}}{\underset{1}{\cancel{250}\ \text{mg}}} \times \overset{1}{\cancel{250}}\ \text{mL}$ $= 65\ \text{mL/hr}$ on a pump	250 mL : 250 mg : : x mL : 65 mg	$\dfrac{\text{x mL}}{65\ \text{mg}} \times \dfrac{250\ \text{mL}}{250\ \text{mg}}$ $\dfrac{65 \times \cancel{250}}{\cancel{250}} = \text{x}$ 65 mL/hr = x

How many hours will the IV run?

$\dfrac{\text{Number mL}}{\text{Number mL/hr}}$

$\dfrac{250\ \text{mL}}{65\ \text{mL/hr}} = 3.8$ or approximately 4 hours

Solve the following problems. Answers appear at the end of this chapter.

1. Order: heparin sodium 800 units/hr IV
   Supply: infusion pump, standard solution of 25,000 units in 250 mL D5W

   a. What is the rate?
   b. How many hours will the IV run?

2. Order: Zovirax (acyclovir) 500 mg in 100 mL D5W IV over 1 hr
   Supply: pump, Zovirax (acyclovir) 500 mg in 100 mL
   What is the rate?

3. Order: Amicar (aminocaproic acid) 24 g in 1,000 mL D5W over 24 hr IV
   Supply: infusion pump, vials of Amicar (aminocaproic acid) labelled 5 g/20 mL
   What is the rate?

4. Order: Cardizem (diltiazem) 125 mg in 100 mL D5W at 10 mg/hr IV
   Supply: infusion pump, vial of Cardizem (diltiazem) labelled 5 mg/mL
   What is the rate?

5. Order: Lasix (furosemide) 100 mg in 100 mL D5W; infuse 4 mg/hr
   Supply: infusion pump, vial of Lasix (furosemide) labelled 10 mg/mL
   What is the rate?

6. Order: regular insulin 15 units/hr IV
   Supply: standard solution of 125 units in 250 mL NS, infusion pump

   a. What is the drip rate?
   b. How many hours will this IV run?

7. Order: nitroglycerin 50 mg in 250 mL D5W over 24 hr via pump
   What is the drip rate?

8. Order: heparin 1200 units/hr IV
   Supply: infusion pump, standard solution of 25,000 units in 500 mL D5W

   a. What is the rate?
   b. How many hours will the IV run?

9. Order: regular insulin 23 units/hr IV
   Supply: infusion pump, standard solution of 250 units in 250 mL NS

   a. What is the rate?
   b. How many hours will the IV run?

10. Order: Streptase (streptokinase) 100,000 international units/hr for 24 hr IV
    Supply: infusion pump, standard solution of 750,000 international units in 250 mL NS
    What is the rate?

mg/min—Rule and Calculation

The order will indicate the amount of drug added to IV fluid and also the amount of drug to administer. These medications are administered through an IV infusion pump in mL/hr.

Example   Order: Bretylol (bretylium) 1 mg/min IV

Supply: infusion pump, standard solution of 1 g in 500 mL D5W (1000 mg in 500 mL)

The order calls for 1 mg/min. You need mL/hr for the pump.

Convert the order to mg/hr, by multiplying the drug amount by 60 (60 minutes =1 hour). 1 mg/min × 60 = 60 mg/hr

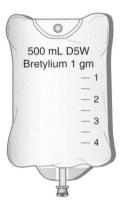

500 mL D5W
Bretylium 1 gm

Formula Method	Proportion Expressed as Two Ratios	Proportion Expressed as Two Fractions
$\dfrac{\overset{30}{\cancel{60 \text{ mg/hr}}}}{\underset{\underset{1}{2}}{\cancel{1000 \text{ mg}}}} \times \cancel{500} \text{ mL} = 30 \text{ mL/hr}$	500 mL : 1000 mg : : x mL : 60 mg	$\dfrac{x \text{ mL}}{60 \text{ mg}} \times \dfrac{500 \text{ mL}}{1000 \text{ mg}}$

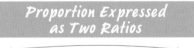

$$\frac{30000}{1000} = x$$

$$30 \text{ mL/hr} = x$$

Set pump at 30 mL/hr.

How many hours will the IV run?

$$\frac{\text{Number mL}}{\text{Number mL/hr}}$$

$$\frac{500 \text{mL}}{30 \text{mL/hr}} = 16.6 \text{ or approximately 17 hours}$$

Example   Order: lidocaine 2 mg/min IV

Supply: infusion pump, standard solution of 2 g in 500 mL D5W (2000 mg in 500 mL)

The order calls for 2 mg/min. We need mL/hr for the pump.

Multiply 2 mg/min × 60 = 120 mg/hr

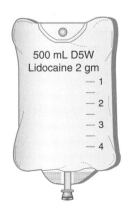

500 mL D5W
Lidocaine 2 gm

Formula Method	Proportion Expressed as Two Ratios	Proportion Expressed as Two Fractions

$$\frac{\overset{30}{\cancel{120 \text{ mg/hr}}}}{\underset{\underset{1}{4}}{\cancel{2000 \text{ mg}}}} \times \cancel{500} \text{ mL} = 30 \text{ mL/hr}$$

500 mL : 2000mg : : x mL : 120 mg

$$\frac{\text{x mL}}{120 \text{ mg}} \underset{\times}{\times} \frac{500 \text{ mL}}{2000 \text{ mg}}$$

$$\frac{6000}{2000} = x$$

$$30 \text{ mL/hr} = x$$

Set pump at 30 mL/hr.

How many hours will the IV run?

$$\frac{\text{Number mL}}{\text{Number mL/hr}}$$

$$\frac{500 \text{ mL}}{30 \text{mL/hr}} = 16.6 \text{ or approximately 17 hours}$$

SELF TEST 2 | **Infusion Rates for Drugs Ordered in mg/min**

Solve the following problems. Answers appear at the end of the chapter.

1. Order: lidocaine 1 mg/min IV
   Supply: 2 g in 250 mL D5W, infusion pump

   a. What is the drip rate?
   b. How many hours will the IV run?

2. Order: Pronestyl (procainamide) 3 mg/min IV
   Supply: Pronestyl (procainamide) 1 g in 250 D5W, infusion pump

   a. What is the drip rate?
   b. How many hours will the IV run?

3. Order: Bretylol (bretylium) 2 mg/min IV
   Supply: Bretylol (bretylium) 1 g in 500 mL D5W, infusion pump

   a. What is the drip rate?
   b. How many hours will the IV run?

4. Order: Cordarone (amiodarone) 1 mg/min for 6 hr
   Supply: Cordarone (amiodarone) 450 mg in 250 mL D5W, infusion pump
   What is the drip rate?

5. Order: Pronestyl (procainamide) 1 mg/min IV
   Supply: Pronestyl (procainamide) 2 g in 500 mL D5W, infusion pump

   a. What is the drip rate?
   b. How many hours will the IV run?

Medications Ordered in mcg/min, mcg/kg/min, or milliunits/min

Intensive care units administer powerful drugs in extremely small amounts called micrograms (1 mg = 1000 mcg). The orders for these drugs often use the patient's weight as a determinant, because these drugs are so potent.

Example	Order: renal dose dopamine 2 mcg/kg/min
	Order: titrate Levophed to maintain arterial mean pressure above 65 mm Hg and below 95 mm Hg

This section shows how to calculate doses in micrograms and in milliunits, and how to use kilograms in determining doses.

mcg/min—Rule and Calculation

Drugs ordered in mcg/min are standardized solutions that may be pre-packaged by the drug manufacturer. They are administered using infusion pumps that deliver medication in mL/hr.

To calculate drugs ordered in mcg/min, first determine how much of the drug is in 1 mL of solution (see beginning of this chapter). If the drug is supplied in mg, convert it to mcg; then divide that amount by 60 to get mcg/min. The final number tells you how much of the drug is in 1 mL of fluid. You can then use one of the three methods to solve for the infusion rate, on the basis of the ordered dosage.

Solving mcg/min requires four steps:

1. Reduce the numbers in the standard solution to mg/mL.

2. Change mg to mcg.

3. Divide by 60 to get mcg/min.

4. Use either the formula, the ratio, or the proportion method to solve for mL/hr.

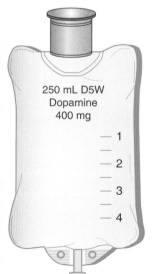

Example	Order: Intropin (dopamine) 400 mcg/min IV

Supply: Infusion pump, standard solution 400 mg in 250 mL D5W

Step 1. Reduce the numbers in the standard solution.

$$\frac{400 \text{ mg}}{250 \text{ mL}} = 1.6 \text{ mg in 1 mL}$$

Step 2. Change mg to mcg.

$$1.6 \text{ mg} \times 1000 = 1600 \text{ mcg/mL}$$

Step 3. Divide by 60 to get mcg/min.

$$\frac{1600 \text{ mcg}}{60 \text{ min}} = 26.67 \text{ mcg/min}$$

(round to hundredths)

Step 4. Solve for mL/hr (round to nearest whole number).

Formula Method	Proportion Expressed as Two Ratios	Proportion Expressed as Two Fractions
$\dfrac{400 \text{ mcg/min}}{26.67 \text{ mcg/min}} \times 1 \text{ mL}$ $= 15 \text{ mL/hr}$	$1 \text{ mL} : 26.67 \text{ mcg/min} :: x \text{ mL} : 400 \text{ mcg/min}$	$\dfrac{1 \text{ mL}}{26.67 \text{ mcg/min}} \times \dfrac{x \text{ mL}}{400 \text{ mcg/min}}$

$$400 = 26.67x$$
$$\frac{400}{26.67} = 15 \text{ mL/hr} = x$$

Set the pump: total number mL = 250; mL/hr = 15

Example   Order: Aramine (metaraminol) 60 mcg/min IV

Supply: infusion pump, standard solution 50 mg in 250 mL D5W

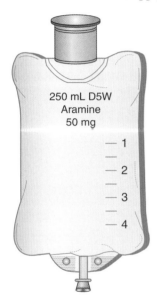

250 mL D5W
Aramine
50 mg

— 1
— 2
— 3
— 4

Step 1. Reduce the numbers in the standard solution.

$$\frac{50 \text{ mg}}{250 \text{ mL}} = 0.2 \text{ mg/mL}$$

Step 2. Change mg to mcg.

0.2 mg = 200 mcg/1 mL

Step 3. Divide by 60 to get mcg/min.

3.33 mcg/min

(Round to hundredths.)

Step 4. Solve. Round to the nearest whole number.

Formula Method	Proportion Expressed as Two Ratios	Proportion Expressed as Two Fractions
$\dfrac{60 \text{ mcg/min}}{3.33 \text{ mcg/min}} \times 1 \text{ mL} = 18 \text{ mL/hr}$	$1 \text{ mL} : 3.33 \text{ mcg/min} :: x \text{ mL} : 60 \text{ mcg/min}$	$\dfrac{1 \text{ mL}}{3.33 \text{ mcg/min}} \times \dfrac{x}{60 \text{ mcg/min}}$

$$60 = 3.33x$$
$$\frac{60}{3.33} = 18 \text{ mL/hr} = x$$

Set the pump: total number mL = 250; mL/hr = 18

mcg/kg/min—Rule and Calculation

Example Order: Intropin (dopamine) 2 mcg/kg/min

Supply: infusion pump, standard solution 200 mg in 250 mL D5W; client weighs 80 kg

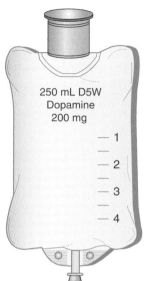

Note that this order is somewhat different. You are to give 2 mcg/kg body weight.

$$\begin{array}{r} 80 \text{ kg} \\ \times 2 \text{ mcg} \\ \hline 160 \text{ mcg} \end{array}$$ The order now is 160 mcg/min.

250 mL D5W
Dopamine
200 mg

— 1

— 2

— 3

— 4

1. Reduce the numbers in the standard solution.

   $$\frac{200 \text{ mg}}{250 \text{ mL}} = 0.8 \text{ mg/mL}$$

2. Change mg to mcg.

   $$0.8 = 800 \text{ mcg/mL}$$

3. Divide by 60 to get mcg/min.

   $$\frac{800}{60} = 13.33$$

   (Round to hundredths.)

4. Solve. Round to the nearest whole number.

Formula Method	Proportion Expressed as Two Ratios	Proportion Expressed as Two Fractions
$\frac{160 \text{ mcg/min}}{13.33 \text{ mcg/min}} \times 1 \text{ mL} = 12 \text{ mL}$	1 mL:13.33 mcg/min::x mL:160 mcg/min	$\frac{x \text{ mL}}{160 \text{ mcg/min}} \times \frac{1 \text{ mL}}{13.33 \text{ mcg/min}}$

$$160 = 13.33x$$

$$\frac{160}{13.33} = 12 \text{ mL} = x$$

Set the pump: total number mL = 250; mL/hr = 12 mL/hr

Milliunits/min—Rule and Calculation

In obstetrics, a Pitocin (oxytocin) drip can initiate labour. The standard solution of Pitocin is prepared by adding 10 units of oxytocin to 1000 mL of 0.9% sodium chloride. The initial dose should be 0.5 to 1 milliunits/min. At 30- to 60-minute intervals, the dose can be gradually increased in increments of 1 to 2 milliunits/min until the desired contraction pattern has been established. Always follow hospital or institutional policy. Because 1 unit = 1000 milliunits (mU), you solve these problems in the same way as mcg/min.

Example   Order: Pitocin (oxytocin) drip commence at 1 mU/min

Supply: infusion pump, standard solution 10 units Pitocin in 1000 mL NS

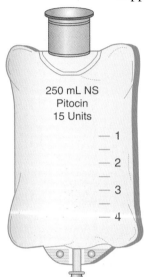

250 mL NS
Pitocin
15 Units

1. Reduce the number in the standard solution.

$$\frac{10 \text{ units}}{1000 \text{ mL}} = 0.01 \text{units/mL}$$

2. Change units of Pitocin to milliunits.

1 unit = 1000 milliunits

0.01 x 1000 = 10 milliunits/mL

3. Divide by 60 to get milliunits/min.

$$\frac{10}{60} = 0.167 \text{ milliunits/min}$$

4. Solve. Round to the nearest whole number.

Formula Method	Proportion Expressed as Two Ratios	Proportion Expresse as Two Fractions
$\frac{1 \text{ milliunits/min}}{0.167 \text{ milliunit/min}} \times 1 \text{ mL} = 2 \text{ mL/hr}$	1 mL : 0.167 milliunit/min : : x mL : 1 milliunit/min	$\frac{1 \text{ mL}}{0.167 \text{ milliunit}} \times \frac{?}{1 \text{ mi}}$

$$\frac{\text{mL} \times 1 \text{ milliunit/min}}{0.167 \text{ milliunit/min}} = x$$

$$\frac{1 \text{ mL}}{0.167} = 5.98 = x$$

Set pump at 6 mL/hr
(1 milliunit/min = 6 mL/hr)

Example   Order: Increase Pitocin q30-60 min by 1-milliunit/min increments until labour is established.

1 milliunit = 6 mL/hr; therefore, increase the IV rate 6 mL/hr q30min until labour is established.

Calculate the number of mL to infuse and the rate of infusion. Answers appear at the end of the chapter.

1. Order: Intropin (dopamine) double strength, 800 mcg/min IV
   Supply: standard solution 800 mg in 250 mL D5W, infusion pump

2. Order: Levophed (norepinephrine), 12 mcg/min IV
   Supply: standard solution of 4 mg in 250 mL D5W, infusion pump

3. Order: Dobutrex (dobutamine) 5 mcg/kg/min IV
   Supply: patient weight, 100 kg; standard solution of 1 g in 250 mL D5W, infusion pump

4. Order: Dobutrex (dobutamine) 7 mcg/kg/min IV
   Supply: patient weight, 70 kg; standard solution of 500 mg in 250 mL D5W, infusion pump

5. Order: nitroglycerin 10 mcg/min IV
   Supply: standard solution of 50 mg in 250 mL D5W, infusion pump

6. Order: Pitocin drip (oxytocin) 0.5 milliunit/min IV
   Supply: infusion pump, standard solution 10 units in 1000 mL NS

7. Order: Isuprel (isoproterenol) titrated at 4 mcg/min IV
   Supply: infusion pump, solution 2 mg in 250 mL D5W

8. Order: Brevibloc (esmolol) 50 mcg/kg/min IV
   Supply: infusion pump, 2.5 g in 250 mL D5W; weight, 58 kg

9. Order: Nipride (nitroprusside) 2 mcg/kg/min IV
   Supply: patient weight, 80 kg; nipride 50 mg in 250 mL D5W, infusion pump

10. Order: Inocor (amrinone) 200 mcg/min
    Supply: Inocor (amrinone) 0.1 g in 100 mL NS, infusion pump

Body Surface Nomogram

Antineoplastic drugs used in cancer chemotherapy have a narrow therapeutic range. Calculation of these drugs is based on BSA in square metres—a method considered more precise than mg/kg/body weight. BSA is the measured or calculated area of the body.

There are several mathematical formulas to calculate body surface area. One often used is:

$$\sqrt{\frac{weight\,(kg) \times height\,(cm)}{3600}} = \text{BSA}$$

Average BSA:

"Normal" BSA: 1.7 m^2

Average BSA for men: 1.9 m^2

Average BSA for women: 1.6 m^2

You can estimate BSA by using a three-column chart called a nomogram (Fig. 9-2). Mark the patient's height in the first column and the patient's weight in the third column. Then draw a line between these two marks. The point at which the line intersects the middle column indicates estimated body surface in metres squared. You'll use a different BSA chart for children, because of differences in growth (see Chapter 10).

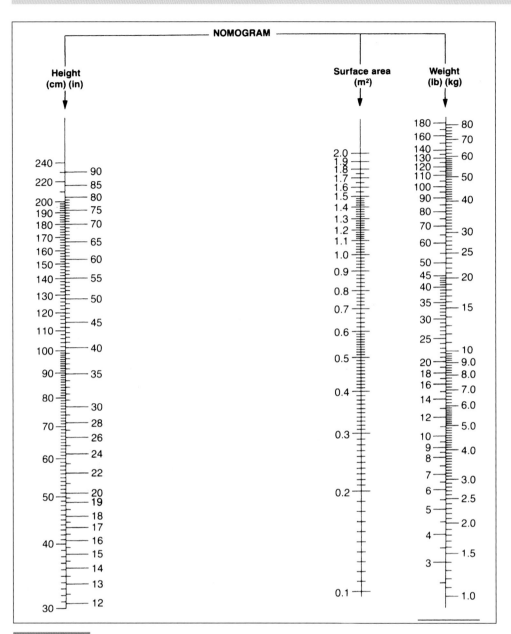

NOMOGRAM

FIGURE 9-2

Body surface area (BSA) is critical when calculating dosages for pediatric patients or for drugs that are extremely potent and need to be given in precise amounts. The nomogram shown here lets you plot the patient's height and weight to determine the BSA. Here's how it works:

1. Locate the patient's height in the left column of the nomogram and the weight in the right column.

2. Use a ruler to draw a straight line connecting the two points. The point where the line intersects the surface area column indicates the patient's BSA in square metres.

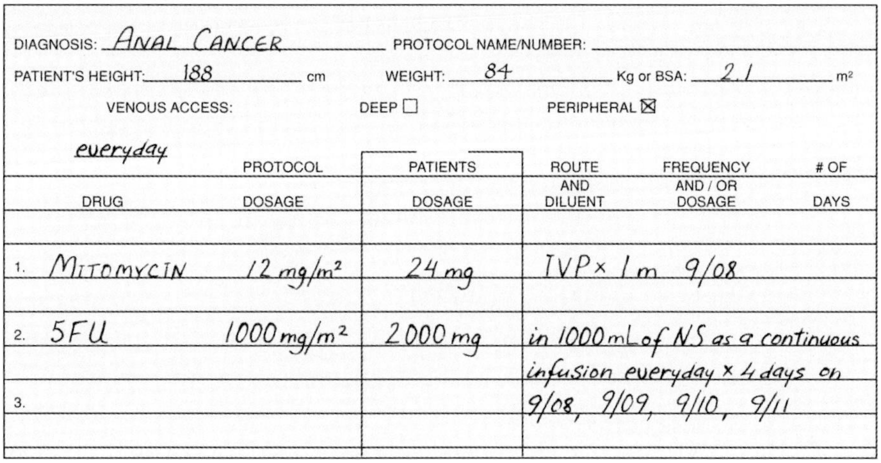

DIAGNOSIS: ANAL CANCER PROTOCOL NAME/NUMBER:

PATIENT'S HEIGHT: 188 cm WEIGHT: 84 Kg or BSA: 2.1 m²

VENOUS ACCESS: DEEP ☐ PERIPHERAL ☒

everyday

DRUG	PROTOCOL DOSAGE	PATIENTS DOSAGE	ROUTE AND DILUENT	FREQUENCY AND / OR DOSAGE	# OF DAYS
1. MITOMYCIN	12 mg/m²	24 mg	IVP × 1 m 9/08		
2. 5FU	1000 mg/m²	2000 mg	in 1000 mL of NS as a continuous infusion everyday × 4 days on 9/08, 9/09, 9/10, 9/11		
3.					

FIGURE 9-3

Portion of doctor's order form for chemotherapy. The doctor or healthcare provider writes the patient's height and weight and calculates the BSA as 2.1 m^2. The protocol dosage is the guide used to determine the patient's dose. For mitomycin, the protocol is 12 $mg/m^2 \times 2\ m^2 = 24$ mg. For 5FU, the protocol dose is 1000 $mg/m^2 \times 2\ m^2 = 2000$ mg.

The oncologist, a physician who specializes in treating cancer, lists the patient's height, weight, and BSA; gives the protocol (drug requirement based on BSA in m^2); and then gives the order.

Figure 9-3 shows a partial order sheet for chemotherapy. Both the pharmacist and the nurse validate the order before preparation.

To determine BSA in m^2, you can use a special calculator, obtained from companies manufacturing antineoplastics. Many websites also calculate BSA; see, for example, www.manuelsweb.com/bsa.htm www.users.med.cornell.edu/~spon/picu/calc/bsacalc.htm

m^2—Rule and Calculation

Oncology drugs are prepared by a pharmacist or specially trained technician who is gowned, gloved, and masked and works under a laminar flow hood; these precautions protect the pharmacist or technician and also ensure sterility. When the medication reaches the unit, the nurse bears two responsibilities: checking the doses for accuracy before administration and using an infusion pump for IV orders.

Example

H, 183 cm; W, 79 kg; BSA, 2.0 m^2

Order: Platinol (cisplatin) 160 mg (80 mg/m^2) IV in 1 L NS with 2 mg magnesium sulfate over 2 hr

1. Check the BSA using the nomogram in Figure 9-2. It is correct. Protocol calls for 80 mg/m^2; 160 mg is correct.
2. The IV is prepared by the pharmacy. Determine the rate of infusion.
   1 L = 1000 mL

$$\frac{\text{Number mL}}{\text{Number hr}} = \text{mL/hr} \qquad \frac{\overset{500}{\cancel{1000}}}{\underset{1}{\cancel{2}}} = 500\ \text{mL/hr}$$

Set the pump: total number mL, 1000; mL/hr, 500

Solve the following problems. Answers appear at the end of this chapter. Use the nomogram in Figure 9-2 to double-check the BSA.

1. H, 183 cm; W, 75 kg; BSA, 1.96 m^2
Order: Doxil (doxorubicin) 39 mg (20 mg/m^2) in D5W 250 mL to infuse over ½ hr

   a. Is dose correct?
   b. How should the pump be set?

2. H, 165 cm; W, 70 kg; BSA, 1.77 m^2
Order: Lomustine (CCNU) 230 mg po (130 mg/m^2) once q6wk

   a. Is dose correct?
   b. Lomustine (CCNU) comes in tabs of 100 mg and 10 mg. What is the dose?

3. H, 187 cm; W, 77 kg; BSA, 2.0 m^2
Order: Cerubidine (daunorubicin) 80 mg (40 mg/m^2) in D5W over 1 hr IV
Supply: IV bag labelled 80 mg in 80 mL D5W; infuse in rapidly flowing IV

   a. Is dose correct?
   b. How should the pump be set? (See IVPB administration in Chapter 8.)

4. H, 170 cm; W, 85 kg; BSA, 2.0 m^2
Order: Vepesid (etoposide) 400 mg po every day × 3 (200 mg/m^2)
Supply: capsules of 50 mg

   a. Is dose correct?
   b. How many capsules should be poured?

5. H, 160 cm; W, 54 kg; BSA, 1.6 m^2
Order: Taxol (paclitaxel) 216 mg (135 mg/m^2) in D5W ½ L glass bottle over 3 hr

   a. Is dose correct?
   b. How should the pump be set?

Patient-Controlled Analgesia (PCA)

PCA, an IV method of pain control, allows a patient to self-administer a preset dose of pain medication. The physician or healthcare provider prescribes the narcotic dose and concentration, the basal rate, the lockout time, and the total maximum hourly dose (Fig. 9-4).

Basal rate is the amount of medication that is infused continuously each hour. *PCA dose* is the amount of medication infused when the patient activates the button control. *Lockout time* or *delay*—a feature that prevents overdosage—is the interval during which the patient cannot initiate another dose after giving a self-dose. *Total hourly dose* is the maximum amount of medication the patient can receive in an hour. The physician or healthcare provider writes all this information on an order form.

Figure 9-5 shows a narcotic PCA medication record. Morphine concentration is 1 mg/mL. The pharmacy dispenses a 100-mL NS bag with 100 mL morphine. The patient continuously receives 0.5 mg by infusion pump and can give 1 mg by pressing the PCA button. Eight minutes must elapse before another PCA dose can be delivered. Note that at 1200h, the nurse charted that the patient made three attempts but received only two injections. This indicates that 8 minutes had not elapsed before one of the attempts.

The nurse's responsibility is to assess the patient every hour, noting how the patient scores his or her pain, the number of PCA attempts, and the total hourly dose received, as well as the cumulative dose, the patient's level of consciousness, side effects, and respirations.

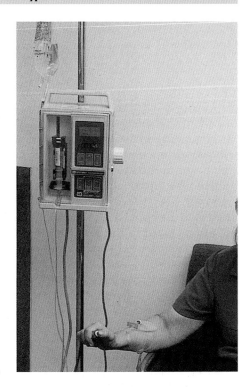

Patient-controlled analgesia allows the client to self-administer medication, as necessary, to control pain. (From Roach, S. S. [2004]. *Introductory clinical pharmacology* [7th ed.]. Philadelphia: Lippincott Williams & Wilkins, p. 173.)

AVERY MEDICAL CENTRE
Narcotic PCA
Medication Administration Record

Check appropriate order:

  X Morphine 1 mg/1 mL:50 mL
  ____ Fentanyl. Concentration:_____ Volume: _____
  ____ Demerol 10 mg/1 mL:50 mL
  ____ Other: _____ Concentration _____ Volume:_____

Dose: _*1*_ mg/mL
Lockout:_*8*_ min
1 hour limit: _*8*_ mg/mL
Basal *0.5* mg/hr

Infusion started by: _____ RN
       (zero out prior shift volume with each new bag/syringe)
Settings confirmed by: _____ RN
Date/Time discontinued: _____
Discontinued by: _____ RN
Total Amount Administered: _____
Waste returned to pharmacy: _____

Pharmacist: Witness: Witness:

Date	0600	0800	1000	1200	1400	1600
Number of attempts	3	2	2	3		
Number of injections	3	2	2	2		
Basal dose	0.5	0.5	0.5	0.5		
Total mL	3.5	4.5	4.5	2.5		
Cumulative mL	3.5	8	12.5	15		
Pain score	5	5	5	6		
Level of consciousness	1	1	1	1		
Respiratory rate (per minute)	16	20	16	22		
Nurse's initials	GP	GP	GP	GP		

Level of Consciousness: 1-alert, 2-drowsy, 3-sleeping, 4-confused, 5-difficult to arouse

Nurse's signature _____ Initial _____
Nurse's signature _____ Initial _____
Nurse's signature _____ Initial _____
Nurse's signature _____ Initial _____

Sample PCA medication record.

Heparin and Insulin Protocols

Many hospitals and other institutions now use protocols to give the nurse more autonomy in determining the rate and amount of drug the patient is receiving. These protocols are based on a parameter, usually a lab test ordered by healthcare provider. After receiving the lab test results, the nurse uses the protocol to determine the change (if any) in the dosage amount and when subsequent lab testing is to be done.

Two drugs used in protocols are heparin and insulin.

Heparin Protocol

Heparin, an anticoagulant, is titrated according to the results of the lab test, aPTT (activated partial thromboplastin time). Weight-based heparin protocol calculates the dose of heparin based on the patient's weight.

Sample heparin protocol:

Heparin drip: 25,000 units in 500 mL D5W

Bolus: 80 units/kg

Starting Dose: 18 units/kg/hr

Titrate according to the following chart:

aPTT (seconds)	<45 seconds	45-48 seconds	49-66 seconds	67-70 seconds	71-109 seconds	110-130 seconds	>130 seconds
Bolus	Bolus with 40 units/kg	Bolus with 40 units/kg	No bolus	No bolus	No bolus	No bolus	No bolus
Rate adjustment	Increase rate by 3 units/kg/hr	Increase rate by 2 units/kg/hr	Increase rate by 1 unit/kg/hr	No change	No change	Decrease rate by 1 unit/kg/hr	Stop infusion for 1 hour. Decrease rate by 2 units/kg/hr
Next lab	aPTT in 6 hours	aPTT in 6 hours	aPTT in 6 hours	aPTT next AM	aPTT next AM	aPTT in 6 hours	aPTT in 6 hours

Example

Example: patient weight is 70 kg.

1. Calculation for bolus dose: 80 units/kg.

   Multiply 80 units $\times$ 70 kg = 5600 units/kg

2. Infusion rate.

   First calculate what the dose will be

   Starting dose is 18 units/kg/hr

   Multiply 18 $\times$ 70 kg = 1260 units/kg

   Now use the calculation similar to that on p. 238

Formula Method	Proportion Expressed as Two Ratios	Proportion Expressed as Two Fractions
$\frac{1260 \text{ units}}{25{,}000 \text{ units}} \times 500 \text{ mL} = 25.2 \text{ mL/hr}$	500 mL : 25000 units : : x mL : 1260 units	$\frac{500 \text{ mL}}{25000 \text{ units}} \times \frac{x \text{ mL}}{1260 \text{ units}}$

$$\frac{500 \times 1260}{25000} = x$$

$$25.2 \text{ mL/hr} = x$$

Set the pump at 25 mL/hr.

3. The aPTT result 6 hours after the infusion started is 50. According to the table, increase the drip by 1 u/kg/hr.

   First, calculate the dose

   1 unit $\times$ 70 kg = 70 units/kg

   Then set up the same formula:

Formula Method	Proportion Expressed as Two Ratios	Proportion Expressed as Two Fractions
$\frac{70 \text{ units}}{25{,}000 \text{ units}} \times 500 \text{ mL} = 1.4 \text{ mL}$	500 mL : 25000 units : : x mL : 70 units	$\frac{500 \text{ mL}}{25000 \text{ units}} \times \frac{x \text{ mL}}{70 \text{ units}}$

$$500 \times 70 = 25000 x$$

$$\frac{35000}{25000} = x$$

$$1.4 \text{ mL} = x$$

4. Increase the infusion rate by 1.4 mL.

   25.2 + 1.4 = 26.6 mL/hr. Set the pumps at 27 mL/hr

   Recheck the aPTT in 6 hours and titrate according to the result

SELF TEST 5

Use the chart on page 248 to solve the following problems. Use heparin 25,000 units in 500 mL as your IV solution. The patient's weight is 70 kg. Beginning infusion rate for each problem is 25.2 mL/hr. Answers appear at the end of the chapter.

1. The patient's aPTT is 45 seconds.

   a. Is there a bolus dose? If so, what is the dose?
   b. Is there a change in the infusion rate? Calculate the new infusion rate.

2. The patient's aPTT is 40 seconds.

   a. Is there a bolus dose? If so, what is the dose?
   b. Is there a change in the infusion rate? Calculate the new infusion rate.

3. The patient's aPTT is 110 seconds.

   a. Is there a bolus dose? If so, what is the dose?
   b. Is there a change in the infusion rate? Calculate the new infusion rate.

4. The patient's aPTT is 140 seconds.

   a. Is there a bolus dose? If so, what is the dose?
   b. Is there a change in the infusion rate? Calculate the new infusion rate.

Insulin Infusion Protocol

Intended only for use in intensive care settings, insulin infusions are initiated on adult patients with hyperglycemia. The rate of the infusion is titrated according to blood glucose measured hourly using a glucometer. Considerations made prior to the initiation of the infusion include absence of any neurologic injury and enteral or parenteral nutrition. Additionally, insulin infusion is not used in patients experiencing diabetic emergencies, such as diabetic ketoacidosis (DKA) or hyperglycemic hyperosmolar states. Insulin infusion protocols always contain actions to be taken if hypoglycemia occurs. For example, some protocols indicate that physician must be notified and 1 ampoule of D50W given IVP if blood glucose is less than 4.0 mmol/L. Always follow hospital or institutional policy. This section provides a partial example of an insulin infusion protocol.

Critical Care Insulin Infusion Protocal

GOAL: Maintain serum glucose between 4.5–8.0 mmol/L

1. **Initiating an insulin infusion**

   Prepare an infusion of Humulin R insulin 50 units in 100 mL of 0.9% sodium chloride (concentration 0.5 units/mL). *NB – all doses are of Humulin R.*

Glucose Level	4.5–8.0 mmol/L	8.1–11.0 mmol/L	11.1–14.0 mmol/L	14.1–17.0 mmol/L	17.1–20.0 mmol/L	20 >mmol/L
Action	Monitor only	Start infusion 2 units/hr	2 units IVP Start infusion 2 units/hr	4 units IVP Start infusion 2 units/hr	8 units IVP Start infusion 2 units/hr	Call MD

2. Ongoing Infusion Titration

Check glucose q1h.

Glucose Level	Infusion rate 1–5 units/hr	Infusion rate 6–10 units/hr	Infusion rate 11–16 units/hr	Infusion rate > 16 units/hr
4.0–4.4 mmol/L	Discontinue infusion Recheck glucose in q30min x2 When glucose >6 restart infusion. Reduce rate by 1 unit/hr	Discontinue infusion Recheck glucose in q30min x3 When glucose >6 restart infusion. Reduce rate by 2 units/hr	Discontinue infusion Recheck glucose in q30min x4 When glucose >6 restart infusion. Reduce rate by 3 unit/hr	
4.5–8.0 mmol/L (Desired range)		Monitor and maintain glucose in desired range		
8.1–11.4 mmol/L	Increase infusion 1unit/hr	Increase infusion 2 units/hr	Increase infusion 3 units/hr	Call MD for new order
11.5–14.0 mmol/L	2 units IVP Increase infusion 1 unit/hr	2 units IVP Increase infusion 2 units/hr	2 units IVP Increase infusion 3 units/hr	
14.1–17.0 mmol/L	4 units IVP Increase infusion 1 unit/hr	4 units IVP Increase infusion 2 units/hr	4 units IVP Increase infusion 3 units/hr	
17.1–20.0 mmol/L	8 units IVP Increase infusion 1 unit/hr	8 units IVP Increase infusion 2 units/hr	8 units IVP Increase infusion 3 units/hr	
> 20.1 mmol/L		Call MD For New Order		

Example   1800h—Blood glucose is 12.2 mmol/L.

1. Initiation—give 2 units of Humulin R IVP.

2. Calculate the infusion rate to administer 2 units/hr.

Formula Method	Proportion Expressed as Two Ratios	Proportion Expressed as Two Fractions
$\dfrac{2 \text{ units/hr} \times 1 \text{ mL}}{0.5 \text{ units}}$	1 mL: 0.5 units :: x: 2 units/hr	$\dfrac{1 \text{ mL}}{0.5 \text{ units}} \times \dfrac{\text{x mL}}{2 \text{ units/hr}}$

$$1 \text{ mL} \times 2 \text{ units/hr} = 0.5 \text{ units } 1 \text{ mL x } 2 \text{ units/hr}$$
$$\frac{1 \text{ mL} \times 2 \text{ units}}{0.5 \text{ units/hr}} = 1 \text{ mL x } 2 \text{ units}$$
$$4 \text{ mL/hr} = x$$

3. Initiation—refer to "Initiating an Insulin Infusion Protocol"

Locate blood glucose at top of table. Follow instructions.

Set pump at 4 mL/hr. Recheck blood glucose in 1 hour.
1900h—Blood glucose is 8.4 mmol/L

4. Titrate IV infusion—refer to "Ongoing Infusion Titration"

Find current infusion rate at top of table. Locate current glucose level on left of table. Follow instructions.
Increase infusion 1 unit/hr. (2 units/hr + 1 unit/hr = 3 units/hr)
Calculate the new infusion rate.

Formula Method	Proportion Expressed as Two Ratios	Proportion Expressed as Two Fractions
$\dfrac{3 \text{ units/hr} \times 1 \text{ mL}}{0.5 \text{ units}}$	1 mL: 0.5 units :: x: 3 units/hr	$\dfrac{1 \text{ mL}}{0.5 \text{ units}} = \dfrac{x \text{ mL}}{3 \text{ units/hr}}$

$$1 \text{ mL} \times 3 \text{ units/hr} = 0.5 \text{ units} \ 1 \text{ mL} \times 2 \text{ units/hr}$$
$$\frac{1 \text{ mL} \times 3 \text{ units}}{0.5 \text{ units/hr}} = 1 \text{ mL} \times 2 \text{ units}$$
$$6 \text{ mL/hr} = x$$

Set IV pump at 6 mL/hr. Recheck blood glucose in 1 hour.

2000h—Blood glucose is 4.7 mmol/L

5. No change to infusion rate (6 mL/hr). Recheck blood glucose in 1 hour.

SELF TEST 6

Using Insulin Infusion Protocol above, complete the following calculations for your patient.

1. The insulin infusion is at 11 units/hr. Your patient's blood glucose is 11.4 mmol/L.

   a. Indicate action to be taken as per protocol.
   b. Calculate new infusion rate.

2. The insulin infusion is at 14 units/hr. Your patient's blood glucose is 4.3 mmol/L.

   Indicate action to be taken as per protocol.

3. Insulin infusion has been stopped for 60 minutes. Your patient's blood glucose is 6.3 mmol/L. The insulin infusion was at 14 units/hr.

   a. Indicate action to be taken as per protocol.
   b. Calculate new infusion rate.

Solve these problems. Answers are given at the end of the chapter.

1. Order: start Normadyne (labetalol) 0.5 mg/min on pump
   Supply: infusion pump, standard solution of 200 mg in 200 mL D5W
   What is the pump setting?

2. Order: aminophylline 250 mg in 250 mL D5W at 75 mg/hr IV
   Supply: infusion pump, vial of aminophylline labelled 250 mg/10 mL

   a. How much drug is needed?
   b. What is the pump setting?

3. Order: Bretylol (bretylium) 2 g in 500 mL D5W at 4 mg/min IV
   Supply: infusion pump, standard solution of 2 g in 500 mL D5W
   What is the pump setting?

4. Order: Zovirax (acyclovir) 400 mg in 100 mL D5W over 2 hr
   Supply: infusion pump, 500-mg vials of Zovirax (acyclovir) with 10 mL diluent; makes
               50 mg/mL

   a. How much drug is needed?
   b. What is the pump setting?

5. Order: Abbokinase (urokinase) 5,000 units/hr over 5 hr IV
   Supply: infusion pump, vials of 5,000 units
   Directions: Dissolve Abbokinase (urokinase) in 1 mL sterile water. Add to 250 mL D5W.

   a. How much drug is needed?
   b. What is the pump setting?

6. Order: magnesium sulfate 4 g in 100 mL D5W to infuse over 30 min IV
   Supply: infusion pump, 50% solution of magnesium sulfate

   a. How much drug is needed?
   b. What is the pump setting?

7. Order: nitroglycerin 80 mcg/min IV
   Supply: infusion pump, standard solution of 50 mg in 250 mL D5W
   What is the pump setting?

8. Order: Dobutrex (dobutamine) 6 mcg/kg/min IV
   Supply: infusion pump, solution 500 mg/250 mL D5W; weight, 82 kg
   What is the pump setting?

9. Order: Pitocin (oxytocin) 2 milliunits/min IV
   Supply: infusion pump, solution of 9 units in 150 mL NS
   a. What is the pump setting?

10. H, 152.4 cm; W, 50 kg; BSA, 1.45 m^2
    Order: Platinol (cisplatin) 116 mg (80 mg/m^2) in 1 L NS to infuse over 4 hr

    a. Is dose correct?
    b. How should the pump be set?

CRITICAL THINKING: TEST YOUR CLINICAL SAVVY

A 65-year-old patient with a 10-year history of congestive heart failure and type 1 diabetes is admitted to the ICU with chest pain of more than 24 hours. The patient is receiving heparin, insulin, calcium gluconate, and potassium chloride, all intravenously.

a. Why would an infusion pump be needed with these medications?

b. Why would medications that are based on body weight require the use of a pump? Why would medications based on BSA require an infusion pump?

c. Can any of these medications be regulated with standard roller clamp tubing? What would be the advantage? What would be the contraindication?

d. What other information would you need to calculate the drip rates of these medications?

e. Why would it be necessary to calculate how long each infusion will last?

Putting It Together

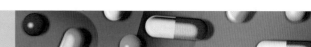

Mrs. R is a 79-year-old female with dyspnea without chest pain, fever, chills, or sweats. No evidence for bleeding. Admitted through the ER with BP 82/60, afebrile, sinus tachycardia at 110/min. She underwent emergency dialysis and developed worsening dyspnea and was transferred to the ICU. BP on admission to ICU was 70/30, tachypneic on 100% nonrebreather mask. No c/o chest discomfort or abdominal pain. Dyspnea worsened and patient became bradycardic and agonal respirations developed. A Code Blue was called and the patient was resuscitated after intubation. Spontaneous pulse and atrial fibrillation were noted.

Past Medical History: cardiomegaly, severe cardiomyopathy, chronic atrial fibrillation, unstable angina, hypertension, chronic kidney disease with hemodialysis, TIA in 3/07.

Allergies: calcium channel blockers

Current Vital Signs: pulse 150/min, blood pressure is 90/40, RR 18 via the ventilator. Afebrile. Weight: 90 kg

Medication Orders

Zosyn (piperacillin/tazobactam) *antibiotic* 0.75 G IV in 50 mL q8h
Protonix (pantoprazole) *antiulcer* 40 mg IV q12h. dilute in 10 mL NS and give slow IV push
Neo-Synephrine (phenylephrine) *vasopressor* drip 30 mg in 500 mL D5W
    100 mcg/min titrate for SBP > 90
Levophed (norepinephrine) *vasopressor* in 4 mg in 500 mL D5W
    Titrate SBP > 90 start at 0.5 mcg/min
½ NS 1000 mL at 150 mL/hr
Heparin (*anticoagulant*) 12 units/kg/hr. no loading dose. IV solution 25,000 units in 500 mL D5W
    Titrate to keep aPTT 49-70
Aspirin (*antiplatelet*) 81 mg po/N/G daily
Lanoxin (digoxin) *cardiac glycoside* 0.25 mg IV daily
Diprivan (propofol) *sedative* 10 mg/mL
    Titrate 5-50 mcg/kg/min for sedation

(continued)

Putting It Together

Calculations

1. Calculate how many mcg/mL of Neo-Synephrine.

2. Calculate the rate on the infusion pump of Neo-Synephrine 100 mcg/min.

3. Calculate how many mcg/mL of Levophed.

4. Calculate the rate on the infusion pump of Levophed 0.5 mcg/min.

5. Calculate the dose of heparin.

6. Calculate the rate on the infusion pump of the heparin dose. When is the next aPTT due?

7. Diprivan is mixed in 100 mL. How many mg are mixed to equal 10 mg/mL?

8. Calculate the rate on the infusion pump of Diprivan, using the range 5–50 mcg/kg/min.

Critical Thinking Questions

1. Do any of the patient's medical conditions warrant changes in the medication orders?

2. Why would two vasopressors be given together?

3. What is the reason for giving the patient Diprivan?

4. What medication may help atrial fibrillation yet be contraindicated in this patient?

5. What is a possible reason for the sinus tachycardia of 150/min?

6. What is the reason for giving a drug slow IV push, such as the Protonix?

Answers in Appendix B.

PROFICIENCY TEST 1   Special IV Calculations

Name: _____

Solve these problems. Answers are given in Appendix A.

1. Order: regular insulin 15 units/hr IV
   Supply: infusion pump, standard solution 125 units in 250 mL NS
   What is the pump setting?

2. Order: heparin sodium 1500 units/hr IV
   Supply: infusion pump, standard solution 25,000 units in 500 mL D5W IV
   What is the pump setting?

3. Order: Bretylol (bretylium) 2 g in 500 mL D5W at 2 mg/min IV
   Supply: infusion pump, standard solution of 2 g in 500 mL D5W
   What is the pump setting?

4. Order: Cardizem (diltiazem) 125 mg in 100 mL D5W at 5 mg/hr IV
   Supply: infusion pump, vial of Cardizem (diltiazem) labelled 5 mg/mL

   a. What is the pump setting?
   b. How much drug is needed?

5. Order: lidocaine 4 mg/min IV
   Supply: infusion pump, standard solution of 2 g in 500 mL D5W
   What is the pump setting?

6. Order: KCl 40 mEq/L at 10 mEq/hr IV
   Supply: infusion pump, vial of KCl labelled 20 mEq/10 mL in D5W 1000 mL

   a. How much KCl should be added?
   b. What is the pump setting?

7. Order: Pronestyl (procainamide) 1 mg/min IV
   Supply: infusion pump, standard solution of 2 g in 500 mL D5W
   What is the pump setting?

8. Order: Fungizone (amphotericin) B 50 mg in 500 mL D5W over 6 hr IV
   Supply: infusion pump, vial of 50 mg

   a. How should the drug be added to the IV?
   b. What is the pump setting?

9. Order: Pitressin (vasopressin) 18 units/hr IV, solution 200 units in 500 mL D5W
   Supply: infusion pump, vial of Pitressin (vasopressin) labelled 20 units/mL

   a. How much drug is needed?
   b. What is the pump setting?

10. Order: Dobutrex (dobutamine) 250 mcg/min IV
    Supply: infusion pump, solution of 500 mg in 500 mL D5W
    What is the pump setting?

11. Order: renal dose Intropin (dopamine) 2.5 mcg/kg/min
    Supply: infusion pump, solution 400 mg in 250 mL D5W; W, 60 kg
    What is the pump setting?

(continued)

12. Order: Pitocin (oxytocin) 2 milliunits/min IV
    Supply: infusion pump, solution of 5 units in 500 mL NS
    What is the pump setting?

13. H, 160 cm; W, 65 kg; BSA, 1.7 m^2
    Order: Ara-C 170 mg (100 mg/m^2) in 1 L D5W over 24 hr

    a. Is dose correct?
    b. How should the pump be set?

14. Order: Nipride (nitroprusside) 5 mcg/kg/min IV
    Supply: patient wgt = 90 kg; Nipride (nitroprusside) 50 mg in 250 mL D5W, infusion
                pump
    What is the pump setting?

15. Order: epinephrine 2 mcg/min
    Supply: epinephrine 4 mg in 250 mL D5W, infusion pump
    What is the pump setting?

16. Patient's aPTT is 45 seconds. Use the heparin protocol chart on page 248. Patient's weight is
    90 kg. Heparin 25,000 units in 500 mL. Rate is currently 32 mL/hr.

    a. Is there a bolus dose? If so, what is the dose?
    b. Is there a change in the infusion rate? Calculate the new infusion rate.

17. Patient's aPTT is 40 seconds. Use the heparin protocol chart on page 248. Patient's weight is
    90 kg. Heparin 25,000 units in 500 mL. Rate is currently 32 mL/hr.

    a. Is there a bolus dose? If so, what is the dose?
    b. Is there a change in the infusion rate? Calculate the new infusion rate.

18. Patient's aPTT is 110 seconds. Use the heparin protocol chart on page 248. Patient's weight is
    90 kg. Heparin 25,000 units in 500 mL. Rate is currently 32 mL/hr.

    a. Is there a bolus dose? If so, what is the dose?
    b. Is there a change in the infusion rate? Calculate the new infusion rate.

19. Use regular insulin 50 units in 100 mL NS. Use the insulin protocol on p. 251 for changes.

    Patient's blood glucose is 6.8 mmol/L. Repeat blood glucose in 1 hour is 7.1 mmol/L.

    a. What is the infusion rate?
    b. Is there a change in the rate? If so, what is the new rate?

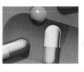

Answers to Self Tests

Self Test 1 Infusion Rates

Formula Method	Proportion Expressed as Two Ratios	Proportion Expressed as Two Fractions
1. $\dfrac{\overset{8}{\cancel{800} \text{ units/hr}}}{\underset{\underset{1}{\cancel{100}}}{\cancel{25,000} \text{ units}}} \times \overset{1}{\cancel{250}} \text{ mL}$ $= 8$ mL/hr on a pump	$250 \text{ mL} : 25000 \text{ units} :: \text{x mL} : 800 \text{ units}$	$\dfrac{\text{x mL}}{800 \text{ units}} \times \dfrac{250 \text{ mL}}{25000 \text{ units}}$

$$200000 = 25000x$$

$$\frac{200000}{25000} = x$$

$$8 \text{ mL/hr} = x$$

$\dfrac{\text{number mL}}{\text{number mL/hr}}$

$\dfrac{250 \text{ mL}}{8 \text{ mL/hr}}$ $\begin{array}{r} 31.2 \\ 8 \overline{)250.0} \\ \underline{24} \\ 10 \\ \underline{8} \\ 2.0 \end{array}$ approximately 31 hours; hospital policy states that IV bags be changed after 24 hours

2. Add 500 mg acyclovir to 100 mL D5W using a reconstitution device (see Chapter 8).

$\dfrac{\text{number mL}}{\text{number hr}} = \text{mL/hr}$

$\dfrac{100 \text{ mL}}{1 \text{ hr}}$ No math is necessary. Set the pump at 100 mL/hr.

3. **a.** Add amicar to IV.

Formula Method	Proportion Expressed as Two Ratios	Proportion Expressed as Two Fractions
$\dfrac{24 \text{ g}}{\cancel{5} \text{ g}} \times \overset{4}{\cancel{20}} \text{ mL} = 96 \text{ mL}$	$20 \text{ mL} : 5 \text{ g} :: \text{x mL} : 24 \text{ g}$	$\dfrac{\text{x mL}}{24 \text{ g}} \times \dfrac{20 \text{ mL (cc)}}{5 \text{ g}}$

$$24 \times 20 = 5x$$

$$\frac{480}{5} = x$$

$$96 \text{ mL} = x$$

(*Note:* Adding 96 mL to 1000 mL D5W = 1096 mL. This is too much fluid.)

Use five vials. Empty four completely.
Take 16 mL from the last vial.
20 mL × 4 vials = 80 mL + 16 mL = 96 mL
Remove 96 mL D5W from the IV bag before adding the amicar. This results in 1000 mL.

b. $\frac{\text{number mL}}{\text{number hr}} = \text{mL/hr}$

$$\frac{1000 \text{ mL}}{24 \text{ hr}} \quad \begin{array}{r} 41.6 \\ \overline{)1000.0} \\ \underline{96} \\ 40 \\ \underline{24} \\ 16.0 \\ \underline{14.4} \end{array}$$

Set pump at 42 mL/hr.

4. a. Add diltiazem to IV.

Formula Method	Proportion Expressed as Two Ratios	Proportion Expressed as Two Fractions
$\dfrac{\overset{25}{\cancel{125 \text{ mg}}}}{\cancel{5 \text{ mg}}} \times 1 \text{ mL} = 25 \text{ mL}$	1 mL : 5 mg : : x mL : 125 mg	$\dfrac{x \text{ mL}}{125 \text{ mg}} \times \dfrac{1 \text{ mL}}{5 \text{ mg}}$

$$\frac{125}{5} = x$$

$$25 \text{ mL} = x$$

(*Note:* Adding 25 mL to 100 mL D5W = 125 mL. This is too much fluid. Remove 25 mL D5W from the IV bag before adding the diltiazem. This results in 100 mL.)

b. Add 25 mL to IV bag.

Formula Method	Proportion Expressed as Two Ratios	Proportion Expressed as Two Fractions
$\dfrac{\overset{2}{\cancel{10 \text{ mg}}}}{\underset{1}{\cancel{\underset{5}{125 \text{ mg}}}}} \times \overset{4}{\cancel{100}} \text{ mL} = 8 \text{ mL/hr}$	100 mL : 125 mg : : x mL : 10 mg	$\dfrac{x \text{ mL}}{10 \text{ mg}} \times \dfrac{100 \text{ mL}}{125 \text{ mg}}$

$$\frac{1000}{125} = x$$

$$8 \text{ mL/hr} = x$$

5. a. Add furosemide to IV.

Formula Method	Proportion Expressed as Two Ratios	Proportion Expressed as Two Fractions
$\dfrac{\overset{10}{\cancel{100 \text{ mg}}}}{\underset{1}{\cancel{10 \text{ mg}}}} \times 1 \text{ mL} = 10 \text{ mL}$	1 mL : 10 mg : : x mL : 100 mg	$\dfrac{x \text{ mL}}{100 \text{ mg}} \times \dfrac{1 \text{ mL}}{10 \text{ mg}}$

$$100 = 10x$$

$$10 \text{ mL} = x$$

(*Note:* Adding 10 mL to 100 mL D5W = 110 mL. This is too much fluid. Remove 10 mL D5W from the IV bag before adding the furosemide. This results in 100 mL.)

Add 10 mL to the IV bag.

b. Because the solution is 100 mg/100 mL (1:1) and the order reads 4 mg/hr, the pump should be set at 4 mL/hr.

Formula Method	Proportion Expressed as Two Ratios	Proportion Expressed as Two Fractions
$\dfrac{4 \text{ mg/hr}}{\underset{1}{100 \text{ mg}}} \times \overset{1}{100} \text{ mL} = 4 \text{ mL/hr}$	$100 \text{ mL} : 100 \text{ mg} :: x \text{ mL} : 4 \text{ mg}$	$\dfrac{x \text{ mL}}{4 \text{ mg}} \times \dfrac{100 \text{ mL}}{100 \text{ mg}}$

$$400 = 100x$$
$$4 \text{ mL/hr} = x$$

6. a.

Formula Method	Proportion Expressed as Two Ratios	Proportion Expressed as Two Fractions
$\dfrac{15 \text{ units}}{125 \text{ units}} \times 250 \text{ mL}$ $0.12 \times 250 \text{ mL} = 30 \text{ mL/hr}$	$250 \text{ mL} : 125 :: x \text{ mL} : 15 \text{ units}$	$\dfrac{x \text{ mL}}{15 \text{ units}} \times \dfrac{250 \text{ mL}}{125}$

$$3750 = 125x$$
$$30 \text{ mL/hr} = x$$

b. The total volume of medication is 125 units and the client receives 15 units/hr.

$$\dfrac{125}{15} \quad 15 \overline{\smash{\big)}\,125.00}^{\,8.33} = \text{approximately 8 hours}$$
$$\underline{120}$$
$$5.0$$
$$\underline{4.5}$$
$$50$$

7. Nitroglycerin is prepared by the pharmacy as a standard solution of 50 mg in 250 mL/hr. We only need to calculate mL/hr.

Rule: $\dfrac{\text{number mL}}{\text{number hr}} = \text{mL/hr}$

$$\dfrac{250 \text{ mL}}{24 \text{ hr}} \quad 24 \overline{\smash{\big)}\,250.0}^{\,10.4}$$
$$\underline{24}$$
$$10\ 0$$
$$\underline{9\ 6}\qquad \text{Set pump at 10 mL/hr.}$$

8. a.

Formula Method	Proportion Expressed as Two Ratios	Proportion Expressed as Two Fractions
$\dfrac{1200 \text{ units}}{\underset{5}{25000 \text{ units}}} \times \overset{1}{500} \text{ mL} = 24 \text{ mL/hr}$	$500 \text{ mL} : 25{,}000 \text{ units} :: x \text{ mL} : 1200 \text{ units}$	$\dfrac{x \text{ mL}}{1200 \text{ units}} \times \dfrac{500 \text{ mL}}{25{,}000 \text{ units}}$

$$600000 = 25{,}000x$$
$$\dfrac{600000}{25000} = x$$
$$24 \text{ mL/hr} = x$$

b. Rule: $\frac{\text{number mL}}{\text{number mL/hr}}$

$\frac{500 \text{ mL}}{24 \text{ mL/hr}} = 20.8$ or approximately 21 hours

9. a.

Formula Method	Proportion Expressed as Two Ratios	Proportion Expressed as Two Fractions
$\frac{23 \text{ units/hr}}{250 \text{ units}} \times 250 \text{ mL} = 23 \text{ mL/hr}$	250 mL : 250 units : : x mL : 23 units	$\frac{x \text{ mL}}{23 \text{ units}} \times \frac{250 \text{ mL}}{250 \text{ units}}$

$23 \text{ mL/hr} = x$

b. Rule: $\frac{\text{number mL}}{\text{number mL/hr}}$

$\frac{250 \text{ mL}}{23 \text{ mL/hr}} = 10.8$ or approximately 11 hours

10.

Formula Method	Proportion Expressed as Two Ratios	Proportion Expressed as Two Fractions
$\frac{100\,000 \text{ units}}{750\,000 \text{ units}} \times 250 \text{ mL} = 33 \text{ mL/hr}$	250 mL : 750000 units : : x mL : 100000 units	$\frac{x \text{ mL}}{100000 \text{ units}} \times \frac{250 \text{ mL}}{750000 \text{ units}}$

$\frac{2500}{75} = x$

$33 \text{ mL/hr} = x$

Self Test 2 Infusion Rates for Drugs Ordered in mg/min

1. a. Order: 1 mg/min = 60 mg/hr (1 mg/min × 60 minutes)

Solution: 2 g in 250 mL

2 g = 2000 mg

Formula Method	Proportion Expressed as Two Ratios	Proportion Expressed as Two Fractions
$\frac{\overset{1}{60 \text{ mg/hr}}}{\underset{8}{2000 \text{ mg}}} \times 250 \text{ mL}$ $= 7.5 \text{ mL/hr or } 8 \text{ mL/hr}$	250 mL : 2000 mg : : x mL : 60 mg	$\frac{x \text{ mL}}{60 \text{ mg}} \times \frac{250 \text{ mL}}{2000 \text{ mg}}$

$75000 = 2000 \text{ x}$

$7.5 \text{ mL} = x$

Set pump at 8 mL/hr.

b. $\frac{\text{number mL}}{\text{number mL/hr}}$

$\frac{250 \text{ mL}}{8 \text{ mL/hr}} = 31.25$ or approximately 31 hours; hospital policy requires that IV bags be changed every 24 hours

2. a. Order: 3 mg/min = 180 mg/hr (3 mg/min × 60 minutes)

Solution: 1 g in 250 mL

1 g = 1000 mg

Formula Method	Proportion Expressed as Two Ratios	Proportion Expressed as Two Fractions
$\dfrac{180\,\text{mg/hr}}{\underset{4}{\cancel{1000}}\ \cancel{\text{mg}}} \times \cancel{250}\ \text{mL} = 45\ \text{mL/hr}$	250 mL : 1000 mg : : x mL : 180 mg	$\dfrac{x\ \text{mL}}{180\ \text{mg}} \times \dfrac{250\ \text{mL}}{1000\ \text{mg}}$

$$45000 = 1000\,x$$

$$45 = x$$

Set pump at 45 mL/hr.

$$\dfrac{1\ \text{mL}}{0.27} = \dfrac{x\ \text{mL}}{12\ \text{mcg/min}}$$

b. $\dfrac{12\ \text{mcg/min}}{0.27\ \text{mcg/min}} \times 1\ \text{mL} = 44\ \text{mL/hr}$

$\dfrac{\text{number mL}}{\text{number mL/hr}}$

1 mL : 0.27 mcg/min : : x mL : 12 mcg/min

$\dfrac{250\ \text{mL}}{45\ \text{mL/hr}} = 5.5$ or approximately 6 hours

$$12 = 0.27x$$

3. a. Order: 2 mg/min = 120 mg/hr (2 mg/min × 60 minutes)

$$\dfrac{12}{0.27} = x$$

Solution: 1 g in 500 mL

1 g = 1000 mg

$$44\ \text{mL/hr} = x$$

Formula Method	Proportion Expressed as Two Ratios	Proportion Expressed as Two Fractions
$\dfrac{120\,\text{mg/hr}}{\underset{2}{\cancel{1000}}\ \cancel{\text{mg}}} \times \overset{1}{\cancel{500}}\ \text{mL} = 60\ \text{mL/hr}$	500 mL : 1000 mg : : x mL : 120 mg	$\dfrac{x\ \text{mL}}{120\ \text{mg}} \times \dfrac{500\ \text{mL}}{1000\ \text{mg}}$

$$60000 = 1000\,x$$

$$60\ \text{mL/hr} = x$$

Set pump at 60 mL/hr.

b. $\dfrac{\text{number mL}}{\text{number mL/hr}}$

$\dfrac{500\ \text{mL}}{60\ \text{mL/hr}} = 8.3$ or approximately 8 hours

4. Order: 1 mg/min = 60 mg/hr (1 mg/min × 60 minutes)

Solution: 450 mg in 250 mL

Formula Method	Proportion Expressed as Two Ratios	Proportion Expressed as Two Fractions
$\dfrac{60\,\text{mg/hr}}{\underset{9}{\cancel{450}}\ \cancel{\text{mg}}} \times \overset{5}{\cancel{250}}\ \text{mL} = 33.33$ or 33 mL/hr	250 mL : 450 mg : : x mL : 60 mg	$\dfrac{x\ \text{mL}}{60\ \text{mg}} \times \dfrac{250\ \text{mL}}{450\ \text{mg}}$

$$1500 = 45x$$

$$\dfrac{1500}{45} = x$$

$$33.33 = x$$

Set the pump at 33 mL/hr. Run for 6 hours.

5. a. Order: 1 mg/min = 60 mg/hr (1 mg/min × 60 minutes)

Solution: 2 g in 500 mL

2 g = 2000 mg

Formula Method	Proportion Expressed as Two Ratios	Proportion Expressed as Two Fractions
$\dfrac{60 \text{ mg/hr}}{\underset{4}{2000 \text{ mg}}} \times \overset{1}{500} \text{ mL} =$ 15 mL/hr	500 mL : 2000 mg : : x mL : 60 mg	$\dfrac{\text{x mL}}{60 \text{ mg}} \times \dfrac{500 \text{ mL}}{2000 \text{ mg}}$ 30000 = 2000x 15 mL/hr = x

Set the pump at 15 mL/hr.

b. $\dfrac{\text{number mL}}{\text{number mL/hr}}$

$\dfrac{500 \text{ mL}}{15 \text{ mL/hr}}$ = 33.3 or approximately 33 hours; hospital policy requires that IV bags be changed every 24 hours

Self Test 3 Infusion Rates for Drugs Ordered in mcg/min, mcg/kg/min, milliunits/min

1. Order: 800 mcg/min

Standard solution: 800 mg in 250 mL D5W

Step 1. $\dfrac{800 \text{ mg}}{250 \text{ mL}}$ = 3.2 mg/mL

Step 2. 3.2 mg = 3200 mcg/mL

Step 3. $\dfrac{3200}{60}$ = 53.33 mcg/min

Step 4. Solve for mL/hr:

Formula Method	Proportion Expressed as Two Ratios	Proportion Expressed as Two Fractions
$\dfrac{800 \text{ mcg/min}}{53.33 \text{ mcg/min}} \times 1 \text{ mL}$ = 15 mL/hr	1 mL : 53.33 mcg/min : : x mL : 800 mcg/min	$\dfrac{1 \text{ mL}}{53.33} \times \dfrac{\text{x mL}}{800 \text{ mcg/min}}$ 800 = 53.33x $\dfrac{800}{53.33} = \text{x}$ 15 mL/hr = x

Set the pump: total number mL = 250 (standard solution); mL/hr = 15

2. Order: 12 mcg/min

Standard solution: 4 mg in 250 mL D5W

Step 1. $\frac{4 \text{ mg}}{250 \text{ mL}} = 0.016 \text{ mg/mL}$

Step 2. 0.016 mg = 16 mcg/mL

Step 3. $\frac{16 \text{ mcg}}{60 \text{ min}} = 0.27 \text{ mcg/min}$

Step 4. Solve for mL/hr:

Formula Method	*Proportion Expressed as Two Ratios*	*Proportion Expressed as Two Fractions*
$\frac{12 \text{ mcg/min}}{0.27 \text{ mcg/min}} \times 1 \text{ mL} = 44 \text{ mL/hr}$	1 mL : 0.27 mcg/min :: x mL : 12 mcg/min	$\frac{1 \text{ mL}}{0.27} \times \frac{x \text{ mL}}{12 \text{ mcg/min}}$

$$12 = 0.27x$$

$$\frac{12}{0.27} = x$$

Set the pump: total number mL = 250; mL/hr = 44   44 mL/hr = x

3. Order: 5 mcg/kg/min

Weight, 100 kg

Standard solution: 1 g in 250 mL

To obtain the order in mcg:

multiply 100 kg × 5 mcg/kg/min

100 kg
× 5 mcg/kg/min
500 mcg/min (order)

Step 1. 1 g = 1000 mg

$\frac{1000 \text{ mg}}{250 \text{ mL}} = 4 \text{ mg/mL}$

Step 2. 4 mg = 4000 mcg/mL

Step 3. $\frac{4000}{60} = 66.67 \text{ mcg/min}$

Step 4. Solve for mL/hr:

Formula Method	Proportion Expressed as Two Ratios	Proportion Expressed as Two Fractions
$\dfrac{500 \text{ mcg/min}}{66.67 \text{ mcg/min}} \times 1 \text{ mL} = 7.49$ or 8 mL/hr	$1 \text{ mL} : 66.67 \text{ mcg/min} :: x \text{ mL} : 500 \text{ mcg/min}$	$\dfrac{1 \text{ mL}}{66.67} \times \dfrac{x \text{ mL}}{500 \text{ mcg/min}}$

$$500 = 66.67x$$

$$\frac{500}{66.67} = x$$

$$7.5 \text{ or } 8 = x$$

Set the pump: total # mL = 250 (standard solution); mL/hr = 7.5 or 8 mL

4. Order: 7 mcg/kg/min

Standard solution: 500 mg in 250 mL D5W

Patient's wgt, 70 kg

The patient weighs $\dfrac{\begin{array}{r} 70 \text{ kg} \\ \times\, 7 \text{ mcg/kg/min} \end{array}}{490 \text{ mcg/min}}$

Step 1. $\dfrac{500 \text{ mg}}{250 \text{ mL}} = ? \text{ mg/mL}$

Step 2. $2 \times 1000 = 2000 \text{ mcg/mL}$

Step 3. $\dfrac{2000}{60} = 33.33 \text{ mcg/min}$

Step 4. Solve for mL/hr:

Formula Method	Proportion Expressed as Two Ratios	Proportion Expressed as Two Fractions
$\dfrac{490 \text{ mcg/min}}{33.33 \text{ mcg/mL/min}} \times 1 \text{ mL} = x$ $x = 14.7 \text{ or } 15 \text{ mL/hr}$	$1 \text{ mL} : 33.33 \text{ mcg/min} :: x \text{ mL} : 490 \text{ mcg/min}$	$\dfrac{1 \text{ mL}}{33.33} \times \dfrac{x \text{ mL}}{490 \text{ mcg/min}}$

$$490 = 33.33x$$

$$\frac{490}{33.33} = x$$

$$14.7 \text{ or } 15 \text{ mL/hr} = x$$

Set the pump: total number mL = 250 (standard solution); mL/hr = 15

5. Order: 10 mcg/min

Standard solution: 50 mg in 250 mL

Step 1. $\dfrac{50 \text{ mg}}{250 \text{ mL}} = 0.2 \text{ mg/mL}$

Step 2. $0.2 \times 1000 = 200 \text{ mcg/mL}$

Step 3. $\dfrac{200 \text{ mcg}}{60 \text{ mL}} = 3.33 \text{ mcg/min}$

Step 4. Solve for mL/hr:

Formula Method	Proportion Expressed as Two Ratios	Proportion Expressed as Two Fractions
$\dfrac{10 \text{ mcg/min}}{3.33 \text{ mcg/min}} \times 1 \text{ mL} = x$ $x = 3 \text{ mL/hr}$	1 mL : 3.33 mcg/min :: x mL : 10 mcg/min	$\dfrac{1 \text{ mL}}{3.33} \times \dfrac{x \text{ mL}}{10 \text{ mcg/min}}$ $10 = 3.33x$ $\dfrac{10}{3.33} = 3.33$

Set the pump: total number mL = 250; mL/hr = 3   3 mL/hr = x

6. Order: 0.5 milliunit/min

   Standard solution: 10 units in 1000 mL NS

   Step 1. $\dfrac{10 \text{ units}}{1000 \text{ mL}} = 0.01$ units/mL

   Step 2. 1 unit = 1000 milliunits

          0.01 units = 10 milliunits

   Step 3. $\dfrac{10}{60} = 0.167$ milliunit/min

   Step 4. Solve for mL/hr:

Formula Method	Proportion Expressed as Two Ratios	Proportion Expressed as Two Fractions
$\dfrac{0.5 \text{ milliunit/min}}{0.167 \text{ milliunit/min}} \times 1 \text{ mL}$	1 mL : 0.167 milliunit :: × 10.5 milliunit	$\dfrac{1 \text{ mL}}{0.167 \text{ milliunit/min}} = \dfrac{x}{0.5 \text{ milliunit/min}}$

Set pump at 3 mL/hr $\dfrac{0.5 \text{ mL}}{0.167} = 2.99 = x$

7. Order: 4 mcg/min

   Solution: 2 mg in 250 mL

   Step 1. $\dfrac{2 \text{ mg}}{250 \text{ mL}} = 0.008$ mg/mL

   Step 2. $0.008 \times 1000 = 8$ mcg/mL

   Step 3. $\dfrac{8 \text{ mcg}}{60 \text{ mL}} = 0.133$ mcg/min

   Step 4. Solve for mL/hr:

Formula Method	Proportion Expressed as Two Ratios	Proportion Expressed as Two Fractions
$\dfrac{4 \text{ mcg/min}}{0.133 \text{ mcg/min}} \times 1 \text{ mL} = x$ $x = 30 \text{ mL/hr}$	1 mL : 0.133 mcg/min :: x mL : 4 mcg/min	$\dfrac{1 \text{ mL}}{0.133} \times \dfrac{x \text{ mL}}{4 \text{ mcg/min}}$ $4 = 0.133x$ $\dfrac{4}{0.133} = x$

Set the pump: total number mL = 250; mL/hr = 30   30 mL = x

8. Order: 50 mcg/kg/min

Solution: 2.5 g in 250 mL

Weight: 58 kg

$$58 \text{ kg} \times 50 \text{ mcg} = 2900 \text{ mcg} \left(\text{order}\right)$$

Step 1. 2.5 g = 2500 mg

$$\frac{2500 \text{ mg}}{250 \text{ mL}} = 10 \text{ mg/mL}$$

Step 2. $10 \times 1{,}000 = 10{,}000$ mcg/mL

Step 3. $\frac{10000}{60} = 166.67$ mcg/min

Step 4. Solve for mL/hr:

Formula Method	Proportion Expressed as Two Ratios	Proportion Expressed as Two Fractions
$\frac{2900 \text{ mcg/min}}{166.67 \text{ mcg/min}} \times 1 \text{ mL} = 17 \text{ mL/hr}$	$1 \text{ mL} : 166.67 \text{ mcg/min} :: x \text{ mL} : 2900 \text{ mcg/min}$	$\frac{1 \text{ mL}}{166.67} \times \frac{x \text{ mL}}{2900 \text{ mcg/min}}$

$$2900 = 166.67x$$

Set the pump: total number mL = 250; mL/hr = 17

$$\frac{2900}{166.67} = x$$

$$17 \text{ mL} = x$$

9. Order: 2 mcg/kg/min

Solution: 50 mg in 250 mL

Weight: 80 kg

$$80 \text{ kg} \times 2 \text{ mcg} = 160 \text{ mcg}\left(\text{order}\right)$$

Step 1. $\frac{50 \text{ mg}}{250 \text{ mL}} = 0.2$ mg/mL

Step 2. 0.2 mg = 200 mcg

$$0.2 = 200 \text{ mcg/mL}$$

Step 3. $\frac{200 \text{ mg}}{60 \text{ mL}} = 3.33$ mcg/mL

Step 4. Solve for mL/hr:

Formula Method	Proportion Expressed as Two Ratios	Proportion Expressed as Two Fractions
$\frac{160 \text{ mcg/min}}{3.33 \text{ mcg/min}} \times 1 \text{ mL} = x$ $x = 48$	$1 \text{ mL} : 3.33 \text{ mcg/min} :: x \text{ mL} : 160 \text{ mcg/min}$	$\frac{1 \text{ mL}}{3.33} \times \frac{x \text{ mL}}{160 \text{ mcg/min}}$

$$160 = 3.33x$$

$$\frac{160}{3.33} = x$$

Set the pump: total number mL = 250; mL/hr = 48

$$48 = x$$

10. Order: 200 mcg/min

Solution: 0.1 g in 100 mL

100 mg in 100 mL

Step 1. $\frac{100 \text{ mg}}{100 \text{ mL}} = 1$ mg/mL

Step 2. 1 mg = 1000 mcg

1000 mcg/1 mL

Step 3. $\frac{1000 \text{ mg}}{60} = 16.67$ mcg/min

Step 4. Solve for mL/hr:

Formula Method	Proportion Expressed as Two Ratios	Proportion Expressed as Two Fractions
$\frac{200 \text{ mcg/min}}{16.67 \text{ mcg/min}} \times 1$ mL $= x$ $x = 11.99$ or 12 mL/hr	1 mL : 16.67 : : x mL : 200 mcg/min	$\frac{1 \text{ mL}}{16.67} \times \frac{x \text{ mL}}{200 \text{ mcg/min}}$ $200 = 16.67x$ $\frac{200}{16.67} = x$ $12 = x$

Set the pump: total number mL = 100; mL/hr = 12

Self Test 4 Use of Nomogram

1. a. Dose is correct; 20 mg/m^2 $\times$ 1.96 = 39 mg

   b. Order calls for 250 mL over ½ hour, but pump is set in mL/hr. Double 250 mL.

   Setting: total number mL = 250; mL/hr = 500.

   The pump will deliver 250 mL in ½ hour.

2. a. Correct; 130 mg/m^2 $\times$ 1.77 = 230 mg

   b. Pour two 100-mg tabs and three 10-mg tabs.

3. a. Correct; 40 mg/m^2 $\times$ 2 = 80 mg

   b. Rapidly flowing IV is the primary line. Set the secondary pump: total number mL, 80; mL/hr, 80 (see Chapter 8 for IVPB).

4. a. Correct; 200 mg/m^2 $\times$ 2 = 400 mg

Formula Method	Proportion Expressed as Two Ratios	Proportion Expressed as Two Fractions
$\frac{\overset{8}{400 \text{ mg}}}{50 \text{ mg}} \times 1$ capsule = 8 capsules	1 capsule : 50 mg : : x capsules : 400 mg	$\frac{x \text{ capsule}}{400 \text{ mg}} \times \frac{1 \text{ capsule}}{50 \text{ mg}}$ $400 = 50x$ 8 capsules $= x$

5. a. Correct; 135 mg/m^2 $\times$ 1.6 = 216 mg

   b. ½ L = 500 mL over 3 hr; $\frac{500}{3}$ $\frac{166.6}{\smash{\overline{)500}}} = 167$

   Set the pump: total number mL = 500; mL/hr = 167

Self Test 5

1. **a.** Bolus with 40 units/kg
   $40 \times 70 = 2800$ units

   b. increase rate by 2 units/kg per hour
   $2 \times 70 = 140$ units

Formula Method	Proportion Expressed as Two Ratios	Proportion Expressed as Two Fractions
$\frac{140 \text{ units}}{25000 \text{ units}} \times 500 \text{ mL} = x$ $x = 2.8$ mL	$500 \text{ mL} : 25000 \text{ units} :: x \text{ mL} : 140 \text{ units}$	$\frac{500 \text{ mL}}{25000 \text{ units}} \times \frac{x \text{ mL}}{140 \text{ units}}$

$$\frac{500 \times 140}{25000} = x$$

$$2.8 \text{ mL} = x$$

Increase rate by 2.8 mL

$25.2 + 2.8 = 28$ mL/hr

2. **a.** Bolus with 40 units/kg
   $40 \times 70 = 2800$ units

   b. Increase rate by 3 units/kg/hr
   $3 \times 70 = 210$ units

Formula Method	Proportion Expressed as Two Ratios	Proportion Expressed as Two Fractions
$\frac{210 \text{ units}}{25000 \text{ units}} \times 250 \text{ mL} = x$ $x = 4.2$ mL	$500 \text{ mL} : 25000 \text{ units} :: x \text{ mL} : 210 \text{ units}$	$\frac{500 \text{ mL}}{25000 \text{ units}} \times \frac{x \text{ mL}}{210 \text{ units}}$

$$\frac{500 \times 210}{25000} = x$$

$$4.2 \text{ mL} = x$$

Increase rate by 4.2 mL

$25.2 + 4.2 = 29.4$ mL/hr

3. **a.** No bolus

   b. Decrease rate by 1 unit/kg/hr
   $1 \times 70 = 70$ units

Formula Method	Proportion Expressed as Two Ratios	Proportion Expressed as Two Fractions
$\frac{70 \text{ units}}{25000 \text{ units}} \times 500 \text{ mL} = x$ $x = 1.4$ mL	$500 \text{ mL} : 25000 \text{ units} :: x \text{ mL} : 70 \text{ units}$	$\frac{500 \text{ mL}}{25000 \text{ units}} \times \frac{x \text{ mL}}{70 \text{ units}}$

$$\frac{70 \times 500}{25000} = x$$

$$1.4 \text{ mL} = x$$

Decrease drip by 1.4 mL

$25.2 - 1.4 = 23.8$ mL/hr

4. a. No bolus

b. Stop infusion for 1 hour
   Decrease rate by 2 units/kg/hr
   $2 \times 70 = 140$ units

Formula Method	Proportion Expressed as Two Ratios	Proportion Expressed as Two Fractions
$\frac{140 \text{ units}}{25000 \text{ units}} \times 500 \text{ mL} = x$ $x = 2.8$ mL	500 mL : 25000 units :: x mL : 140 units	$\frac{500 \text{ mL}}{25000 \text{ units}} \times \frac{x \text{ mL}}{140 \text{ units}}$

$$\frac{500 \times 140}{25000} = x$$

$$2.8 \text{ mL} = x$$

Decrease rate by 2.8 mL
$25.2 - 2.8 = 22.4$ mL/hr

Self Test 6 Answer

1. a. Increase infusion 3 units/hr.

   $11 \text{ units/hr} + 3 \text{ units/hr} = 14 \text{ units/hr}$

Formula Method	Proportion Expressed as Two Ratios	Proportion Expressed as Two Fractions
$\frac{14 \text{ units/hr}}{0.5 \text{ units}} \times 1 \text{ mL}$	1 mL : 0.5 units :: x 14 units/hr 1 mL $\times$ 14 units/hr $=$ 0.5 units x	$\frac{1 \text{ mL}}{0.5 \text{ units}} \times \frac{x \text{ mL}}{14 \text{ units/hr}}$

$$\frac{1 \text{ mL} \times 14 \text{ units}}{0.5 \text{ units/hr}} = x$$
$$28 \text{ mL/hr} = x$$

b. Set IV Pump at 28 mL/hr. Recheck blood glucose in 1 hour.

2. Discontinue (stop) infusion. Recheck glucose in q30min x 4.

3. a. Restart infusion. Reduce rate by 3 units/hr (14 units – 3 units = 11 units).

Formula Method	Proportion Expressed as Two Ratios	Proportion Expressed as Two Fractions
$\frac{11 \text{ units/hr}}{0.5 \text{ units}} \times 1 \text{ mL}$	1 mL : 0.5 units :: x 11 units/hr	$\frac{1 \text{ mL}}{10.5 \text{ units}} \times \frac{x \text{ mL}}{11 \text{ units/hr}}$

$$\frac{1 \text{ mL} \times 11 \text{ units}}{0.5 \text{ units/hr}} = x$$
$$22 \text{ mL/hr} = x$$

b. Set IV pump at 22 mL/hr. Recheck blood glucose in 30 minutes.

Self Test 7 Infusion Problems

1. A pump is needed. This is set in mL/hr. The order calls for 0.5 mg/min. Because there are 60 minutes in an hour, multiply 0.5 mg × 60 = 30 mg/hr. The standard solution is 200 mg in 200 mL. This is a 1:1 solution, so 30 mg/hr = 30 mL/hr. You can also solve using the three methods:

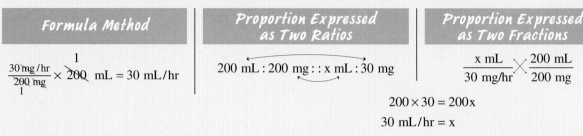

Formula Method	Proportion Expressed as Two Ratios	Proportion Expressed as Two Fractions
$\dfrac{\overset{1}{\cancel{30\,\text{mg/hr}}}}{\underset{1}{\cancel{200\,\text{mg}}}} \times \overset{1}{\cancel{200}}\ \text{mL} = 30\ \text{mL/hr}$	$200\ \text{mL} : 200\ \text{mg} :: x\ \text{mL} : 30\ \text{mg}$	$\dfrac{x\ \text{mL}}{30\ \text{mg/hr}} \times \dfrac{200\ \text{mL}}{200\ \text{mg}}$

$$200 \times 30 = 200x$$
$$30\ \text{mL/hr} = x$$

Total number mL = 200; mL/hr = 30

2. Aminophylline comes 250 mg/10 mL. Remove 10 mL from the IV bag and add 10 mL drug. Order is 75 mg/hr. You have 250 mg in 250 mL (a 1:1 solution); therefore, set the pump at 75 mL/hr. You can also solve using the three methods:

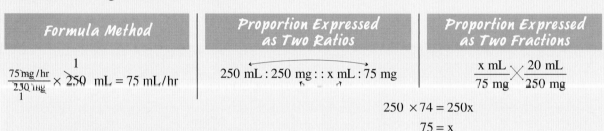

Formula Method	Proportion Expressed as Two Ratios	Proportion Expressed as Two Fractions
$\dfrac{\overset{1}{\cancel{75\,\text{mg/hr}}}}{\underset{1}{\cancel{250\,\text{mg}}}} \times \cancel{250}\ \text{mL} = 75\ \text{mL/hr}$	$250\ \text{mL} : 250\ \text{mg} :: x\ \text{mL} : 75\ \text{mg}$	$\dfrac{x\ \text{mL}}{75\ \text{mg}} \times \dfrac{20\ \text{mL}}{250\ \text{mg}}$

$$250 \times 74 = 250x$$
$$75 = x$$

Total number mL = 250; mL/hr = 75

3. 2 g = 2000 mg

A pump is needed and is set in mL/hr. Order calls for 4 mg/min. There are 60 minutes in an hour: 60 × 4 = 240 mg/hr

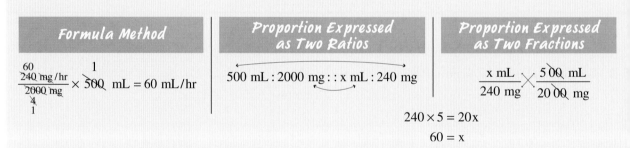

Formula Method	Proportion Expressed as Two Ratios	Proportion Expressed as Two Fractions
$\dfrac{\overset{60}{\cancel{240\,\text{mg/hr}}}}{\underset{\underset{1}{4}}{\cancel{2000\,\text{mg}}}} \times \overset{1}{\cancel{500}}\ \text{mL} = 60\ \text{mL/hr}$	$500\ \text{mL} : 2000\ \text{mg} :: x\ \text{mL} : 240\ \text{mg}$	$\dfrac{x\ \text{mL}}{240\ \text{mg}} \times \dfrac{500\ \text{mL}}{2000\ \text{mg}}$

$$240 \times 5 = 20x$$
$$60 = x$$

Total number mL = 500; mL/hr = 60

4. Add acyclovir. Calculate the amount:

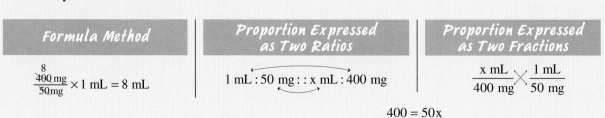

Formula Method	Proportion Expressed as Two Ratios	Proportion Expressed as Two Fractions
$\dfrac{\overset{8}{\cancel{400\,\text{mg}}}}{\cancel{50\,\text{mg}}} \times 1\ \text{mL} = 8\ \text{mL}$	$1\ \text{mL} : 50\ \text{mg} :: x\ \text{mL} : 400\ \text{mg}$	$\dfrac{x\ \text{mL}}{400\ \text{mg}} \times \dfrac{1\ \text{mL}}{50\ \text{mg}}$

$$400 = 50x$$
$$8 = x$$

Remove 8 mL fluid from the IV bag and add 8 mL of drug. 8 mL × 50 mg/mL = 400 mg. This is now 400 mg/100 mL.

$$\frac{\text{number mL}}{\text{number hr}} = \text{mL/hr}$$

$$\frac{\overset{50}{\cancel{100}}\text{ mL}}{\underset{1}{\cancel{2}}\text{ hr}} = 50 \text{ mL/hr on a pump}$$

Total number mL = 100; mL/hr = 50

5. 5000 units/hr × 5 hr = 25,000 units in 250 mL D5W. Need five vials. Dissolve each with 1 mL sterile water. 5 vials = 25,000 units in 5 mL. Add to 250 mL D5W.

   Calculate the mL/hr:

Formula Method	Proportion Expressed as Two Ratios	Proportion Expressed as Two Fractions
$\dfrac{\overset{}{\cancel{5000}\text{ units/hr}}}{\underset{1}{\underset{100}{\cancel{25,000}\text{ units}}}} \times \cancel{250}\text{ mL}$ = 50 mL/hr on a pump	250 mL : 25000 units : : x mL : 5000 units	$\dfrac{x\text{ mL}}{5000\text{ units}} \times \dfrac{\overset{1}{\cancel{250}}\text{ mL}}{\underset{100}{\cancel{25,000}}\text{ units}}$ $5000 = 100x$ $50\text{ mL/hr} = x$

Total number mL = 250; mL/hr = 50

6. Logic: magnesium sulfate comes in a 50% solution; 50 g in 100 mL = 0.5 g in 1 mL

   Calculate the mL/hr:

Formula Method	Proportion Expressed as Two Ratios	Proportion Expressed as Two Fractions
$\dfrac{4\text{ g}}{0.5\text{ g}} \times 1\text{ mL} =$ $x = 8\text{ mL}$	1 mL : 0.5 g : : x mL : 4 g	$\dfrac{x\text{ mL}}{4\text{ g}} = \dfrac{1\text{ mL}}{0.5\text{ g}}$ $4\text{ g} = 0.5x$ $8\text{ mL} = x$

Add 8 mL MgSO$_4$ to 100 mL D5W. Infuse over 30 minutes. The pump is set in mL/hr (60 minutes).

$$\frac{60\text{ minutes}}{30\text{ minutes}} = 2$$

Multiply 100 mL × 2 = 200 mL/hr

Total number mL = 100 mL

7. Order: 80 mcg/min

   Supply: 50 mg in 250 mL

   Step 1. $\dfrac{50\text{ mg}}{250\text{ mL}} = 0.2$ mg/mL

   Step 2. $0.2 \times 1000 = 200$ mcg/mL

   Step 3. $\dfrac{200}{60} = 3.33$ mcg/min

Step 4. Solve for mL/hr:

Formula Method	Proportion Expressed as Two Ratios	Proportion Expressed as Two Fractions
$\dfrac{80 \text{ mcg/min}}{3.33 \text{ mcg/min}} \times 1 \text{ mL} = x = 24$	1 mL : 3.33 mcg/min : : x mL : 80 mcg/min	$\dfrac{1 \text{ mL}}{3.33} \times \dfrac{x \text{ mL}}{80 \text{ mcg/min}}$

$$80 = 3.33x$$

$$\frac{80}{3.33} = x$$

$$24 = x$$

Set pump: total number mL = 250; mL/hr = 24

8. Order: 6 mcg/kg/min

   Solution: 500 mg/250 mL

   wgt: 82 kg

   a. 6 mcg/kg × 82 kg = 492 mcg

   Step 1. $\dfrac{500 \text{ mg}}{250 \text{ mL}} = 2 \text{ mg/mL}$

   Step 2. $2 \times 1000 = 2000 \text{ mcg/mL}$

   Step 3. $\dfrac{2000}{60} = 33.33 \text{ mcg/min}$

   Step 4. Solve for mL/hr:

Formula Method	Proportion Expressed as Two Ratios	Proportion Expressed as Two Fractions
$\dfrac{492 \text{ mcg/min}}{33.33 \text{ mcg/min}} \times 1 \text{ mL} = 14.7 \text{ or } 15$ 15 mL/hr	1 mL : 492 mcg/min : : x mL : 33.33 mcg/min	$\dfrac{1 \text{ mL}}{33.33} \times \dfrac{x \text{ mL}}{492 \text{ mcg/min}}$

$$492 = 33.33x$$

$$\frac{492}{33.33} = x$$

14.7 or 15 mL/hr = x

Set pump: total number mL = 250; mL/hr = 15

9. Order: 2 milliunits/min

   Supply: 9 units in 150 mL NS

   Step 1. $\dfrac{9 \text{ units}}{150 \text{ mL}} = 0.06 \text{ units/mL}$

Step 2. 1 unit = 1000 milliunits
         $0.06 \times 1000 = 60$ milliunits/mL

Step 3. $\frac{60}{60} = 1$ milliunit/mL

Step 4. Solve for mL/hr:

Formula Method	Proportion Expressed as Two Ratios	Proportion Expressed as Two Fractions
$\dfrac{2 \text{ milliunits/min}}{1 \text{ milliunit/min}} \times 1 \text{ mL}$	1 mL : 1 milliunit : : x mL : 2 milliunits	$\dfrac{1 \text{ mL}}{1 \text{ milliunit}} \times \dfrac{\text{x mL}}{2 \text{ milliunits}}$

$$2 = x$$

Set pump: total number mL = 150 mL; mL/hr = 2

10. a. Correct; $1.45 \text{ m}^2 \times 80 \text{ mg/m}^2$

b. 1 L = 1000 mL

$$\frac{\text{number mL}}{\text{number hr}} = \frac{\overset{250}{\cancel{1000} \text{ mL}}}{\underset{1}{\cancel{4} \text{ hr}}} = 250 \text{ mL/hr}$$

Set the pump: total number mL = 1000; mL/hr = 250

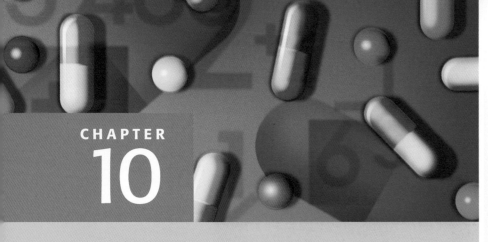

LEARNING OBJECTIVES

1. Dosage based on mg/kg body weight; body surface area

2. Determining a safe dose

3. mg/kg body weight calculations

4. BSA calculations

5. Calculating oral and parenteral doses

CHAPTER

10

Dosage Problems for Infants and Children

In previous chapters, we discussed calculations for adult medications administered orally and parenterally. This chapter considers dosage for infants and children. Wide variations in age, weight, growth, and development within this group require special care in computation. Because pediatric doses are lower than adult doses and are narrower in dosage range, a slight error can result in serious harm.

All infants and children should be weighed (grams or kilograms) prior to dosage calculations. In addition, the child's age should be entered into the pharmacy computer system to activate alerts if dosage is unsafe.

Before preparing and administering a pediatric medication, the nurse determines that the dose is safe for the child. Safe means that the amount ordered is neither an overdose (which can produce toxic effects) nor an underdose (which may lead to therapeutic failure). If you notice a discrepancy in the dose, consult the physician or healthcare provider who ordered the drug.

Children's medications are usually given either by mouth in a liquid form or IV. This chapter also includes subcutaneous and IM injections, which are used primarily for immunizations. Pediatric injections are calculated to the nearest hundredth and are often administered using a 1-mL precision (formerly called tuberculin) syringe. For pediatric IV therapy, microdrip, Buretrols, other volume control sets or infusion pumps are used. In the pediatric setting, you often find infusion pumps that can be set in tenths or hundredths. Most institutions have guidelines for pediatric infusions; if no guidelines are available, consult a reliable pediatric reference. Adult guidelines are not safe for children.

Chapter 13 gives a brief overview of pediatric medication administration. For more information related to this topic, such as needle size and injection sites, check pediatric nursing textbooks. Always follow institutional policy. Administering liquid medication to an infant or toddler often requires gently holding the child and using a syringe or dropper (Fig. 10-1A). School-age children often need to be involved in decision-making when administering medication (Fig. 10-1B).

Because pediatric doses must be accurate, it's advisable to use a calculator. The nurse still bears the responsibility, however, of knowing what numbers to enter into the calculator so as to calculate the correct amount. Oftentimes a pediatric medication that requires a calculated dose is prepared and double-checked by pharmacy staff; however, if nurses must prepare pediatric doses that require dosage calculations, it is recommended that calculations and doses be double-checked by a second RN to ensure the same answer is obtained.

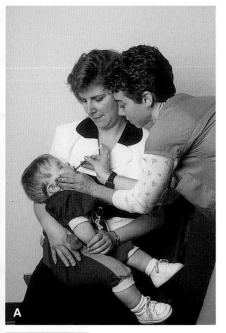
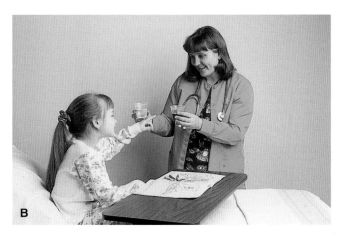

FIGURE 10-1

(A) Administration of liquid medication to infants and toddlers requires gently holding the child and administering with a syringe or dropper. **(B)** Administration of liquid medication to school-age children involves giving them choices, for example, what type of liquid to mix with a medication that is distasteful. (Used with permission from Pillitteri, A. [2007]. *Maternal and child health nursing* [5th ed.]. Philadelphia: Lippincott Williams & Wilkins, pp. 1145 and 1080.)

Dosage Based on mg/kg and Body Surface Area

The dose of most pediatric drugs is based on mg/kg body weight or BSA in metres squared. This section shows you how to use a nomogram to calculate BSA, how to estimate the safety of a dose, and finally, how to determine the dose. To ensure accuracy, use a calculator. All infants and children should be weighed prior to dosage calculation.

To convert grams (g) to kilograms (kg), divide weight in grams by 1000.
e.g., 4900 g ÷ 1000 = 4.9 kg.

Steps and Rule—mg/kg Body Weight

Example   Pediazole (erythromycin and sulfisoxazole) 2.5 mL po q6h is ordered for a child weighing 8 kg. Figure 10-2 shows the label for Pediazole (erythromycin and sulfisoxazole), which comes a dry powder. The usual dose information on the label states calculation of the safe dose is based on *either* the erythromycin component (50 mg/kg/day) *OR* the sulfisoxazole component (150 mg/kg/day to a maximum of 6 g/day) given in three or four equally divided doses for 10 days.

We need to calculate the low and high safe doses of one of the components (both will be shown), determine whether the dose ordered is safe, and prepare the dose. These are the steps:

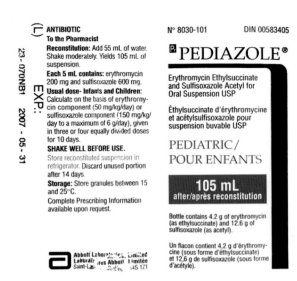

FIGURE 10-2

Label for Pediazole. (Used with permission of Abbott Laboratories.)

STEP 1.	Determine the safe dose range in milligrams per kilograms. Using a reference, determine the safe dose range in milligrams per kilograms.
STEP 2.	Determine whether the ordered dose is safe by comparing the order with the safe dose range listed in the reference.
STEP 3.	Calculate the dose needed.

Step 1a. Determine the safe dose range. The bottle shows that the safe dose of erythromycin is 50 mg/kg/day in three or four equally divided doses.

50 mg/kg/day

$\times$ 8 kg

400 mg/day in three or four divided doses

400/4 = 100   400/3 = 133.33

So the safe dose of erythromycin would be 100 mg q6h or 133 mg q8h.

Step 1b. Determine the safe dose range. The bottle shows that the safe dose of sulfisoxazole is 150 mg/kg/day (to a maximum of 6 g/day) in three or four equally divided doses.

150 mg/kg/day

x 8 kg

1200 mg/day in three or four divided doses (below 6000 mg maximum per day)

1200/4 = 300   1200/3 = 400

So the safe dose of sulfisoxazole would be 300 mg q6h or 400 mg q8h.

Step 2. Is the dose safe? The bottle labels states that each 5 mL contains erythromycin 200 mg and sulfisoxazole 600 mg. Calculate the amount of drug in the prescribed 2.5 mL q6h and ensure it is within the safe dose range.

a. $\dfrac{200 \text{ mg}}{5 \text{ mL}} \times 2.5 \text{ mL} = x$

100 mg = x

Each 2.5 mL of solution gives 100 mg of erythromycin. The safe dose range is 100 mg q6h so the ordered dose is safe.

b. $\dfrac{600 \text{ mg}}{5 \text{ mL}} \times 2.5 \text{ mL} = x$

$300 \text{ mg} = x$

Each 2.5 mL of solution gives 300 mg of sulfisoxazole. The safe dose range is 300 mg q6h so the ordered dose is safe.

Step 3. Calculate the dose. There is no dose calculation here as the order stated the amount of medication volume to be administered. Prepare the medication following the instructions for reconstitution on the label: "(slowly) add 55 mL of water. Shake moderately (until all powder is dissolved). Yields 105 mL of suspension."

Give the ordered amount - 2.5 mL of Pediazole using an oral syringe (Fig. 10-3).

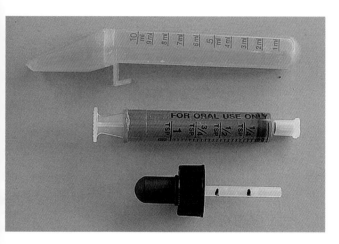

FIGURE 10-3

Examples of equipment used to obtain pediatric doses: (*top*) a medication spoon calculated in mL and teaspoons; (*centre*) an oral syringe calculated in teaspoons; (*bottom*) a safety dropper calibrated in mL.

Example   A 9-month-old child weighing 7.56 kg is ordered Lasix 15 mg po bid (Fig. 10-4). Is the dose safe? What amount should you pour?

Step 1. Determine the safe dose range in mg/kg. The package insert states: "The initial dose of oral Lasix (furosemide) in infants and children is 0.5–1 mg/kg body weight, given as a single dose. Total daily dose not to exceed 2 mg/kg/day in divided dose given 6–12 hours apart."

Initial Dose

$\dfrac{0.5 \text{ mg/kg} \quad \text{to} \quad 1 \text{ mg/kg}}{\times 7.56 \text{ kg} \qquad \times 7.56 \text{ kg}}$

$\quad 3.78 \text{ mg} \quad \text{to} \quad 7.56 \text{ mg}$

Safe Daily Dose

$\dfrac{2 \text{ mg/kg/day}}{\times 7.56 \text{ kg}}$

$\quad 15.12 \text{ mg/day}$

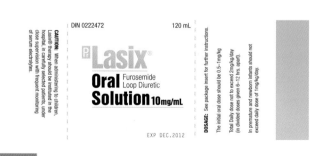

FIGURE 10-4

Label for Lasix (furosemide).

Step 2. Decide whether the ordered dose is safe. The order is 15 mg po bid. 30 mg/day (15 mg ×
2 doses) exceeds the safe dose. Therefore, the dose cannot be given. The nurse must contact
the physician.

Example Lanoxin (digoxin) 25 mcg po × 1 is ordered for a premature infant weighing 1500 g. Is
the dose safe? What amount should be given?

Step 1. Convert grams to kilograms (1000 g = 1 kg).

$$\frac{1500}{1000} = 1.5 \text{ kg}$$

Step 2. Determine the safe dose range in mg/kg.

Drug label states that the safe daily dose range for newborns (birth to 1 month) is 0.008 to 0.018
mg/kg.

Low Dose	*High Dose*
0.008 mg/kg	0.018 mg/kg
× 1.5 kg	× 1.5 kg
0.01 mg	0.03 mg

Step 3. The ordered dose is 25 mcg. Convert to mg.

$$\frac{25 \text{ mcg}}{1000} = 0.025 \text{ mg}$$

The dosage ordered is safe.

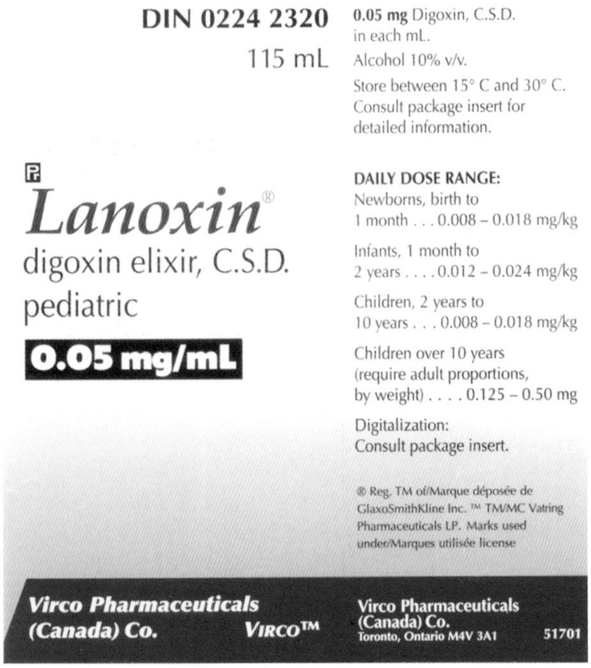

DIN 0224 2320

115 mL

0.05 mg Digoxin, C.S.D.
in each mL.

Alcohol 10% v/v.

Store between 15° C and 30° C.
Consult package insert for
detailed information.

Lanoxin®

digoxin elixir, C.S.D.
pediatric

0.05 mg/mL

DAILY DOSE RANGE:
Newborns, birth to
1 month . . . 0.008 – 0.018 mg/kg

Infants, 1 month to
2 years . . . . 0.012 – 0.024 mg/kg

Children, 2 years to
10 years . . . 0.008 – 0.018 mg/kg

Children over 10 years
(require adult proportions,
by weight) . . . . 0.125 – 0.50 mg

Digitalization:
Consult package insert.

® Reg. TM of/Marque déposée de
GlaxoSmithKline Inc. ™ TM/MC Vatring
Pharmaceuticals LP. Marks used
under/Marques utilisée license

**Virco Pharmaceuticals
(Canada) Co.** Virco™

Virco Pharmaceuticals
(Canada) Co.
Toronto, Ontario M4V 3A1 51701

FIGURE 10-5

Label for Lanoxin. (Courtesy of Virco Pharmaceuticals.)

Step 4.   Calculate the dose. Lanoxin (digoxin) elixir (Fig. 10-5) is supplied 0.05 mg/mL

Formula Method	Proportion Expressed as Two Ratios	Proportion Expressed as Two Fractions
$\dfrac{0.025 \text{ mg}}{0.05 \text{ mg}} \times 1 \text{ mL} = 0.5 \text{ mL}$	$1 \text{ mL} : 0.05 \text{ mg} :: \text{x} : 0.025 \text{ mg}$	$\dfrac{1 \text{ mL}}{0.05 \text{ mg}} \times \dfrac{\text{x}}{0.025 \text{ mg}}$

$$1 \times 0.025 = 0.05x$$

$$\frac{0.025}{0.05} = x$$

$$0.5 \text{ mL} = x$$

Use an oral syringe (1 mL) and draw up 0.5 mL.

Example   A child weighing 30 kg is prescribed epinephrine subcutaneous injection for an allergic reaction. The dosage prescribed is 0.3 mL. Is the dose safe? What amount should be given?

Epinephrine Injection USP
Épinéphrine injectable USP

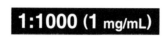

1:1000 (1 mg/mL)

SYMPATHOMIMETIC
Each mL contains: Epinephrine 1 mg, sodium metabisulfite 0.90 mg as an antioxidant, sodium chloride for tonicity, and hydrochloric acid for pH adjustment.
Dosage: Varies with routes of administration: intramuscular, intravenous, intracardiac, endotracheal, or subcutaneous (preferred), and indications.
For allergic manifestations - Adults: 0.2 to 1 mg (0.2 to 1 mL) s.c.   **Children:** 0.01 mL/kg (maximum 0.5 mL) s.c.; may be repeated every 4 hours.
WARNINGS: CONTAINS SODIUM METABISULFITE: USE WITH CAUTION. MAY CAUSE ALLERGIC-TYPE REACTIONS, INCLUDING ANAPHYLACTIC SYMPTOMS OR LIFE THREATENING OR LESS SEVERE ASTHMATIC EPISODES IN CERTAIN SUSCEPTIBLE PERSONS.
See insert for details.
Storage: 15 - 25°C. **Protect from light.** Do not use the solution if its colour is pinkish or darker than slightly yellow, or if it contains a precipitate. Discard unused portion.

SYMPATHOMIMÉTIQUE
Composition de 1 mL: Épinéphrine 1 mg, métabisulfite de sodium 0,90 mg (comme antioxydant), chlorure de sodium pour la tonicité et acide chlorhydrique pour ajuster le pH.
Posologie: Varie selon la voie d'administration, soit intramusculaire, intraveineuse, intracardiaque, endotrachéale ou sous-cutanée (de préférence), et selon les indications.
Dans les cas de manifestations allergiques - Adultes: De 0,2 à 1 mg (de 0,2 à 1 mL) s.-c.   **Enfants:** 0,01 mL/kg (maximum 0,5 mL) s.-c.; peut être répétée aux 4 heures.
MISE EN GARDE: RENFERME DU MÉTABISULFITE DE SODIUM: EMPLOYER AVEC PRUDENCE. PEUT CAUSER DES RÉACTIONS DE TYPE ALLERGIQUE, Y COMPRIS, CHEZ CERTAINES PERSONNES SENSIBLES, DES SYMPTÔMES ANAPHYLACTIQUES OU DES CRISES D'ASTHME POUVANT ALLER JUSQU' À METTRE LA VIE DU PATIENT EN DANGER.
Pour plus de détails, voir le dépliant.
Entreposage: 15 - 25°C. **Craint la lumière.** N'utiliser que si la solution est incolore ou jaune pâle et exempte de précipité. Jetez tout reste.

Hospira Healthcare Corporation
Corporation de Soins de la Santé Hospira
Montréal, Qc H4P 1A5   K183437H

Hospira

8 82135 72411 8

FIGURE 10-6
Label for epinephrine injection. (Used with permission from Hospira.)

Step 1.   Determine the safe dose range in mg/kg.

The drug label (Fig. 10-6) states "0.01 mL/kg subcutaneous. Do not exceed 0.5 mL in a single dose. May be repeated every 4 hours."

Step 2.   The ordered dose is 0.3 mL.

$$\begin{array}{r} 30 \text{ kg} \\ \times\, 0.01 \text{ mL/kg} \\ \hline 0.3 \text{ mL} \end{array}$$

The dosage is safe.

Step 3.   Calculate the dose. No calculation required. Dose is same as ordered amount. Give 0.3 mL subcutaneously.

Example   A child weighing 22.73 kg is ordered promethazine IM 20 mg for excessive postoperative vomiting. Is the dose safe? What amount should be given?

Step 1.   Determine the safe dosage range. The *Nursing Drug Guide* states 1 mg/kg IM q4–6h as needed. The safe dosage range is 12.5–25 mg q4–6h.

Step 2.   The ordered dose is 20 mg.

$$\begin{array}{r} 22.73 \text{ kg} \\ \times \quad 1 \text{ mg/kg} \\ \hline 22.73 \text{ mg} \end{array}$$

A total of 22.73 mg is the calculated dose; however, the ordered dose is within the safe range and can be used.

Step 3.   Calculate the dose.

Promethazine is available 25 mg/mL (Fig. 10-7).

Formula Method	*Proportion Expressed as Two Ratios*	*Proportion Expressed as Two Fractions*
$\frac{20 \text{ mg}}{25 \text{ mg}} \times 1 \text{ mL} = 0.8 \text{ mL}$	$1 \text{ mL} : 25 \text{ mg} :: \text{x} : 20 \text{ mg}$	$\dfrac{1 \text{ mL}}{25 \text{ mg}} \times \dfrac{\text{x}}{20 \text{ mg}}$

$$20 = 25\text{x}$$

$$\frac{20}{25} = \text{x}$$

$$0.8 \text{ mL} = \text{x}$$

Use a 1-mL precision syringe to draw up and administer the dose.

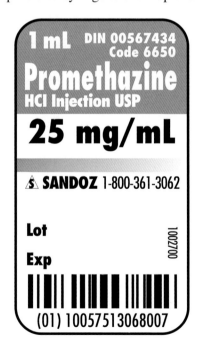

1 mL   DIN 00567434
Code 6650
Promethazine
HCI Injection USP
25 mg/mL
$ **SANDOZ** 1-800-361-3062
Lot
Exp
1002700
(01) 10057513068007

FIGURE 10-7

Label for Promethazine. (Copyright of Sandoz Canada Inc. All rights reserved.)

SELF TEST 1 Dosage Calculations

In these practice problems, determine whether the doses are safe and calculate the amount needed. Answers appear at the end of the chapter.

1. Order: Amoxil (amoxicillin) 60 mg po q8h
    Patient: child weighing 9.09 kg
    Literature: 20 to 40 mg/kg/day in divided doses q8h
    Supply: Amoxil (amoxicillin) 125 mg/5 mL

2. Order: Augmentin (amoxicillin) 175 mg po q8h
    Patient: child weighing 13.18 kg
    Literature: 40 mg/kg/day in divided doses
    Supply: bottle of 125 mg/5 mL

3. Order: ferrous sulfate 200 mg po tid
    Patient: child is 9 years old and weighs 30 kg
    Literature: children 6 to 12 years old, 600 mg divided doses tid
    Supply: bottle of 125 mg/5 mL

4. Order: Tylenol (acetaminophen) 80 mg po q4h prn for temp 100.9°F and above
    Patient: child is 6 years old and weighs 20.5 kg
    Literature: for child 6 to 8 years give four chewable tablets. May repeat four or five times daily. Not to exceed five doses in 24 hours. Is the dose safe?
    Supply: chewable tablets 80 mg

5. Order: Valium (diazepam) 1 mg IM q3–4h prn
    Patient: infant 30 days old
    Literature: child < 6 months IM 1 to 2.5 mg tid or qid
    Supply: vial 5 mg/1 mL

6. Order: Demerol (meperidine) 15 mg subcutaneous q3–4h for relief of pain
    Patient: child is 3 years old and weighs 14 kg
    Literature: Demerol (meperidine) 1.1 mg/kg/dose q3–4h not to exceed 100 mg/day
    Supply: injection 10 mg/mL or 25 mg/mL

7. Order: Dramamine (dimenhydrinate) 25 mg IM q6h as needed
    Patient: child is 10 years old and weighs 30 kg
    Literature: 1.25 mg/kg qid not to exceed 300 mg/day
    Supply: injection labelled 50 mg/mL

8. Order: Cloxapen (cloxacillin) 250 mg po q6h
    Patient: child weighs 21.82 kg
    Literature: for children more than 20 kg, the dose should be 250 to 500 mg q6h.
    Supply: liquid labelled 125 mg in 5 mL

9. Order: Zithromax (azithromycin) po 300 mg × 1 dose
    Patient: child is 10 years old and weighs 30 kg
    Literature: for children 2 to 15 years, 10 mg/kg (not more than 500 mg/day) on day 1.
    Supply: oral suspension 100 mg/5 mL in 15-mL bottle

10. Order: Dilantin (phenytoin) po 60 mg bid
    Patient: infant weighs 5.68 kg
    Literature: 4 to 8 mg/kg/day divided into two doses. Maximum dose is 300 mg/day.
    Supply: Dilantin (phenytoin) suspension 30 mg/5 mL

Determining BSA in m²

A second method to determine pediatric dosage is to calculate BSA (body surface area) in metres squared (m²) using a chart called a nomogram (Fig. 10-8). Height is marked in the left column, weight in the right column. A line is drawn between these two marks. The point at which the line intersects the middle column indicates BSA in m².

There are several mathematical formulas to calculate body surface area. One often used is:

$$\sqrt{\frac{\text{weight (kg)} \times \text{height (cm)}}{3600}} = \text{BSA}$$

Average BSA for children and infants:

9 year old: 1.07 m²

10 year old: 1.14 m²

12-13 year old: 1.33 m²

Neonate: 0.25 m²

2 year old: 0.5 m²

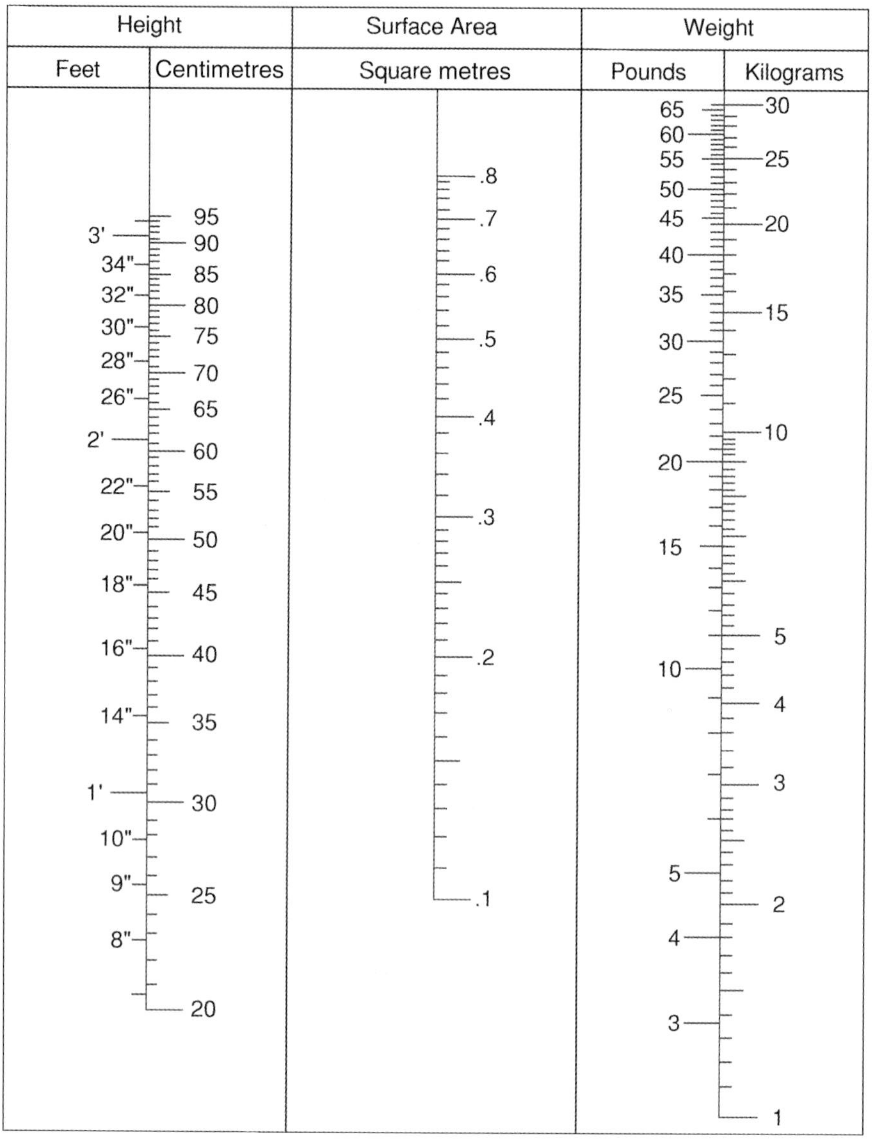

Height		Surface Area	Weight	
Feet	Centimetres	Square metres	Pounds	Kilograms

FIGURE 10-8

Nomogram for infants and toddlers.

Because of differences in growth, charts used for infants and young children are different than those for older children and adults. If a child weighs more than 30 kg or is more than 90 cm tall, use the adult nomogram (Fig. 10-9).

Remember, all infants and children must be weighed in kilograms prior to dosage calculations. (If weighed in grams, divide weight by 1000 to convert to kilograms.)

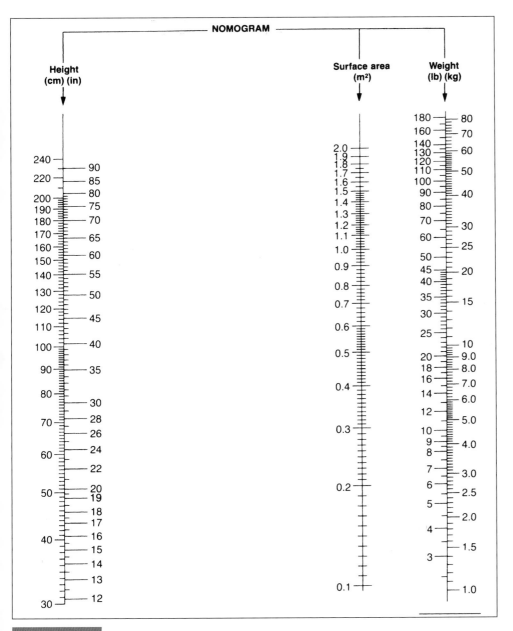

FIGURE 10-9

Nomogram for adults and children. To determine the surface area, draw a straight line between the point representing the patient's height on the left vertical scale to the point representing the patient's weight on the right vertical scale. The point at which this line intersects the middle vertical scale represents the surface area in square metres.

Example

1. An infant with a height of 30 cm and weighing 6.2 kg has a BSA of 0.19 m^2.
2. A child with a height of 128 cm weighing 60 kg has a BSA of 1.55 m^2.

BSA is used mainly in calculating chemotherapy dosages. Determining BSA can be done with a special calculator or using the internet. One useful website for calculating BSA is www.halls.md/body-surface-area/bsa.htm

SELF TEST 2   Determining BSA

Convert height and weight to BSA in m^2 using Figure 10-8 or 10-9. Answers appear at the end of this chapter.

Height	*Weight*	*BSA in m^2*
1. 92 cm	12 kg	
2. 80 cm	13 kg	
3. 128 cm	34 kg	
4. 43 cm	4.1 kg	

STEPS AND RULE—m² MEDICATION ORDERS

STEP 1. Find the BSA in m^2.

STEP 2. Determine the safe dose using a reference.

STEP 3. Decide whether the ordered dose is safe.

STEP 4. Calculate the dose needed.

Example

A 2-year-old child weighing 12.58 kg, height, 90 cm, is prescribed leucovorin calcium 5.5 mg po q6h × 72 hr.

Literature states dose of leucovorin for rescue after methotrexate therapy is 10 mg/m^2/dose q6h × 72 hours.

Supply: 1 mg/mL reconstituted by the pharmacy

Step 1.   Use Figure 10-8.

Height, 90 cm; weight, 12.58 kg

BSA = 0.55

Step 2.   Safe dose is 10 mg/m^2/dose q6h.

$$\begin{array}{r} 10 \text{ mg} \\ \times\, 0.55 \text{ m}^2 \\ \hline 5.5 \text{ mg} = \text{safe dose q6h} \end{array}$$

Step 3.   Order is 5.5 mg q6h. Dose is safe.

Step 4.

Formula Method	Proportion Expressed as Two Ratios	Proportion Expressed as Two Fractions
$\dfrac{5.5\:\text{mg}}{1\:\text{mg}} \times 1\:\text{mL} = 5.5\:\text{mL}$	$1\:\text{mL} : 1\:\text{mg} :: x : 5.5\:\text{mg}$	$\dfrac{1\:\text{mL}}{1\:\text{mg}} \diagup\diagdown \dfrac{x}{5.5\:\text{mg}}$

$$5.5 = x$$

Give 5.5 mL po q6h.

Example   A 6-year-old child weighing 18.5 kg, height, 112.5 cm, is prescribed methotrexate 7.5 mg po twice weekly.

Literature states methotrexate 7.5 to 30 mg/m²/dose twice weekly

Supply: 2.5-mg tablets

Step 1:   Use Figure 10-9.

Height, 112.5 cm; weight, 18.5 kg

BSA = 0.75

Step 2.   Safe dose is 7.5 to 30 mg/m²/dose twice weekly

$$
\begin{array}{ll}
7.5\:\text{kg} & 30\:\text{mg} \\
\underline{\times\,0.75\:\text{m}^2} & \underline{\times\,0.55\:\text{m}^2} \\
5.625\:\text{mg} & 16.5\:\text{mg}
\end{array}
$$

Step 3:   Order is 7.5 mg po twice weekly. Dose is safe.

Step 4:

Formula Method	Proportion Expressed as Two Ratios	Proportion Expressed as Two Fractions
$\dfrac{\overset{3}{7.5\:\text{mg}}}{\underset{1}{2.5\:\text{mg}}} \times 1\:\text{tablet} = 3\:\text{tablets}$	$1\:\text{tablet} : 2.5\:\text{mg} :: x : 7.5\:\text{mg}$	$\dfrac{1\:\text{tablet}}{2.5\:\text{mg}} \diagup\diagdown \dfrac{x}{7.5\:\text{mg}}$

$$7.5 = 2.5x$$

$$\frac{7.5}{2.5} = x$$

$$3\:\text{tablets} = x$$

Give 3 tablets po twice weekly.

In these problems, determine whether the dose is safe, using the nomogram in Figure 10-8 or 10-9 and calculating. Answers appear at the end of the chapter.

1. Child: 8 years; height, 127 cm; weight, 25 kg
   Order: Tambocor (flecainide) 50 mg po q8h
   Literature: dose 100 to 200 mg/m^2/24 hr divided q8–12h
   Supply: 50-mg tablets

2. Child: 12 years; height, 150 cm; weight, 40 kg
   Order: methotrexate 12.5 mg po q week
   Literature: 10 mg/m^2/dose as needed weekly to control fever and joint inflammation in rheumatoid arthritis
   Supply: 2.5-mg tablets

3. Infant: 12 months; height, 76.2 cm; weight, 10 kg
   Order: Deltasone (prednisone) 5 mg po q12h
   Literature: immunosuppressive dose 6–30 mg/m^2/24 hr
   Supply: 5 mg/5 mL syrup

4. Child: 10 years; height, 112 cm; weight, 35 kg
   Order: Marinol (dronabinol) po 5 mg × 1
   Literature: dose 5 mg/m^2 1 to 3 hours before chemotherapy
   Supply: 2.5 mg capsules

5. Child: 12 years; height, 154 cm; weight, 46 kg
   Order: Quinaglute (quinidine) po 250 mg/dose
   Literature: dose 900 mg/m^2/day in 5 divided doses
   Supply: 200-mg, 300-mg tablets

Administering Intravenous Medications

IV medications are administered when a child cannot maintain an oral fluid intake, has fluid electrolyte imbalances, or requires IV medication. Dosages for IV medications are calculated in mg/kg.

IVP (IV push) medications are calculated according to weight and are then administered, using the correct dilution and administration time. This information is in a drug handbook or hospital policy. Continuous IV medications are also calculated according to weight and are then infused through an infusion pump.

IVPB (IV piggyback) medications are administered in small amounts of diluent. Consult a pediatric reference or institutional manual to determine the minimum and maximum safe amounts of diluent. Drugs for IVPB must be initially diluted following the manufacturer's directions. Once you make the initial dilution, withdraw from the vial the amount of drug required to obtain the dose.

Buretrols or other volume control units are used to administer IV fluids (Fig. 10-10). Buretrols are calibrated; they hold only 100 to 150 mL at a time, thus reducing the possibility of fluid overload. In the pediatric setting, Buretrols are usually filled with only 1 hour's worth of IV fluid, so the nurse is responsible for checking the IV every hour to make sure the child is not receiving too much or too little of fluid or medication. Drugs for IVPB that have been diluted can be added to a Buretrol (Fig. 10-11).

For smaller children and infants requiring IVPB medications, the medication is usually added to only 10–20 mL in the Buretrol. This amount of fluid will fill the tubing from the Buretrol to the patient. When the Buretrol is empty of the IV medication, most of the drug will still be in the tubing. For this reason, you need to add an IV flush of 20 mL to the Buretrol after the medication is infused to ensure that the patient receives the drug.

Infusion pumps provide a second safeguard (Fig. 10-12). To ensure that pediatric patients receive accurate dosing, you can set infusion pump rates in tenths and hundredths. In neonatal areas, syringe pumps can deliver IV fluid ranging from 1 to 60 mL.

This section considers the calculation of pediatric doses for IV and IVPB administration.

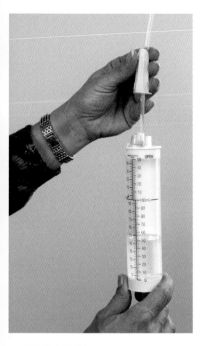

FIGURE 10-10

Volume control infusion device (Buretrol). (Used with permission from Taylor, C. [2008]. *Fundamentals of nursing* [6th ed.]. Philadelphia: Lippincott Williams and Wilkins, p. 853.)

FIGURE 10-11

Adding medication to a volume control infusion device (Buretrol). (Used with permission from Taylor, C. [2008]. *Fundamentals of nursing* [6th ed.]. Philadelphia: Lippincott Williams and Wilkins, p. 854.)

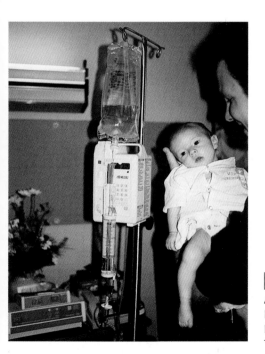

FIGURE 10-12

An infusion pump with a volume control unit. (With permission from Pillitteri, A. [2002]. *Maternal and child health nursing* [4th ed.]. Philadelphia: Lippincott Williams & Wilkins, p. 1106.)

STEPS TO SOLVING PARENTERAL PEDIATRIC MEDICATIONS IVP

STEP 1. Determine the safe dose range in mg/kg using a drug reference.

STEP 2. Decide whether the ordered dose is safe by comparing the order with the safe dosage range listed in the reference.

STEP 3. Calculate the dose needed.

STEP 4. Check the reference for diluent and duration for administration.

To determine how fast to push the medication, you can take the volume calculated and divide by the minutes. Then take that number and divide by 4; the answer tells you approximately how much to push in over 15 seconds. Or you can divide that number by 6, and the answer is approximately how much to push in over 10 seconds. The important point is to push the drug slowly over the time period required and to monitor the IV infusion site.

Example

Child: 5 years; weight, 20 kg

Order: Zantac (ranitidine) 30 mg IV bid

Literature: 2–4 mg/kg q12h IV up to 300 mg/day

Dilute with 5 or 10 mL with 5% dextrose or 0.9% sodium chloride and injected over at least 2 minutes.

Supply: See label (Fig. 10-13).

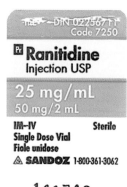

FIGURE 10-13

Label for Ranitdine. (Copyright of Sandoz Canada Inc. All rights reserved.)

Step 1.   Determine the safe dose range.

2 mg/kg	4 mg/kg
× 20 kg	× 20 kg
40 mg	80 mg

Step 2.   The dose is safe. It meets the mg/kg rule and does not exceed 300 mg/day.

30 mg bid = total 60 mg/day

Step 3. Calculate the dose.

Formula Method	Proportion Expressed as Two Ratios	Proportion Expressed as Two Fractions
$\dfrac{\overset{6}{\cancel{30}\text{ mg}}}{\underset{5}{\cancel{25}\text{ mg}}} \times 1\text{ mL} = 1.2\text{ mL}$	$1\text{ mL} : 25\text{ mg} :: x : 30\text{ mg}$	$\dfrac{1\text{ mL}}{25\text{ mg}} \times \dfrac{x}{30\text{ mg}}$

$$\frac{30}{25} = x$$

$$1.2\text{ mL} = x$$

Step 4. Dilute 10 mL suggested diluent. Inject over at least 5 minutes.

Example

Child: 10 years; weight, 40 kg.

Order: Furosemide 40 mg IV bid

Literature: 0.5–1 mg/kg q12h IV, no more than 2 mg/kg/day

Furosemide should be injected slowly over a period of 1–2 minutes when given by IV route.

NOTE: Furosemide injection should not be added into the tubing of a running infusion solution.

Supply: See label (Fig. 10-14).

Step 1. Determine the safe dose range.

40 kg

Step 2. The dose is safe. 40 mg bid = 80 mg/day. It meets the mg/kg rule and does not exceed 2 mg/day (80 mg/day).

Maximum dose: 2 mg/kg/day

The dosage is safe.

Low Dose	*High Dose*
$\dfrac{\begin{array}{r}0.05\text{ mg/kg}\\ \times\ 40\text{ kg}\end{array}}{20\text{ mg}}$	$\dfrac{\begin{array}{r}1\text{ mg/kg}\\ \times\ 40\text{ kg}\end{array}}{40\text{ mg}}$

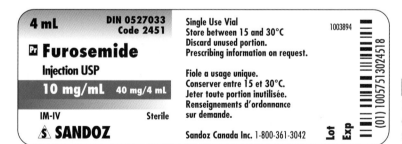

FIGURE 10-14

Label for Furosemide. (Copyright of Sandoz Canada Inc. All rights reserved.)

Step 3. Calculate the dose needed.

Formula Method	Proportion Expressed as Two Ratios	Proportion Expressed as Two Fractions
$\dfrac{\overset{4}{\cancel{40}}\ \text{mg}}{\underset{1}{\cancel{10}}\ \text{mg}} \times 1\ \text{mL} = 4\ \text{mL}$	$1\ \text{mL} : 10\ \text{mg} :: x : 40\ \text{mg}$	$\dfrac{1\ \text{mL}}{10\ \text{mg}} \times \dfrac{x}{40\ \text{mg}}$

$$40 = 10x$$
$$\frac{40}{10} = x$$
$$4\ \text{mL} = x$$

Step 4.   Check the reference for diluent and duration for administration.

STEPS TO SOLVE PARENTERAL PEDIATRIC MEDICATIONS IVPB

1. Decide whether the dose is safe; check a pediatric reference.

2. Decide whether the dilution ordered meets the minimum pediatric safety standard.

3. Prepare the medication according to directions.

4. Draw up the dose and dilute further as needed.

5. Set the pump in mL/hr. If the infusion time is 30 minutes, set the pump for double the amount because the pump delivers mL/hr.

> **Example**   The order is 10 mL over 30 minutes. Set the pump for 20 mL/hr. It will deliver 10 mL in 30 minutes.

6. When the IV is completed, add a flush of 20 mL to the Buretrol to clear the tubing of the medication. Be sure to chart the flush as fluid intake. Follow institutional requirements regarding IV flush.

Example   Child: 4 years; weight, 17 kg

Order: Cefazolin 280 mg IV q8h in 10 mL D5½NS

Literature: Safe dose 25 to 50 mg/kg/day divided in three or four equal doses
Concentration for IV use: 50 mg/mL over 30 minutes

Supply: 1 g powder. Directions: Add 2.5 mL sterile water for injection to make 33.4 mg/mL solution. (Fig. 10-15).

1. Safe dose is 25 to 50 mg/kg/day.

Low Dose	*High Dose*
25 mg/kg/day	50 mg/kg/day
× 17 kg	× 17 kg
425 mg/day	850 mg/day

Order is 280 mg q8h (three doses).

280 mg × 3 = 840 mg

Dose falls within the range and is safe.

Sterile

DIN 02108127
10 x 1 g vials

℞ CEFAZOLIN for Injection, USP

1 g
Cefazolin per vial
ANTIBIOTIC
Intramuscular or intravenous use only

For intramuscular use, add 2.5 mL Sterile Water for Injection for a 334 mg/mL solution.
For direct intravenous (bolus) use, further dilute reconstituted solution to a minimum of 10 mL with Sterile Water for Injection. **SHAKE WELL.**
For intermittent intravenous infusion, further dilute in 50 to 100 mL of one of the recommended intravenous solutions. Use reconstituted solution
within 24 hours when stored at controlled room temperature not exceeding 25°C, or within 72 hours if refrigerated (2°C to 8 °C), protected from light.
Product Monograph available upon request.
Store powder between 15°C and 25°C. Protect from light.
®·Reg'd Trademark of Novopharm Limited, Toronto, Canada M1B 2K9

69397CT-0110 Rev. 03

LOT 360226
EXP 05.2011

FIGURE 10-15

Label for Cefazolin. (Used with permission from Novopharm Limited.)

2. Minimum safe dilution is 50 mg/mL. Dose is 280 mg.

= 6 mL, the minimum dilution. The order of 10 mL D5½NS is safe because it is more than the minimum.

$$
\begin{array}{r}
5.6 \\
50\overline{)280.} \\
\underline{250} \\
300 \\
\underline{300}
\end{array}
$$

3. Prepare the medication according to directions. Add 2.5 mL sterile water to make 33.4 mg mL.

Formula Method	Proportion Expressed as Two Ratios	Proportion Expressed as Two Fractions
$\frac{280\ mg}{334\ mg} \times 1\ mL = 0.84\ mL$	1 mL : 334 mg : : x : 280 mg	$\frac{1\ mL}{334\ mg} \times \frac{x}{280\ mg}$

$$280 = 334x$$

$$\frac{280}{334} = x$$

$$0.84\ mL = x$$

Withdraw 0.84 mL; label the vial and store in the refrigerator.

4. Run about 5 mL D5½NS into the Buretrol. Add the 0.84 mL drug. Add more D5½NS to make 10 mL.

5. Set the pump at 20. This is 20 mL/hr. The pump will deliver 10 mL in 30 minutes.

6. When the IV is completed, add a 20-mL flush of D5½NS to clear the IV tubing of medication.

Example

Infant: 4.3 kg

Order: ampicillin 100 mg IV q6h in 10 mL D5½NS

Literature: The safe dose is 75 to 200 mg/kg/24 hr given q6–8h IV.

Concentration for IV use: 50 mg/mL over 10 to 30 minutes

Supply: Vial of powder labelled 500 mg. Directions: Add 1.8 mL sterile water for injection to make 250 mg/mL; use within 1 hour.

1.   Safe dose is 75 to 200 mg/kg/24 hr given q6–8h.

Low Dose	**High Dose**
75 mg	200 mg
× 4.3 kg	× 4.3 kg
322.5 mg/24 hr	860 mg/24 hr

Order is 100 mg q6h (four doses).

100 mg × 4 doses = 400 mg.

This is within the range. The dose is safe.

2.   Minimum safe dilution is 50 mg/mL (Table 10-1). Dose is 100 mg.

$$50\overline{)100}$$ 2 mL is the minimum dilution; 10 mL is safe.

TABLE 10-1	**Sample of a Dilution Table for Pediatric Antibiotics**	
Antibiotic	**Recommended Final Concentration IV**	**Recommendation Duration of IV**
Ampicillin	50 mg/mL	10–30 min
Ceftazidime	50 mg/mL	10–30 min
Clindamycin	6–12 mg/mL	15–30 min
Garamycin (gentamicin)	2 mg/mL	15–30 min
Penicillin G	Infants: 50,000 units/mL Large child: 100,000 units/mL	10–30 min
Nebupent (pentamidine)	2.5 mg/mL	1 hr

3.   Add 1.8 mL sterile water for injection to 500 mg powder to make 250 mg/mL.

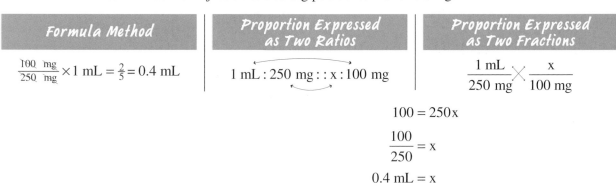

Formula Method	**Proportion Expressed as Two Ratios**	**Proportion Expressed as Two Fractions**
$\frac{100 \ \text{mg}}{250 \ \text{mg}} \times 1 \ \text{mL} = \frac{2}{5} = 0.4 \ \text{mL}$	$1 \ \text{mL} : 250 \ \text{mg} :: x : 100 \ \text{mg}$	$\frac{1 \ \text{mL}}{250 \ \text{mg}} \times \frac{x}{100 \ \text{mg}}$

$$100 = 250x$$

$$\frac{100}{250} = x$$

$$0.4 \ \text{mL} = x$$

Withdraw 0.4 mL from the vial. Discard the remainder (directions say to use within 1 hour).

4.   Add about 5 mL D5½NS to the Buretrol. Add 0.4 mL drug. Add more D5½NS to make 10 mL.

5.   Set the pump at 20. This means 20 mL/hr. The pump will deliver 10 mL in 30 minutes.

6.   When the IV is finished, add a 20-mL flush of D5½NS to the Buretrol to clear the tubing of medication.

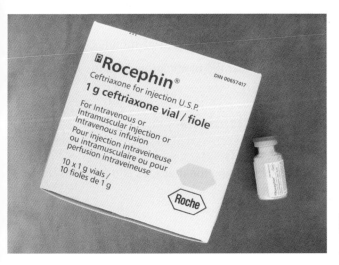

Example

Child: 3 years; weight, 15 kg

Order: Rocephin 600 mg IV q12h in 15 mL D5½NS

Literature: safe dose up to 100 mg/kg/day in two divided doses

Concentration for IV use: 50 mg/mL over 15 minutes

Supply: 1 g powder. Directions: Dilute with 9.6 mL sterile water for injection to make 100 mg/mL; stable for 7 days if refrigerated (Fig. 10-16).

1. Safe dose is up to 100 mg/kg/day.

$$\begin{array}{r} 100 \\ \times\ \ 15 \\ \hline 1500 \end{array}$$ mg/day or 750 mg/day

Order is 600 mg q12h (two doses).

600 mg x 2 = 1200 mg

The dose falls within the range and therefore is safe.

2. Minimum safe dilution is 50 mg/mL. The dose is 600 mg.

600 mg divided by 50 mg/mL gives us 12 mg/mL as a minimal dilution.

The order of 15 mL is safe, because it is more than the minimum.

3. Dilute 1 g with 9.6 mL sterile water to make 100 mg/mL.

Withdraw 6 mL; label the vial and store in the refrigerator.

Formula Method	Proportion Expressed as Two Ratios	Proportion Expressed as Two Fractions
$\frac{600\ \text{mg}}{100\ \text{mg}} \times 1\ \text{mL} = x$	$1\ \text{mL} : 100\ \text{mg} :: x : 600\ \text{mg}$	$\dfrac{1\ \text{mL}}{100\ \text{mg}} \times \dfrac{x}{600\ \text{mg}}$
6 mL		

$$600 = 100x$$

$$\frac{600}{100} = x$$

$$6\ \text{mL} = x$$

4. Run about 5 mL D5½NS into the Buretrol. Add the 6 mL of drug. Add more D5½NS to make 15 mL.

5. Set the pump at 60, which means 60 mL/hr. The pump will deliver 15 mL in 15 minutes.

6. When the IV is completed, add a 20-mL flush of D5½NS to clear the medication from the tubing.

General Guidelines for Continuous IV Medications

1.	Calculate continuous IV medications for children and infants by using the methods and formulas used in Chapter 9.
2.	Base continuous IV dosages on weight in kilograms.
3.	Always use an infusion pump and/or volume control sets.
4.	Use small bags of fluid to prevent fluid overload.
5.	Follow institutional requirements for continuous IV infusions.
6.	To determine the safe dosage range, consult a pediatric text or drug reference.

SELF TEST 4   Parenteral Medication Calculations

In these practice problems, determine whether the dose is safe, calculate the amount needed, and state how the order should be administered. Answers appear at the end of this chapter. Follow the steps used in the examples.

1. Infant: 6 months; weight, 8 kg
    Order: Ceftin (cefuroxime) 200 mg IV q6h in 10 mL D5½NS
    Literature: The safe dose is 50 to 100 mg/kg/24 hr given q6–8h
                   Concentration for IV use: 50 mg/mL over 30 minutes
    Supply: 750-mg vial of powder. Directions: Dilute with 8 mL sterile water for injection
                   to make 90 mg/mL; stable for 3 days if refrigerated.

2. Child: 3 years; weight, 15 kg
    Order: Bactrim (as TMP/SMX) 75 mg IV q12h in 75 mL D5W over 1 hr
    Literature: Safe dose for a child is 8 to 10 mg/kg/24 hr given q12h
                   Concentration for IV use: 1 mL in 15 to 25 mL (supply is a liquid)
    Supply: Vial labelled 80 mg/5 mL

3. Child: 12 years; weight, 40 kg
    Order: Nebcin (tobramycin) 100 mg IV q8h in 50 mL D5½NS
    Literature: The safe dose is 3 to 5 mg/kg/24 hr given q8h
                   Concentration for IV use: 2 mg/mL over 15 to 30 minutes
    Supply: vial 80 mg/2 mL

(continued)

4. Child: 5 years; weight, 18 kg
   Order: Claforan (cefotaxime) 900 mg IV q6h in 25 mL D5½NS
   Literature: The safe dose is 50 to 200 mg/kg/24 hr given q6h
                Concentration for IV use: 50 mg/mL; give over 30 minutes
   Supply: 1 g powder. Directions: Dilute with 10 mL sterile water for injection to make
                95 mg/mL; stable in the refrigerator 10 days.

5. Infant: 3 months; weight, 6 kg
   Order: Unipen (nafcillin) 150 mg IV q8h in 10 mL D5½NS
   Literature: The safe dose is 100 to 200 mg/kg/24 hr given q6h
                Concentration for IV use: 6 mg/mL over 30 to 60 minutes
   Supply: 500-mg vial of powder. Directions: Add 1.7 mL sterile water for injection to
                make 500 mg/2 mL; stable for 48 hr if refrigerated.

6. Child: 8 years; weight, 30 kg
   Order: morphine 2.5 mg IV q4h
   Literature: 0.05 to 0.1 mg/kg/q4h IV. Dilute 2 to 10 mg in at least 5 mL NS. Administer
                over 4 to 5 minutes.
   Supply: morphine injection 1 mg/mL

7. Child: 6 years; weight, 25 kg
   Order: Decadron (dexamethasone) 4 mg IV bid
   Literature: 0.08 to 0.3 mg/kg/day divided q6–12h. Give undiluted IVP over 30 seconds or less.
   Supply: Decadron 4 mg/mL injection

8. Child: 12 years; weight, 45 kg
   Order: Benadryl (diphenhydramine) 25 mg IV q4–6h
   Literature: 12.5 to 25 mg IV q4–6h; maximum dose, 300 mg/24 hr
                Give undiluted IVP over 1 minute.
   Supply: 50 mg/mL injection

9. Infant: 6.82 kg
   Order: Lanoxin (digoxin) maintenance dose IV 50 mcg/day
   Literature: 6 to 7.5 mcg/kg/day. Give undiluted or diluted in 4 mL D5W or NS over
                5 minutes.
   Supply: 0.1 mg/mL injection

10. Child: 9 years; weight, 36.36 kg
   Order: Solu-Medrol (methylprednisolone) IV 60 mg bid
   Literature: 0.5 to 1.7 mg/kg/day divided q12h. Give each 500 mg over 2 to 3 minutes.
   Supply: Solu-Medrol 40 mg/mL

CRITICAL THINKING: TEST YOUR CLINICAL SAVVY

You are working in a pediatric unit and taking care of 5-year-old Georgia Smith. Although she usually has a sweet disposition, she has her moments when she will not do anything she doesn't want to do. She is receiving IV fluids continuously and is ordered an oral medication three times a day that has an aftertaste. Each time the medication is brought to her, she refuses to take it.

a. What are techniques to help her take the medication?
b. Are there other alternatives you could use regarding the medication? How would you implement any of these alternatives?
c. Are there strategies to suggest to the family to promote easier compliance?
d. Besides reducing the possibility of fluid overload, what are some other reasons IV infusion pumps are used with children?

Another patient, 14-year-old Sean McBrady, is unable to swallow pills.

a. What are some alternatives to the medication?
b. Are there contraindications to any of the medication alternatives?
c. What are some ways to get children to swallow pills?
d. What would you suggest to the family to promote easier administration?

Putting It Together

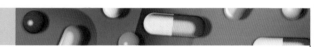

Andy Bee is a 7 year old admitted to the ER with a 6 hour history of wheezing. The mother reports a history of "flu-like" symptoms for 48 hours. He has not had any solid food for 2 days and had minimal fluid intake.

Past Medical History: premature birth at 32 weeks. The child was on a ventilator for 1 week post partum. Small birth weight. Asthma.

Allergies: Penicillin, causing rash and hives.

Current Vital Signs: Blood pressure is 110/80, pulse 120–140/min, respirations 29/min, oxygen saturation 95%, temp 101.8. Weight 30 kg.

Medication Orders

Solu-Medrol (methylprednisolone) *corticosteroid, glucocorticoid* 20 mg IVP x 1 then 10 mg q6h

Proventil (albuterol) *bronchodilator* 0.6 mL in 3 mL NS per nebulizer every 20 minutes x 3

Tylenol (acetaminophen) *antipyretic* liquid 400 mg po for temp >38°C q4h.

NS 10 mL/kg/hr for 1 hour, then 100 mL/hr

(continued)

Putting It Together

Mortin (ibuprofen) *anti-inflammatory* 5 mg/kg po q6h prn for continued temp >38°C if not relieved by Tylenol

Fortaz (ceftazidime) *anti-infective* 2 g IVPB q8h in 50 mL D5½ NS

Lanoxin (digoxin) *cardiac glycoside* 0.72 mg/m² po every day.

Augmentin (amoxicillin/clavulanate) *antiinfective* 150 mg po q8h.

Phenergan (promethazine) *antiemetic* 1 mg/kg IM prn q4–6h for nausea

Calculations

1. Calculate how many mL of Solu-Medrol to give. Available Solu-Medrol vial that yields 20 mg/mL.
   a. One-time dose of 20 mg.
   b. Scheduled dose 10 mg q6h.

2. Calculate how many mL and how many teaspoons of Tylenol elixir to give.
   Available: liquid Tylenol 160 mg/5 mL.
   a. Conversion to mL.
   b. Conversion to tsp.

3. Calculate how many mg of Motrin to give and how many mL to administer. Available: 100 mg/5 mL

4. Calculate how many mL of Fortaz to prepare. Calculate the infusion rate. Available: 2-g vial of powder. Dilute initially with 10 mL sterile water for injection. Infuse 50 mg/mL over 15–30 minutes.

5. Calculate the dose of Digoxin. BSA is 0.9 m².

6. Calculate the dose of Augmentin. Available 125 mg/mL.

7. Calculate how many mg of Phenergan. Is the dose safe? Literature states safe dose 10–25 mg.

8. Calculate the amount of NS to infuse the first hour.

Critical Thinking Questions

1. Should any medication(s) be held and if so why?

2. What medication(s) should be questioned and why?

3. What route of medication may be difficult for this patient? What are some alternatives to medication administration for this patient?

4. Is the amount of NS to infuse abnormally high for this patient? Why or why not?

Answers in Appendix B.

Name: _____

Here is a mix of oral and parenteral pediatric orders. For each problem, determine the safe dose and calculate the amount to give. Answers are given in Appendix A.

1. Newborn: weight, 4 kg
   Order: vitamin K 1 mg IM × 1 dose
   Literature: Prophylaxis and treatment: 0.5 to 1 mg/dose IM, subcutaneous, IV × 1
   Supply: vial 10 mg/mL

2. Infant: 1 yr; 10 kg
   Order: Augmentin (amoxicillin/clavulanate) 125 mg po q8h
   Literature: Safe dose Augmentin (amoxicillin/clavulanate): 20 to 40 mg/kg/24 hours given q8h po
   Supply: 125 mg/5 mL

3. Infant: 10 mo; 10 kg
   Order: benzathine penicillin 500,000 units IM × 1 dose
   Literature: Safe dose 50,000 units/kg × 1 IM. Maximum, 2.4 milliunits
   Supply: vial labelled 600,000 units/mL

4. Infant: 3.6 kg
   Order: gentamicin 9 mg IV q8h in 10 mL D5½NS
   Literature: Safe dose is 2.5 mg/kg/dose q8h
   Concentration for IV 2 mg/mL given over 15 to 30 min
   Supply: vial 40 mg/mL

5. Infant: 6.7 kg
   Order: Colace Syrup (docusate) 10 mg po bid
   Literature: Infants and children under 3: 10 to 40 mg/day
   Supply: 20 mg/5 mL

6. Infant: 5.5 kg
   Order: vancomycin 54 mg IV q8h in 12 mL D5½NS
   Literature: Safe dose is 10 mg/kg q8h IV
   Concentration for IV 5 mg/mL; infuse over 1 hour
   Supply: 500 mg powder
   Directions: Add 10 mL sterile water for injection to give 50 mg/mL; stable in the refrigerator 14 days.

7. Infant: 6.7 kg
   Order: chloral hydrate 350 mg po prior to electroencephalogram
   Literature: Hypnotic for children: 25 to 50 mg/kg/dose po not to exceed 100 mg/kg.
   Supply: 500 mg/5 mL

8. Child: 12 years; height, 152 cm; weight, 40 kg; BSA, 1.32
   Order: methotrexate 10 mg po 1–2×/wk
   Literature: 7.5–30 mg/m^2 1–2×/wk
   Supply: 2.5-mg tablet

9. Child: 8 yr; 24 kg
   Order: Fortaz (ceftazidime) 2 g IVPB q8h in 50 mL D5½NS
   Literature: Safe dose is 2 to 6 g/24 hr given q8–12h IV
   Concentration for IV 50 mg/mL over 15 to 30 minutes
   Supply: 2-g vial of powder
   Dilute initially with 10 mL sterile water for injection.

10. Child: 15.9 kg
    Order: Demerol (meperidine) HCl 20 mg IV stat
    Literature: Children: usual dose 1 to 1.5 mg/kg/dose q3–4h prn. Maximum dose, 100 mg.
    Supply: 50 mg/mL

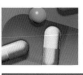

Answers to Self Tests

Self Test 1 Dosage Calculations

1. Step 1. Low dose

$$\begin{array}{r} 9.09 \text{ kg} \\ \times\ 20 \text{ mg} \\ \hline 181.8 \text{ mg/day} \end{array}$$

High dose

$$\begin{array}{r} 9.09 \text{ kg} \\ \times\ 40 \text{ mg} \\ \hline 363.6 \text{ mg/day} \end{array}$$

Step 2. 60 mg × 3 doses = 180 mg/day
The order is safe, although on the low side.

Step 3.

Formula Method	Proportion Expressed as Two Ratios	Proportion Expressed as Two Fractions
$\dfrac{60\text{mg}}{125\text{mg}} \times 5 \text{ mL} = 2.4 \text{ mL}$	5 mL : 125 mg : : x : 60 mg	$\dfrac{5 \text{ mL}}{125 \text{ mg}} \times \dfrac{\text{x}}{60 \text{ mg}}$

$$60 \times 5 = 125\text{x}$$
$$\frac{300}{125} = \text{x}$$
$$2.4 \text{ mL} = \text{x}$$

Give 2.4 mL po q8h.

2. Step 1.

$$\begin{array}{r} 40 \text{ mg} \\ \times\ 13.18 \text{ kg} \\ \hline 527.27 \text{ mg/day (calculator)} \end{array}$$

Step 2. 175 mg × 3 doses = 525 mg/day. The order is safe.

$$\begin{array}{r} 175 \text{ mg} \\ \times\ \ \ \ 3 \text{ doses} \\ \hline 525 \text{ mg/day} \end{array}$$

Step 3.

Formula Method	Proportion Expressed as Two Ratios	Proportion Expressed as Two Fractions
$\dfrac{\overset{7}{\cancel{175}} \text{ mg}}{\underset{25}{\cancel{125}} \text{ mg}} \times \overset{1}{\cancel{5}} \text{ mL} = 7$	5 mL : 125 mg : : x : 175 mg	$\dfrac{5 \text{ mL}}{125 \text{ mg}} \times \dfrac{\text{x}}{175 \text{ mg}}$

$$5 \times 175 = 125\text{x}$$
$$\frac{875}{125} = \text{x}$$
$$7 \text{ mL} = \text{x}$$

Give 7 mL po q8h.

3. It was not necessary to use a rule. The literature was clear. Children 6 to 12 years should receive 600 mg divided into three doses, which equals 200 mg/dose. The ordered dose is safe.

Formula Method	Proportion Expressed as Two Ratios	Proportion Expressed as Two Fractions
$\frac{200}{125} \times 5 = \frac{1000}{125}$ $125\overline{)1000.}$ 8.0 mL	5 mL : 125 mg : : x : 200 mg	$\frac{5\ mL}{125\ mg} \times \frac{x}{200\ mg}$

$$5 \times 200 = 125x$$

$$\frac{1000}{125} = x$$

$$8\ mL = x$$

Give 8 mL po tid.

4. Tylenol 80 mg seems low. Literature says a child of 6 years should receive four chewable tablets. This would be 320 mg. Check with the physician or healthcare provider.

5. The literature states that children under 6 months can receive 1 to 2.5 mg IM three to four times a day. The individual dose for the infant is 1 mg. This is safe, but the physician wrote q3–4h prn for the time. This would allow six to eight doses per 24 hours. The nurse can give the first dose but should clarify the times with the physician or healthcare provider.

Formula Method	Proportion Expressed as Two Ratios	Proportion Expressed as Two Fractions
$\frac{1\ mg}{5\ mg} \times 1\ mL = 0.2\ mL\ IM$	1 mL : 5 mg : : x : 1 mg	$\frac{1\ mL}{5\ mg} \times \frac{x}{1\ mg}$

$$1 = 5x$$

$$\frac{1}{5} = x$$

$$0.2\ mL = x$$

Give 0.2 mL IM.

6. Step 1.   14 kg
              $\times$ 1.1 mg/kg
              15.4 mg

Step 2. 15.4 mg q3h = 15.4 × 8 doses = 123.2/day. This range exceeds the 100 mg/day maximum. Contact the physician to change the order to q4h only.

15.4 mg q4h = 15.4 mg × 6 doses = 92.4 mg/day. This range is safe.

Formula Method	Proportion Expressed as Two Ratios	Proportion Expressed as Two Fractions
$\frac{\overset{3}{15}\ mg}{\underset{2}{10}\ mg} \times 1\ mL = 1.5\ mL$	1 mL : 10 mg : : x : 15 mg	$\frac{1\ mL}{10\ mg} \times \frac{x}{15\ mg}$

$$15 = 10x$$

$$\frac{15}{10} = x$$

$$1.5\ mL = x$$

Formula Method	Proportion Expressed as Two Ratios	Proportion Expressed as Two Fractions
$\dfrac{\overset{3}{\cancel{15}} \text{ mg}}{\underset{5}{\cancel{25}} \text{ mg}} \times 1 \text{ mL} = 0.6 \text{ mL}$	$1 \text{ mL} : 25 \text{ mg} :: x : 15 \text{ mg}$	$\dfrac{1 \text{ mL}}{25 \text{ mg}} \diagdown \dfrac{x}{15 \text{ mg}}$

$$15 = 25x$$
$$0.6 \text{ mL} = x$$

Give the 0.6-mL dose subcutaneously because it is less liquid to inject.

7. Step 1. $\begin{array}{r} 30 \text{ kg} \\ \times\, 1.25 \text{ mg/kg} \\ \hline 37.5 \text{ mg} \end{array}$

   Step 2. $\begin{array}{r} 25 \\ \times\, 4 \ \ (q6h) \\ \hline 100 \ \ \text{mg/day} \end{array}$

The dose does not exceed 300 mg/day.
However, the dose ordered is less than the recommended dose. Check with the physician or healthcare provider.

Formula Method	Proportion Expressed as Two Ratios	Proportion Expressed as Two Fractions
$\dfrac{\overset{1}{\cancel{25}} \text{ mg}}{\underset{2}{\cancel{50}} \text{ mg}} \times 1 \text{ mL} = 0.5 \text{ mL}$	$1 \text{ mL} : 50 \text{ mg} :: x : 25 \text{ mg}$	$\dfrac{1 \text{ mL}}{50 \text{ mg}} \diagdown \dfrac{x}{25 \text{ mg}}$

$$25 = 50x$$
$$\frac{25}{50} = x$$
$$0.5 \text{ mL} = x$$

Give 0.5 mL IM.

8. a. For children more than 20 kg, the dose is 250 to 500 mg q6h. The dose is safe.

Formula Method	Proportion Expressed as Two Ratios	Proportion Expressed as Two Fractions
$\dfrac{\overset{2}{\cancel{250}} \text{ mg}}{\underset{1}{\cancel{125}} \text{ mg}} \times 5 \text{ mL} = 10 \text{ mL}$	$5 \text{ mL} : 125 \text{ mg} :: x : 250 \text{ mg}$	$\dfrac{5 \text{ mL}}{125 \text{ mg}} \diagdown \dfrac{x}{250 \text{ mg}}$

$$1250 = 125x$$
$$\frac{1250}{125} = x$$
$$10 \text{ mL} = x$$

Give 10 mL po q6h.

9. a.   30 kg
          $\times$10 mg/kg
         ─────────
          300 mg

The literature states not more than 500 mg/day. The dose is safe.

b.

Formula Method	Proportion Expressed as Two Ratios	Proportion Expressed as Two Fractions
$\dfrac{\overset{3}{\cancel{300}}\ \text{mg}}{\underset{1}{\cancel{100}}\ \text{mg}}\times 5\ \text{mL} = 15\ \text{mL}$	5 mL : 100 mg : : x : 300 mg	$\dfrac{5\ \text{mL}}{100\ \text{mg}}\times\dfrac{\text{x}}{300\ \text{mg}}$

$$1500 = 100x$$
$$\frac{1500}{100} = x$$
$$15\ \text{mL} = x$$

Give 15 mL $\times$ 1 dose.

10. a.   5.68 kg   5.68 kg
        $\times$ 4 mg/kg $\times$ 8 mg/kg
       ──────────   ──────────
        22.72 mg   45.44 mg

The dose (60 mg) is too high. Check with the physician.

Self Test 2 Determining BSA

1. 0.55 m^2 (adult nomogram)   **3.** 1.1 m^2 (adult nomogram)

2. 0.54 m^2 **4.** 0.22 m^2

Self Test 3 Use of the Nomogram

1. Step 1. Find the BSA in m^2 = 0.94.

Step 2. Determine safe dose.

   Low Dose   *High Dose*
      100 mg   200 mg
   $\times$ 0.94 $\times$ 0.94
   ────────   ────────
       94 mg   188 mg

The safe dose is 94 to 188 mg over 24 hr.

Step 3. Is the order safe?

50 mg q8h = 50 mg $\times$ 3 = 150 mg/24 hr

The dose is safe.

Step 4. Order is 50 mg; supply is 50 mg. Give 1 tablet q8h.

2. Step 1. Find the BSA in m^2 = 1.29.

Step 2. The safe dose is   10 mg
                   $\times$ 1.29
                  ─────────
                   12.9 mg

Step 3. Is the order safe? Yes; 12.5 mg is below the maximum.

Step 4.

Formula Method	Proportion Expressed as Two Ratios	Proportion Expressed as Two Fractions
$\dfrac{\overset{5}{\cancel{12.5\ mg}}}{\underset{1}{\cancel{2.5\ mg}}} \times 1$ tablet = 5 tablets	1 tablet : 2.5 mg : : x : 12.5 mg	$\dfrac{1\ tablet}{2.5\ mg} \times \dfrac{x}{12.5\ mg}$

$$12.5 = 2.5x$$
$$\frac{12.5}{2.5} = x$$

Give 5 tablets po every week.

5 tablets = x

3. Step 1. Find the BSA in m^2 = 0.46.

   Step 2. The safe dose is 6.30 mg/m^2/24 hr.

Low Dose	*High Dose*
6 mg	30 mg
$\times$ 0.46	$\times$ 0.46
2.76 mg	13.8 mg

   The safe dose is 2.8 mg to 13.8 mg over 24 hr.

   Step 3. Order is 5 mg $\times$ 12 hr = 10 mg. The dose is safe.

   Step 4. Order is 5 mg; supply is 5 mg/5 mL. Give 5 mL po q12h.

4. Step 1. Find the BSA in m^2 = 1.1

   Step 2. Determine the safe dose.

   5 mg
   $\times$ 1.1
   5.5 mg

   Step 3. Is the order safe?

   Yes. The order is 5 mg.

   Step 4.

Formula Method	Proportion Expressed as Two Ratios	Proportion Expressed as Two Fractions
$\dfrac{\overset{2}{\cancel{5\ mg}}}{\underset{1}{\cancel{2.5\ mg}}} \times 1$ capsule = 2 capsules	1 capsule : 2.5 mg : : x : 5 mg	$\dfrac{1\ capsule}{2.5\ mg} \times \dfrac{x}{5\ mg}$

$$5 = 2.5x$$
$$\frac{5}{2.5} = x$$

Give 2 capsules po $\times$ 1.

2 capsules = x

5. Step 1. Find the BSA in m^2 = 1.4

   Step 2. Determine the safe dose.

   900 mg
   $\times$ 1.4
   1260 mg/day

   Step 3. 250 mg $\times$ 5 = 1250 mg/day. The order is safe.

Step 4. Calculate using both dosage supplies.

Formula Method	Proportion Expressed as Two Ratios	Proportion Expressed as Two Fractions
$\dfrac{\overset{5}{\cancel{250}} \text{ mg}}{\underset{4}{\cancel{200}} \text{ mg}} \times 1 \text{ tablet} = 1.25 \text{ tablet}$	$1 \text{ tablet} : 200 \text{ mg} :: x : 250 \text{ mg}$	$\dfrac{1 \text{ tablet}}{200 \text{ mg}} \times \dfrac{x}{250 \text{ mg}}$

$$250 = 200x$$
$$\frac{250}{200} = x$$
$$1.25 \text{ tablets} = x$$

Formula Method	Proportion Expressed as Two Ratios	Proportion Expressed as Two Fractions
$\dfrac{\overset{5}{\cancel{250}} \text{ mg}}{\underset{6}{\cancel{300}} \text{ mg}} \times 1 \text{ tablet} = 0.83 \text{ tablet}$	$1 \text{ tablet} : 300 \text{ mg} :: x : 250 \text{ mg}$	$\dfrac{1 \text{ tablet}}{300 \text{ mg}} = \dfrac{x}{250 \text{ mg}}$

Use the 200-mg tablets to give 1.25 tablets.

$$250 = 300x$$
$$\frac{250}{300} = x$$
$$0.83 \text{ tablet} = x$$

Self Test 4 Parenteral Medication Calculations

1. Step 1. The safe dose is 50 to 100 mg/kg/24 hr.

Low Dose	*High Dose*
50 mg	100 mg
× 8 kg	× 8 kg
400 mg/24 hr	800 mg/24 hr

Order is 200 mg q6h (4 doses).

200 mg × 4 = 800 mg/24 hr. Dose is safe.

Step 2. Minimum safe dilution is 50 mg/mL.

$$50 \overline{)200 \text{ mg}} \quad \text{4 mL is the minimum dilution}$$

A total of 10 mL is safe.

Step 3. Dilute 750 mg with 8 mL sterile water to make 90 mg/mL.

Formula Method	Proportion Expressed as Two Ratios	Proportion Expressed as Two Fractions
$\dfrac{200 \text{ mg}}{90 \text{ mg}} \times 1 \text{ mL} = 2.2 \text{ mL (calculator)}$	$1 \text{ mL} : 90 \text{ mg} :: x : 200 \text{ mg}$	$\dfrac{1 \text{ mL}}{90 \text{ mg}} \times \dfrac{x}{200 \text{ mg}}$

$$200 = 90x$$
$$\frac{200}{90} = x$$
$$2.2 \text{ mL} = x$$

Withdraw 2.2 mL of the drug into a syringe. Label the remainder and store in the refrigerator.

Step 4. Add about 5 mL D5½NS to the Buretrol.

Add the 2.2 mL of drug. Add more D5¼NS to make 10 mL.

Step 5. Set the pump at 20. This means 20 mL/hr. The pump will deliver 10 mL in 30 minutes.

Step 6. When the IV is finished, add a 20-mL flush of D5½NS to clear the tubing of medication.

2. Step 1. The safe dose is 8 to 10 mg/kg/24 hours given q12h.

Low Dose	*High Dose*
8 mg	10 mg
× 15 kg	× 15 kg
120 mg/24 hr	150 mg/24 hr

Order is 75 mg q12h (two doses) = 150 mg/24 hr. The dose is safe.

Step 2. The minimum safe dilution is 1 mL in 15 to 25 mL. The drug comes as a liquid, 80 mg/5 mL.

Formula Method	**Proportion Expressed as Two Ratios**	**Proportion Expressed as Two Fractions**
$\frac{75 \text{ mg}}{80 \text{ mg}} \times 5 \text{ mL} = 4.7 \text{ mL (calculator)}$	5 mL : 80 mg :: x : 75 mg	$\frac{5 \text{ mL}}{80 \text{ mg}} \times \frac{x}{75 \text{ mg}}$
$375 = 80x$		$375 = 80x$
$\frac{375}{80} = x$		$\frac{375}{80} = x$
		$4.7 \text{ mL} = x$

Step 3. 75 mL D5W is a safe concentration (more than 70.5 mL).

Step 4. Draw up 4.7 mL drug into a syringe. Discard the remainder.

Step 5. Add about 50 mL D5W to the Buretrol. Add the 4.7 mL medication. Now add D5W until 75 mL is reached. Order is to administer over 1 hr. Set the pump at 75.

Step 6. When the IV is completed, add a 20-mL flush of D5W to clear the tubing of medication.

3. Step 1. The safe dose range is 3 to 5 mg/kg/24 hr given q8h.

Low Dose	*High Dose*
3 mg	5 mg
× 40 kg	× 40 kg
120 mg/24 hr	200 mg/24 hr

Order is 100 mg q8h (3 doses).

100 mg × 3 = 300 mg. Dose is not safe. Contact the physician or healthcare provider.

4. Step 1. The safe dose is 50 to 200 mg/kg/24 hr given q6h.

Low Dose	*High Dose*
50 mg	200 mg
× 18 kg	× 18 kg
900 mg/24 hr	3600 mg/24 hr

The order is 900 mg q6h (4 doses).

900 mg × 4 = 3600 mg/24 hr

The dose is safe.

Step 2. The minimum safe dilution is 50 mg/mL.

$$50 \text{ mg} \overline{)900 \text{ mg}} \quad \frac{18}{}$$

18 mL is the minimum safe dilution.

25 mL is safe.

Step 3. 1-g powder.

Dilute with 10 mL to make 95 mg/mL.

Formula Method	Proportion Expressed as Two Ratios	Proportion Expressed as Two Fractions
$\dfrac{900 \text{ mg}}{95 \text{ mg}} \times 1 \text{ mL} = 9.5 \text{ mL drug}$	$1 \text{ mL} : 95 \text{ mg} :: x : 900 \text{ mg}$	$\dfrac{1 \text{ mL}}{95 \text{ mg}} \diagdown \dfrac{x}{900 \text{ mg}}$

$$900 = 95x$$

$$\frac{900}{95} = x$$

Draw up the 9.5 mL in a syringe.　　　　　　$9.5 \text{ mL} = x$

Discard the remainder; the amount is too small to keep.

Step 4. Add about 10 mL of D5½NS to the Buretrol. Add the 9.5 mL medication. Add D5½NS to make a total of 25 mL.

Step 5. Set the pump at 50. The pump will deliver 25 mL in 30 minutes.

Step 6. When the IV is finished, add a flush of 20 mL D5½NS to clear the tubing of medication.

5. Step 1. The safe dose is 100 to 200 mg/kg/24 hr.

Low Dose	High Dose
100 mg	200 mg
× 6 kg	× 6 kg
600 mg/24 hr	1200 mg/24 hr

Order is 150 mg q8h (three doses) = 450 mg/24 hr

The dose is below range and is q8h. The literature states q6h.

Step 2. The minimum safe dilution is 6 mg/mL.

The order is 150 mg.

$$6\overline{)150}\ \ \underset{}{\overset{25}{}} = 25 \text{ mL}$$

The dilution of 10 mL does not meet concentration requirements. It should be 25 mL. Consult with the physician or healthcare provider regarding the dose, times of administration, and dilution.

6. Step 1. Determine the safe dose.

Low Dose	High Dose
0.05 mg	0.1 mg
× 30 kg	× 30 kg
1.5 mg	3 mg

Step 2. The dose is safe.

Step 3. Supply: 1 mg = 1 mL

2.5 mg = 2.5 mL

Step 4. Dilute in at least 5 mL NS and administer over 4 to 5 minutes.

7. Step 1. Determine the safe dose.

Low Dose	High Dose
0.08 mg	0.3 mg
× 25 kg	× 25 kg
2 mg/day	7.5 mg/day

Step 2. The dose is slightly high. Consult the physician or healthcare provider. 4 mg bid = 8 mg/day.

Step 3. Supply is 4 mg/mL. Give 1 mL after notifying physician of higher dose.

Step 4. Give 1 mL undiluted over 30 seconds or less.

8. Step 1. Determine the safe dose.

Ordered dose (25 mg) is within 12.5–25-mg range.

Step 2. The dose is safe.

q4h: 25 mg × 6 hours = 150 mg

q6h: 25 mg × 4 hours = 100 mg

It does not exceed 300 mg/24 hr.

Step 3.

Formula Method	Proportion Expressed as Two Ratios	Proportion Expressed as Two Fractions
$\dfrac{\overset{1}{\cancel{25}}\ \text{mg}}{\underset{2}{\cancel{50}}\ \text{mg}} \times 1\ \text{mL} = 0.5\ \text{mL}$	$1\ \text{mL} : 50\ \text{mg} :: x : 25\ \text{mg}$	$\dfrac{1\ \text{mL}}{50\ \text{mg}} \times \dfrac{x}{25\ \text{mg}}$

$$25 = 50x$$

Step 4. Give 0.5 mL undiluted IVP over 1 minute.

$$\frac{25}{50} = x$$

9. Step 1. Determine the safe dose.

$$0.5\ \text{mL} = x$$

Low Dose	High Dose
6 mcg/kg	7.5 mcg/kg
× 6.82 kg	× 6.82 kg
40.92 mcg/day	51.15 mcg/day

Step 2. The dose is safe (50 mcg/day).

Step 3. Calculate the dose.

0.1 mg = 100 mcg/1 mL

Formula Method	Proportion Expressed as Two Ratios	Proportion Expressed as Two Fractions
$\dfrac{\overset{1}{\cancel{50}}\ \text{mcg}}{\underset{2}{\cancel{100}}\ \text{mcg}} \times 1\ \text{mL} = 0.5\ \text{mL}$	$1\ \text{mL} : 100\ \text{mcg} :: x : 50\ \text{mg}$	$\dfrac{1\ \text{mL}}{100\ \text{mcg}} \times \dfrac{x}{50\ \text{mcg}}$

$$50 = 100x$$

$$\frac{50}{100} = x$$

$$0.5\ \text{mL} = x$$

Step 5. Give 0.5 mL undiluted or diluted in 4 mL D5W or NS over 5 minutes.

10. Step 1. Determine the safe dose.

Low Dose	High Dose
0.5 mg/kg	1.7 mg/kg
× 36.36 kg	× 36.36 kg
18.18 mg/day	61.81 mg/day

Step 2. 60 mg bid = 60 mg × 2 = 120 mg/day

The dose is too high. Contact the physician or healthcare provider.

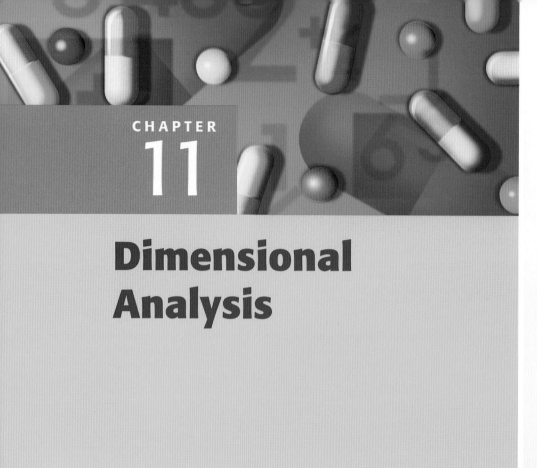

Dimensional Analysis

A fourth method of dosage calculation is called dimensional analysis. This method is used extensively in mathematics and science, especially chemistry calculations. Students often say that once you master dimensional analysis, you tend to use it all the time, because it is simpler and more accurate than the other methods.

The dimensional analysis method uses terminology similar to that of other calculation methods. There are several ways to set up the dimensional analysis equation. As elsewhere in this book, the problems below start with a desired dose, using a supply or "available" amount. First you set up the entire equation with a numerator and a denominator, and then you solve the equation.

After learning dimensional analysis, you may want to go back to the other chapters and solve the problems in the proficiency tests using this new method. The answers to the proficiency tests in this chapter are worked in dimensional analysis as well as in the formula and proportion methods.

Oral Solid Medication Equation and Calculation

Start by calculating an equation for a simple oral solid medication:

Example

Order: Champix (varenicline) 0.75 mg po every day

Supply: Champix 0.5 mg scored tablets (Fig. 11-1)

Write the desired dose first in the numerator:

0.75 mg

Then write the available dose as a fraction:

1 tablet

0.5 mg

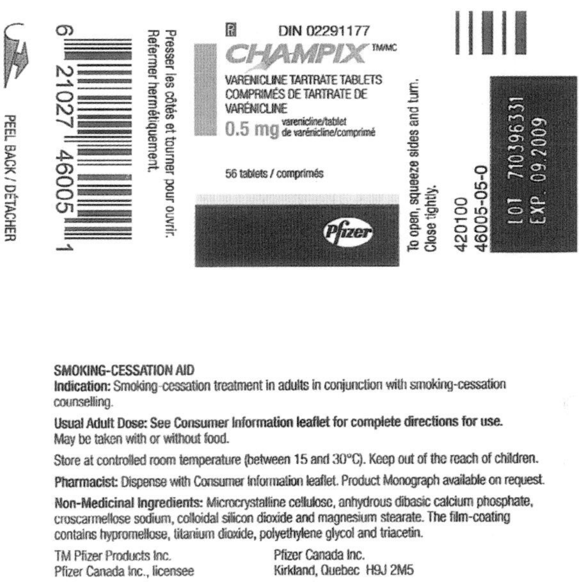

FIGURE 11-1

Label for Champix. (Used with permission of Pfizer Inc.)

Now combine both of these (note that the dimensional analysis setup resembles a proportion expressed as two fractions).

$$\frac{0.75\,\text{mg}}{} \; \Bigg| \; \frac{1\ \text{tablet}}{0.5\ \text{mg}}$$

According to the basic rules of reducing fractions (review Chapter 1 if necessary), the two "mg" designations cancel each other. Reduce the numbers if possible. Divide both numbers by 0.5.

$$\frac{\overset{1.5}{\cancel{0.75\,\text{mg}}}}{} \; \Bigg| \; \frac{1\ \text{tablet}}{\underset{1}{\cancel{0.5\,\text{mg}}}}$$

The setup should now look like this:

$$\frac{1.5}{} \; \Bigg| \; \frac{1\ \text{tablet}}{1}$$

> **FINE POINTS** ● ○ ● ●
>
> When reducing fractions, first attempt to divide the denominator evenly by the numerator.

Multiply the numerators, multiply the denominators, and then divide the product of the numerators by the product of the denominators. In this example, the numbers in the numerator are $1.5 \times 1 = 1.5$. The only number in the denominator is 1. Divide by 1 to get: 1.5 or 1½ tablets.

$$\frac{1.5}{} \; \Bigg| \; \frac{1\ \text{tablet}}{1} \; \Bigg| \; \frac{1.5 \times 1}{1} = 1.5 \text{ or } 1\tfrac{1}{2} \text{ tablets}$$

Give 1½ tablets po every day.

Example

Order: Avapro (irbesartan) 300 mg po every day

Supply: See Figure 11-2.

The dose desired is 300 mg. The supply is 1 tablet = 150 mg.

The equation would look like

$$\frac{300\ \text{mg}}{} \; \Bigg| \; \frac{1\ \text{tablet}}{150\ \text{mg}}$$

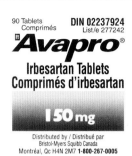
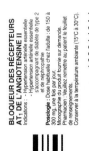

90 Tablets
Comprimés
DIN 02237924
List/e 277242

ANGIOTENSIN II AT₁ RECEPTOR BLOCKER

FIGURE 11-2

Label for Avapro. (Used with permission of Bristol-Meyers Squibb Canada.)

Cancel the "mg." Reduce the fraction. Solve.

$$\frac{\overset{2}{\cancel{300}} \text{ mg}}{1} \cdot \frac{1 \text{ tablet}}{\cancel{150} \text{ mg}} \quad \frac{2 \times 1}{1} = 2 \text{ tablets}$$

Give 2 tablets po every day.

FINE POINTS

Drawing a "circle" around the desired measurement system helps you know what you are solving for. This reminder is especially helpful when the equation becomes more complex.

Oral Liquid Medication Equation and Calculation

Follow the same basic rules of setting up the equation, using either the liquid medication available or the supply dose.

Example

Order: Amoxicillinoral suspension 100 mg po every day × 4 days

Supply: See Figure 11-3.

The equation is

$$\frac{100 \text{ mg}}{} \cdot \frac{5 \text{ mL}}{125 \text{ mg}}$$

Cancel the "mg." Reduce the fraction by dividing both numbers by 50. Continue the equation by multiplying the numerators and/or multiplying the denominators. Solve.

$$\frac{\overset{4}{\cancel{100}} \text{ mg}}{} \cdot \frac{5 \text{ mL}}{\underset{5}{\cancel{125}} \text{ mg}} \cdot \frac{4 \times 5}{5} = 4 \text{ mL}$$

Give 4 mL po every day × 4 days.

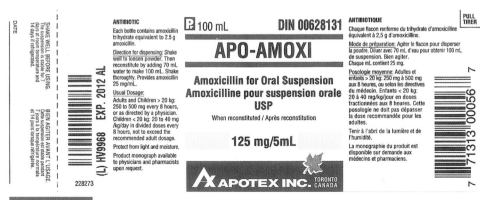

FIGURE 11-3

Label for amoxicillin for oral suspension. (Used with permission of Apotex Inc.)

FIGURE 11-4

Label for midazolam. (Copyright of Sandoz Canada Inc. All rights reserved.)

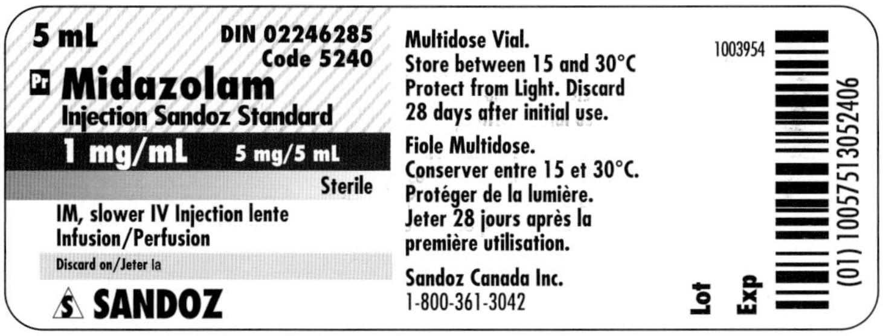

Parenteral Liquid Medication Equation and Calculation

Follow the same rules as with oral liquid.

Example

Order: midazolam 2.5 mg IV q3–4h prn

Supply: See Figure 11-4.

The equation is

$$\begin{array}{c|c} 2.5\text{ mg} & 1\text{ mL} \\ \hline & 1\text{ mg} \end{array}$$

Cancel the "mg." The fraction is already reduced. Solve.

$$\begin{array}{c|c|c} 2.5\ \cancel{\text{mg}} & 1\text{ mL} & 2.5\times 1 \\ \hline & 1\ \cancel{\text{mg}} & 1 \end{array} = 2.5 \text{ or } 2\tfrac{1}{2}\text{ mL}$$

Give 2½ mL IV q3–4h prn. Follow dilution and administration guidelines.

Insulin Equation and Calculation

Follow the same basic setup. The equation is the answer.

Example

Order: Humulin R 10 units subcutaneously now

Supply: See Figure 11-5.

The equation is

$$\begin{array}{c|c} 10\text{ units} & \\ \hline & \end{array} = 10\text{ units}$$

Use an insulin syringe.

Give 10 units subcutaneously.

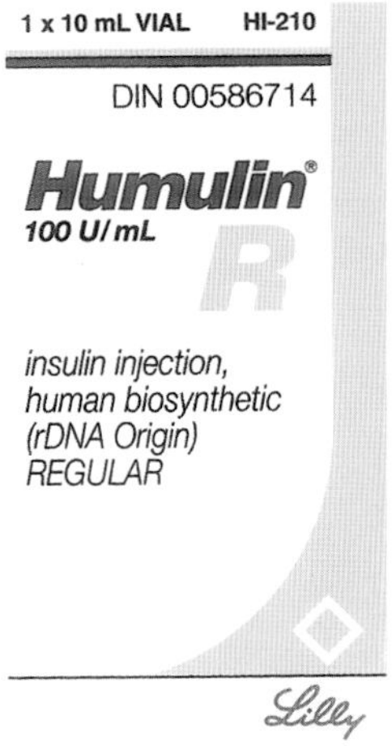

FIGURE 11-5

Label for Humulin R. (Used with permission of Eli Lilly Canada Inc.)

STEPS TO SETTING UP A DIMENSIONAL ANALYSIS PROBLEM

1. Identify the desired dose. Place it in the numerator.

2. Identify the supply or available dose.

3. Identify what you are solving for (this is stated in the problem). Draw a "circle" around this measurement system.

4. Combine steps 1 and 2. Set up the problem so that the measurement systems that you do not need for the answer will cancel each other. This should leave the measurement system desired on the top of the equation.

5. If possible, reduce the fraction. Cancel out any like measurement systems.

6. Multiply the numbers in the numerator. Multiply the numbers in the denominator.

7. Divide the numerator by the denominator.

SELF TEST 1   Calculation of Medications

Solve these problems using dimensional analysis. Answers are given at the end of the chapter. The answers show how to set up the problem and how to solve it.

1. Order: Xanax (alprazolam) 0.5 mg po bid
   Supply: Xanax (alprazolam) 0.25 mg tablets

2. Order: penicillin 800,000 units po q4h × 10 days
   Supply: 1 tablet equals 400,000 units

3. Order: Zithromax (azithromycin) 400 mg po every day × 4 days
   Supply: Zithromax (azithromycin) 200 mg/5 mL

4. Order: Deltasone (prednisone) 10 mg po tid
   Supply: tablets labelled 2.5 mg

5. Order: Lasix (furosemide) 60 mg po every day
   Supply: scored tablets labelled 40 mg

6. Order: Demerol (meperidine) 75 mg IV q4–6h prn
   Supply: Demerol (meperidine) 50 mg/mL

7. Order: Lanoxin (digoxin) 0.5 mg IV q4h × 3 doses
   Supply: Lanoxin (digoxin) 0.25 mg/mL

8. Order: heparin 1500 units subcutaneous bid
   Supply: heparin 5000 units/mL

9. Order: morphine 15 mg IV q4h prn
   Supply: morphine 10 mg/mL

10. Order: Solu-Medrol (methylprednisolone) 80 mg IV every day
    Supply: Solu-Medrol (methylprednisolone) 125 mg/2 mL

Dimensional Analysis Method with Equivalency Conversions

If the dosage desired and the dosage available are not in the same measurement system, an additional step is necessary. By using a conversion factor, you can convert the equation so that it contains only one measurement system.

Conversion factor, a term used in dimensional analysis, means the equivalents necessary to convert between systems of measurement. A conversion factor is a ratio of units that equals 1.

Example   **Metric conversion factors**

$$\frac{1 \text{ g}}{1000 \text{ mg}} \quad \text{or} \quad \frac{1000 \text{ mg}}{1 \text{ g}}$$

$$\frac{1 \text{ mg}}{1000 \text{ mcg}} \quad \text{or} \quad \frac{1000 \text{ mcg}}{1 \text{ mg}}$$

Each of these equals 1.

Example   Order: Synthroid (levothyroxine) 150 mcg po every day

Supply: See Figure 11-6. Use 0.075 mg for this example.

$$\frac{150 \text{ mcg} \quad| \quad 1 \text{ tablet}}{\qquad\qquad| \quad 0.075 \text{ mg}}$$

Add a conversion factor to state the answer in mcg. 1 mg = 1000 mcg, so you include this conversion factor.

$$\frac{150 \text{ mcg} \quad| \quad 1 \text{ tablet} \quad| \quad 1 \text{ mg}}{\qquad\qquad| \quad 0.075 \text{ mg} \quad| \quad 1000 \text{ mcg}}$$

Solve the problem in the same way as previous dimensional analysis examples. Cancel the measurement systems. Then reduce the fraction (dividing 50 into both 150 and 1000).

$$\frac{\overset{3}{\cancel{150}} \text{ mcg} \quad| \quad 1 \text{ tablet} \quad| \quad 1 \text{ mg}}{\qquad\qquad| \quad 0.075 \text{ mg} \quad| \quad \underset{20}{\cancel{1000}} \text{ mcg}} \quad \frac{3 \times 1 \times 1}{0.075 \times 20} = \frac{3}{1.5} = 2 \text{ or 2 tablets}$$

Give 2 tablets po every day.

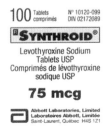
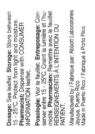

FIGURE 11-6

Label for Synthyroid. (Used with permission of Abbott Laboratories.)

Example   Order: Flumazenil 200 mcg IV over 15 seconds for reversal of anesthesia

Supply: See Figure 11-7.

$$\frac{200\ \text{mcg}}{} \left| \frac{1\ \text{mL}}{0.1\ \text{mg}} \right| \frac{1\ \text{mg}}{1000\ \text{mcg}}$$

Reduce and solve (dividing 200 into both 200 and 1000).

$$\frac{\overset{1}{\cancel{200}}\ \text{mcg}}{} \left| \frac{5\ \text{mL}}{0.5\ \text{mg}} \right| \frac{1\ \text{mg}}{\underset{5}{\cancel{1000}}\ \text{mcg}} \left| \frac{1 \times 1 \times 1}{0.1 \times 5} = \frac{1}{0.5} = 2\ \text{mL} \right.$$

Give 2 mL IV over 15 seconds. Follow institutional requirements for diluting and administering IV drugs.

Place the same units of measurement opposite each other (one in the numerator, the other one in the denominator) in the equation. In this example, the two units of "mg" are placed on opposite sides in the fraction and the two "mcg" are placed on opposite sides. The two "mg" cancel each other and the two "mcg" cancel each other, leaving "mL" as the remaining unit of measurement.

An advantage to dimensional analysis is that you can place any conversion factor within the equation. This helps to reduce errors that may occur because a conversion was not included in the calculation.

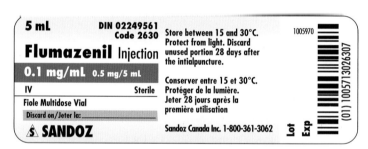

FIGURE 11-7

Label for flumazenil. (Copyright of Sandoz Canada Inc. All rights reserved.)

STEPS TO SETTING UP A DIMENSIONAL ANALYSIS PROBLEM

1. Identify the desired dose. Place it in the numerator.

2. Identify the supply or available dose.

3. Identify what you are solving for (this is stated in the problem). Draw a "circle" around this measurement system.

4. **Identify any conversions needed. Add the conversion factors to the equation. Add these to the equation so that like measurement systems will cancel each other.**

5. Combine steps 1 and 2. Set up the problem so that the measurement systems that you do not need for the answer will cancel each other. This should leave the measurement system desired on the top of the equation.

6. If possible, reduce the fraction. Cancel out any like measurement systems.

7. Multiply the numbers in the numerator. Multiply the numbers in the denominator.

8. Divide the numerator by the denominator.

SELF TEST 2   Calculation of Medications Involving Equivalencies

Solve these problems using dimensional analysis. Answers are given at the end of the chapter. The answers show how to set up the problem and how to solve it.

1. Order: Motrin (ibuprofen) 0.8 g po bid
   Supply: 400-mg tablets

2. Order: Synthroid (levothyroxine) 0.3 mg po every day
   Supply: 300-mcg scored tablets

3. Order: vitamin B_{12} 1 mg IM every week
   Supply: 1000 mcg/mL

4. Order: ampicillin 500 mg IM q6h
   Supply: 1 g/mL

5. Order: epinephrine 0.4 mg subcutaneous × 1
   Supply: 1-mL ampoule 1:1000 (remember, 1:1000 = 1 g in 1000 mL)

6. Order: lidocaine 30 mg subcutaneous
   Supply: ampoule labelled 2% (remember, 2% = 2 g in 1000 mL)

Dimensional Analysis Method with Weight-Based Calculations

Medications that are calculated on the basis of weight will add a further step in the dimensional analysis method: the ordered dose must be multiplied by the weight or BSA.

Example

Order: furosemide 1 mg/kg IV bid for 12-year-old weighing 30 kg

Supply: See Figure 11-8.

Desired dose: 1 mg/kg

Set up the problem so that "kg" is in the denominator.

$$\frac{1 \text{ mg}}{\text{kg}} \Big|$$

Now add the supplied dose.

$$\frac{1 \text{ mg}}{\text{kg}} \Big| \frac{1 \text{ mL}}{10 \text{ mg}}$$

Add the patient's weight in kg.

$$\frac{1 \text{ mg}}{\text{kg}} \Big| \frac{1 \text{ mL}}{10 \text{ mg}} \Big| \frac{30 \text{ kg}}{}$$

Proceed with the rest of the steps. Cancel out "mg" and "kg." Reduce the fraction. Multiply the numerators. Multiply the denominators. Divide the numerator by the denominator

$$\frac{1 \text{ mg}}{\text{kg}} \Big| \frac{1 \text{ mL}}{10 \text{ mg}_{1}} \Big| \frac{\overset{3}{30} \text{ kg}}{} \Big| \frac{1 \times 1 \times 3}{1} = 3 \text{ mL}$$

Give 3 mL IV bid. Follow institutional requirements for diluting and administering IV drugs.

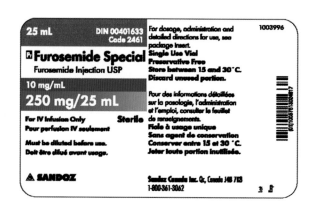

FIGURE 11-8

Label for Furosemide. (Copyright of Sandoz Canada Inc. All rights reserved.)

Example   Order: Demerol (meperidine) 1.5 mg/kg IM q3–4h for pediatric patient weighing 34.1 kg

Supply: See Figure 11-9.

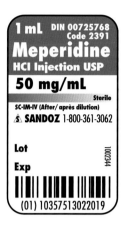

FIGURE 11-9

Label for meperidine. (Copyright of Sandoz Canada Inc. All rights reserved.)

Set up the equation.

$$\frac{1.5 \text{ mg}}{\text{kg}} \left| \frac{1 \text{ mL}}{50 \text{ mg}} \right| \frac{34.1 \text{ kg}}{}$$

Cancel "mg" and "kg". Reduce the fraction. Solve.

$$\frac{1.5 \text{ mg}}{\text{kg}} \left| \frac{1 \text{ mL}}{50 \text{ mg}} \right| \frac{34.1 \text{ kg}}{}$$

$$\frac{1.5 \times 34.1}{50} = 1.02 \text{ or } 1 \text{ mL}$$

Give 1 mL IM q3–4h.

Calculation of Medications Based on BSA

Calculation of medications based on BSA is similar to setting up calculations for medications based on weight.

Example   Order: Zovirax (acyclovir) 500 mg/m^2 infused IV over 1 hour; BSA, 1.1 m^2

Supply: reconstituted vial with concentration of 50 mg/mL

$$\frac{500 \text{ mg}}{\text{m}^2} \left| \frac{1 \text{ mL}}{50 \text{ mg}} \right| \frac{1.1 \text{ m}^2}{}$$

Cancel out the "mg" and the "m^2." Reduce the fraction. Solve.

$$\frac{\overset{10}{\cancel{500} \text{ mg}}}{\cancel{\text{m}^2}} \left| \frac{1 \text{ mL}}{\underset{1}{\cancel{50} \text{ mg}}} \right| \frac{1.1 \text{ m}^2}{} \left| \frac{10 \times 1 \times 1.1}{1} = 11 \text{ mL} \right.$$

Give 11 mL IV over 1 hour.

If the weight-based medication is ordered in several doses, then add another step to the equation with the number of doses ordered. The solution will then be the amount of drug per dose.

Example Order: Solu-Cortef (hydrocortisone) IM 10 mg/m²/day in three divided doses; BSA, 2.0 m²

Available: vial of 25 mg/mL

This example uses: $\dfrac{day}{3\ doses}$

so that the answer will be the amount of drug for each dose.

Set up the equation.

$$\frac{10\ mg}{m^2/day} \left| \frac{1\ mL}{25\ mg} \right| \frac{2.0\ m^2}{} \left| \frac{day}{3\ doses} \right.$$

Cancel "m²," "mg," "day." Reduce the fraction. Solve.

$$\frac{\overset{2}{\cancel{10}}\ \cancel{mg}}{\cancel{m^2/}\ \cancel{day}} \left| \frac{1\ mL}{\underset{5}{\cancel{25}}\ \cancel{mg}} \right| \frac{2.0\ \cancel{m^2}}{} \left| \frac{\cancel{day}}{3\ \cancel{doses}} \right| \frac{2 \times 1 \times 2}{5 \times 3} = \frac{4}{15} = 0.27\ mL/dose$$

Give 0.27 mL IM per dose.

SELF TEST 3 | **Calculation of Medications Using Weight or BSA**

Solve these problems using dimensional analysis. Answers are given at the end of the chapter. The answers show how to set up the problem and how to solve it.

1. Order: Lasix (furosemide) 1 mg/kg IV; weight, 70 kg
   Supply: Lasix (furosemide) 10 mg/mL

2. Order: Augmentin (amoxicillin/clavulanate) 10 mg/kg po bid; weight, 30 kg
   Supply: Augmentin (amoxicillin/clavulanate) 125 mg/5 mL

3. Order: Keflex (cephalexin) 25 mg/kg/day in four divided doses; weight, 22.7 kg
   Supply: Keflex (cephalexin) 250 mg/5 mL
   How much per dose?

4. Order: Decadron (dexamethasone) 0.4 mg/kg/day in four divided doses; weight, 11.4 kg
   Supply: Decadron (dexamethasone) 4 mg/mL
   How much per dose?

5. Order: methotrexate 10 mg/m²/dose every week; BSA, 1.29 m²
   Supply: methotrexate 2.5-mg tablets

Dimensional Analysis Method with Reconstitution of Medications

These calculations are set up with the same method as parenteral calculations. Follow the reconstitution directions and use the result as the dosage available.

Example Order: Rocephin 1 g IV q12h

Supply: Reconstitute with 9.6 mL sterile water to yield 100 mg/mL (Fig. 11-10).
Use the conversion factor of 1 g = 1000 mg.

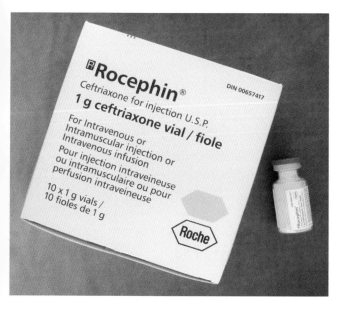

$$\frac{1\ g}{} \left| \frac{1\ \text{mL}}{100\ \text{mg}} \right| \frac{1000\ \text{mg}}{1\ g}$$

Cancel "mg" and "g." Reduce the fraction. Solve.

$$\frac{1\ \cancel{g}}{} \left| \frac{1\ \text{mL}}{\underset{1}{\cancel{100}}\ \cancel{\text{mg}}} \right| \frac{\overset{10}{\cancel{1000}}\ \cancel{\text{mg}}}{1\ \cancel{g}} \left| \frac{1 \times 1 \times 10}{1 \times 1} \right. = 10\ \text{mL}$$

Follow institutional requirements for dilution and administration of IV drugs.

SELF TEST 4 Reconstitution

Solve these problems using dimensional analysis. Answers are given at the end of the chapter. The answers show how to set up the problem and how to solve it.

1. Order: cefonicid 0.5 g IM q12h
   Supply: 1-g vial of powder. Follow reconstitution directions to yield solution 250 mg/mL.

2. Order: penicillin 1 million units IM q6h
   Supply: 5-million-unit vial. Follow reconstitution directions to yield solution
            1 million units/mL.

3. Order: Ancef (cefazolin) 0.3 g IM
   Supply: 500 mg powder. Follow reconstitution directions to yield solution 225 mg/mL.

4. Order: ampicillin/sulbactam 1500 mg IV q8h
   Supply: Unasyn (ampicillin/sulbactam) 1.5-g vial. Follow reconstitution directions to yield
            solution 1.5 g/5 mL.

5. Order: ceftazidime 0.25 g
   Supply: Fortaz (ceftazidime) vial. Follow reconstitution directions to yield solution 500 mg/mL.

Dimensional Analysis Method with Calculation of Intravenous Fluids

Example   Order: D5W 1000 mL over 10 hr

To calculate mL/hr, set up the equation:

$$\frac{1000 \text{ mL}}{10 \text{ hours}}$$

Reduce the fraction.

$$\frac{\overset{100}{\cancel{1000}} \text{ (mL)}}{\underset{1}{\cancel{10}} \text{ (hr)}} \ \frac{100}{1} = 100 \text{ mL/hr}$$

If an infusion pump is used, then the rate will be 100 mL/hr.

If using gravity flow tubing, then the equation will include the drop or tubing factor, and you must convert the "hour" to "minutes." To do this, use the conversion factor:

$$\frac{1 \text{ hour}}{60 \text{ minutes}}$$

Example   Order: D5W 1000 mL over 10 hr

Supply; Drop factor of 20 gtt/mL

$$\frac{1000 \text{ mL}}{10 \text{ hr}} \ \left| \ \frac{20 \text{ (gtt)}}{\text{mL}} \ \right| \ \frac{1 \text{ hr}}{60 \text{ (min)}}$$

Cancel the "mL" and the "hr." Reduce the fraction. Solve.

$$\frac{\overset{100}{\cancel{1000}} \ \cancel{\text{mL}}}{\underset{1}{\cancel{10}} \ \cancel{\text{hr}}} \ \left| \ \overset{1}{\cancel{20}} \text{ (gtt)} \ \right| \ \frac{1 \ \cancel{\text{hr}}}{\underset{3}{\cancel{60}} \text{ (min)}} \ \left| \ \frac{100 \times 1 \times 1}{1 \times 3} = \frac{100}{3} = 33.3 \text{ or } 33 \text{ gtt/min} \right.$$

SELF TEST 5   **Basic IV Calculations and Drop Factors**

Solve these problems using dimensional analysis. Answers are given at the end of the chapter. The answers show how to set up the problem and how to solve it.

1. Order: D5½NS 1000 mL over 8 hr
How many mL/hr?

2. Order: D5W 500 mL over 5 hr
How many mL/hr?

3. Order: NS 250 mL over 5 hr
How many mL/hr?

4. Order: whole blood 500 mL over 4 hr
How many mL/hr?

(continued)

SELF TEST 5 Basic IV Calculations and Drop Factors *(Continued)*

5. Order: NS 250 mL over 2 hr; drop factor, 20 gtt/mL
How many gtt/min?

6. Order: D5W 100 mL over 30 min; drop factor, 15 gtt/mL
How many gtt/min?

7. Order: NS 500 mL over 4 hr; drop factor, 60 gtt/mL
How many gtt/min?

8. Order: D5W 300 mL over 90 min; drop factor 60 gtt/mL
How many gtt/min?

9. Order: NS 1000 mL over 8 hr; drop factor, 20 gtt/mL
How many gtt/min?

10. Order: ½NS 500 mL over 4 hr; drop factor, 10 gtt/mL
How many gtt/min?

Dimensional Analysis Method with Advanced Intravenous Calculations

You can use the dimensional analysis method to calculate medications that are administered with continuous IV infusion. Infusion pumps are always used.

Calculating mL/hr

Example

Order: heparin 1200 units/hr per infusion pump

How many mL/hr? (Infusion pumps are set in mL/hr)

Supply: See Figure 11-11. Heparin 25,000 units in 500 mL ½NS

Set up the equation.

$$\frac{1200 \text{ units}}{\text{hr}} \Bigg| \frac{500 \text{ mL}}{25000 \text{ units}}$$

Cancel "units." Reduce the fraction. Solve.

$$\frac{1200\ \cancel{\text{units}}}{\text{hr}} \Bigg| \frac{\overset{1}{\cancel{500}}\ \text{mL}}{\underset{50}{\cancel{25000}}\ \cancel{\text{units}}} \Bigg| \frac{1200}{50} = 24 \text{ mL/hr}$$

Set pump at 24 mL/hr.

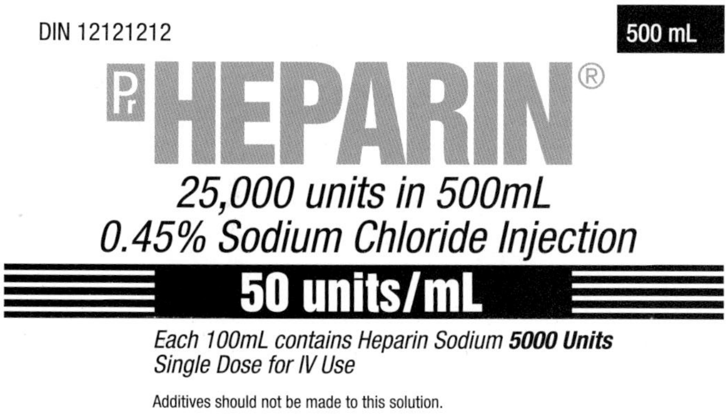
DIN 12121212
500 mL
HEPARIN®
25,000 units in 500mL
0.45% Sodium Chloride Injection
50 units/mL
Each 100mL contains Heparin Sodium 5000 Units
Single Dose for IV Use
Additives should not be made to this solution.

FIGURE 11-11
Label for Heparin IV solution.

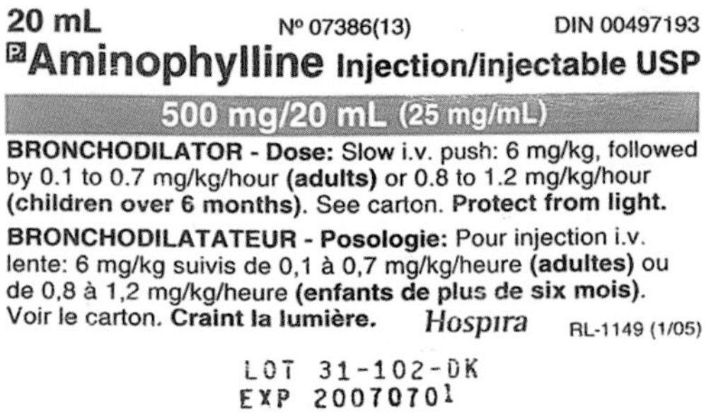

20 mL   №º 07386(13)   DIN 00497193
Ⓟ Aminophylline Injection/injectable USP

500 mg/20 mL (25 mg/mL)

BRONCHODILATOR - Dose: Slow i.v. push: 6 mg/kg, followed
by 0.1 to 0.7 mg/kg/hour **(adults)** or 0.8 to 1.2 mg/kg/hour
(children over 6 months). See carton. Protect from light.

BRONCHODILATATEUR - Posologie: Pour injection i.v.
lente: 6 mg/kg suivis de 0,1 à 0,7 mg/kg/heure **(adultes)** ou
de 0,8 à 1,2 mg/kg/heure **(enfants de plus de six mois).**
Voir le carton. **Craint la lumière.**   *Hospira*   RL-1149 (1/05)

LOT 31-102-DK
EXP 20070701

FIGURE 11-12

Label for aminophylline. (Used with permission
of Hospira.)

Example

Order: aminophylline 30 mg/hr per infusion pump

How many mL/hr?

Supply: See Figure 11-12. Aminophylline 500 mg/500 mL D5W

Set up the equation.

$$\frac{30 \text{ mg}}{\text{hr}} \Bigg| \frac{500 \text{ mL}}{500 \text{ mg}}$$

Cancel "mg." Reduce the fraction. Solve.

$$\frac{30 \text{ mg}}{\text{hr}} \Bigg| \frac{\overset{1}{500} \text{ mL}}{\underset{1}{500} \text{ mg}} \Bigg| \frac{30}{1} = 30 \text{ mL/hr}$$

Set the infusion pump at 30 mL/hr.

Calculating mg/hr or units/hr

You can also use dimensional analysis to determine how much of a given drug is infusing per an infusion
pump.

Example

Order: heparin 10 mL/hr per infusion pump

How many units infusing per hour?

Supply: heparin 25,000 units/500 mL ½NS.

Set up the equation.

$$\frac{10 \text{ mL}}{\text{hr}} \Bigg| \frac{25{,}000 \text{ units}}{500 \text{ mL}}$$

Cancel "mL." Reduce the fraction. Solve.

$$\frac{10 \text{ mL}}{\text{hr}} \Bigg| \frac{\overset{50}{25{,}000} \text{ units}}{\underset{1}{500} \text{ mL}} \Bigg| \frac{10 \times 50}{1} = 500 \text{ units/hr}$$

Example

Order: calcium gluconate 25 mL/hr

How many grams are infusing per hour?

Supply: calcium gluconate 1 g in 100 mL D5W.

Set up the equation.

$$\frac{25 \text{ mL}}{\text{hr}} \left| \frac{1 \text{ g}}{100 \text{ mL}} \right.$$

Cancel "mL." Reduce the fraction. Solve.

$$\frac{\overset{1}{\cancel{25}} \text{ } \cancel{\text{mL}}}{\text{hr}} \left| \frac{1 \text{ g}}{\underset{4}{\cancel{100}} \text{ } \cancel{\text{mL}}} \right| \frac{1}{4} = \frac{1}{4} \text{ or } 0.25 \text{ g/hr}$$

Calculating mL/hr for Drugs Ordered in mg or mcg/min

Vasoactive drugs are ordered in dosages per minute. Use the conversion factor: $\dfrac{60 \text{ min}}{1 \text{ hr}}$

Example

Order: procainamide 3 mg/min per infusion pump

How many mL/hr?

Supply: Procainamide 100 mg/mL 10 mL vial Fig. 11-13. Add to D5W 250 mL

Final concentration: procainamide 1 g/250 mL (4 mg/mL)

Set up the equation. Use the conversion factor $\dfrac{1 \text{ g}}{1000 \text{ mg}}$.

Use $\dfrac{60 \text{ min}}{1 \text{ hr}}$ because the order is in minutes but the answer will be in hours.

$$\frac{3 \text{ mg}}{\text{min}} \left| \frac{250 \text{ mL}}{1 \text{ g}} \right| \frac{1 \text{ g}}{1000 \text{ mg}} \left| \frac{60 \text{ min}}{\text{hr}} \right.$$

Cancel "mg," "g," and "min." Reduce the fraction. Solve.

$$\frac{3 \text{ } \cancel{\text{mg}}}{\cancel{\text{min}}} \left| \frac{\overset{1}{\cancel{250}} \text{ } \cancel{\text{mL}}}{1 \text{ } \cancel{\text{g}}} \right| \frac{1 \text{ } \cancel{\text{g}}}{\underset{4}{\cancel{1000}} \text{ } \cancel{\text{mg}}} \left| \frac{60 \text{ } \cancel{\text{min}}}{\text{hr}} \right| \frac{3 \times 1 \times 1 \times 60}{1 \times 4} = \frac{180}{4} = 45 \text{ mL/hr}$$

Set the infusion pump at 45 mL/hr to deliver 3 mg/min.

Example

Order: nitroglycerine 30 mcg/min per infusion pump

How many mL/hr?

Supply: nitroglycerine 50 mg in 250 mL D5W

Set up the equation. Use the conversion factor: $\dfrac{1 \text{ mg}}{1000 \text{ mcg}}$.

$$\frac{30 \text{ mcg}}{\text{min}} \left| \frac{250 \text{ mL}}{50 \text{ mg}} \right| \frac{1 \text{ mg}}{1000 \text{ mcg}} \left| \frac{60 \text{ min}}{\text{hr}} \right.$$

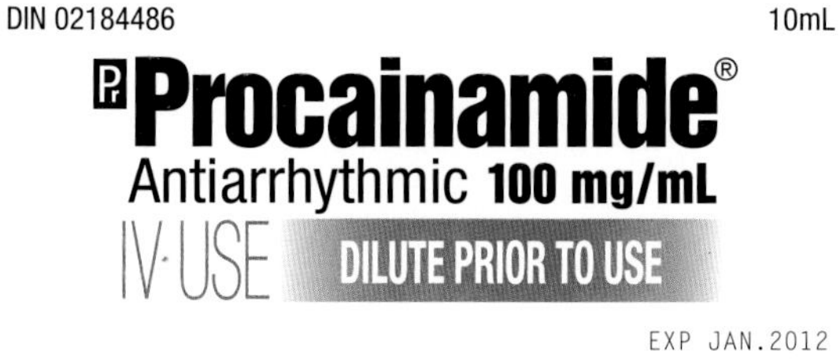

DIN 02184486   10mL

ℙProcainamide®

Antiarrhythmic **100 mg/mL**

IV·USE **DILUTE PRIOR TO USE**

EXP JAN.2012

FIGURE 11-13

Label for procainamide. (Copyright of Sandoz Canada Inc. All rights reserved.)

Cancel "mcg," "mg," and "min." Reduce the fraction. Solve.

$$\frac{30 \ \overset{1}{\cancel{mcg}}}{\cancel{min}} \ \bigg| \ \frac{\overset{1}{\cancel{250}} \ \cancel{(mL)}}{\underset{10}{\cancel{50}} \ \cancel{mg}} \ \bigg| \ \frac{1 \ \cancel{mg}}{\underset{4}{\cancel{1000}} \ \cancel{mcg}} \ \bigg| \ \frac{\overset{12}{\cancel{60}} \ \cancel{min}}{\cancel{(hr)}} \ \bigg| \ \frac{30 \times 1 \times 1 \times 12}{10 \times 4} = \frac{360}{40} = 9 \ mL/hr$$

Set the infusion pump at 9 mL/hr to deliver 30 mcg/minute.

Calculating mL/hr for Drugs Ordered in mcg/kg/min

Vasoactive drugs such as dobutamine, dopamine, nipride, and others are ordered in dosages per kilogram per minute. Use the conversion factor: $\dfrac{60 \ min}{1 \ hr}$ to convert minutes to hours.

Example

Order: infuse dobutamine at 2 mcg/kg/min per infusion pump.

How many mL/hr?

Available: dobutamine 250 mg/500 mL D5W; weight, 70 kg (Fig. 11-14). (Label represents a single dose; this will be mixed in 500 mL.)

Set up the equation. Use the conversion factor: $\dfrac{1 \ mg}{1000 \ mcg}$.

$$\frac{2 \ mcg}{kg/min} \ \bigg| \ \frac{500 \ mL}{250 \ (mg)} \ \bigg| \ \frac{1 \ mg}{1000 \ mcg} \ \bigg| \ \frac{70 \ kg}{} \ \bigg| \ \frac{60 \ min}{hr}$$

Cancel "mcg," "mg," "kg," and "min." Reduce the fraction. Solve.

$$\frac{2 \ \cancel{mcg}}{\cancel{kg} / \cancel{min}} \ \bigg| \ \frac{\overset{1}{\cancel{500}} \ \cancel{(mL)}}{\cancel{250} \ \cancel{mg}} \ \bigg| \ \frac{1 \ \cancel{mg}}{\underset{2}{\cancel{1000}} \ \cancel{mcg}} \ \bigg| \ \frac{7 \ \cancel{0} \ \cancel{kg}}{} \ \bigg| \ \frac{60 \ \cancel{min}}{\cancel{(hr)}}$$

$$= \frac{2 \times 1 \times 1 \times 7 \times 60}{25 \times 2} = \frac{840}{50}$$

$$= 16.8 \ or \ 17 \ mL/hr$$

Set the infusion pump at 17 mL/hr to deliver 2 mcg/kg/min for a 70-kg patient.

10 vials x 20 mL

DIN 02242010
Code 2180

℞ Dobutamine Injection USP | Latex-Free Stopper*

12.5 mg/mL   250 mg/20 mL   **Sterile**

| For intravenous infusion only. Must be diluted prior to use. |

Sympathomimetic–IV Infusion After Dilution–Single Use Vial
For dosage, administration and detailed directions for use, see package insert. **Usual Adult Dosage Range :** 2.5 to 10 µg/kg/min. Not recommended for use in children. **Administration:** Must be diluted to at least 50 mL with a compatible intravenous solution. Once diluted, use within 24 hours. **Store between 15 and 30˚C. Protect from light. Discard unused portion.** Product Monograph on request.

Ⓢ **SANDOZ**   LOT : 144177 EXP : 2009–07

FIGURE 11-14

Label for dobutamine. (Copyright of Sandoz Canada Inc. All rights reserved.)

⬤▭ Heparin and Insulin Intravenous Calculations

Heparin Protocol

Weight-based heparin calculations will use a protocol such as the one in Chapter 9 (p. 248). One advantage to the dimensional analysis method is that two calculations will be combined into one equation (see step 2 below).

Sample heparin protocol:

Heparin drip: 25,000 units in 500 mL

Bolus: 80 units/kg

Starting Dose: 18 units/kg/hr

Example

Patient weight is 70 kg.

1. Calculation for bolus dose: 80 units/kg

   The dimensional analysis equation will look like:

   $$\frac{80 \text{ units}}{1 \text{ kg}} \Bigg| \; 70 \text{ kg}$$

   Cancel "kg." Multiply the numerators. Solve.

   $$\frac{80 \text{ units}}{1 \text{ kg}} \Bigg| \frac{70 \text{ kg}}{} \Bigg| \frac{80 \times 70}{} = 5600 \text{ units}$$

2. Infusion rate. The answer will be in mL/hr on an infusion pump.

   Heparin drip: 25000 units in 500 mL.

   Set up the equation:

   $$\frac{80 \text{ units}}{\text{kg/hr}} \Bigg| \frac{500 \text{ mL}}{25000 \text{ units}} \Bigg| \; 70 \text{ kg}$$

   Cancel "kg," "units." Reduce the fraction. Solve.

   $$\frac{18 \text{ units}}{\text{kg/hr}} \Bigg| \frac{\overset{1}{500} \text{ mL}}{\underset{50}{25\,000} \text{ units}} \Bigg| \; 70 \text{ kg} \Bigg| \frac{18 \times 70}{50} = 25.2 \text{ mL/hr}$$

3. The aPTT result 6 hours after the infusion started is 50. According to the table (p. 254), we increase the drip by 1 unit/kg/hr.

   Set up the equation:

   $$\frac{1 \text{ unit}}{\text{kg/hr}} \Bigg| \frac{500 \text{ mL}}{25000 \text{ units}} \Bigg| \; 70 \text{ kg}$$

   Cancel "kg," "units." Reduce the fraction. Solve.

   $$\frac{1 \text{ unit}}{\text{kg/hr}} \Bigg| \frac{\overset{1}{500} \text{ mL}}{\underset{50}{25000} \text{ units}} \Bigg| \; 70 \text{ kg} \Bigg| \frac{70}{50} = 1.4 \text{ mL/hr}$$

   Increase the drip by 1.4 mL : 25.2 + 1.4 = 26.6 mL/hr

   Repeat aPTT in 6 hours and titrate per protocol

Insulin Protocol

Continuous insulin infusions based on blood sugar will use a protocol such as the one in Chapter 9 (p. 251).

Sample insulin protocol:

"If blood glucose > 11.0 mmol/L; give IV Humulin R insulin bolus 2 units."

Initiate infusion rate at the calculated dose:

"Start infusion at 2 units Humulin R per hour"

Supply: Humulin R insulin 50 units in 100 mL 0.9% sodium chloride. (concentration 0.5 units/mL)

Example Blood glucose 12.1 mmol/L

1. Calculate the bolus dose

   The dimensional analysis equation will be:

   $$\frac{1 \text{ mL}}{0.5 \text{ units}} \quad \bigg| \quad 2 \text{ units}$$

   Cancel "units." Multiple the numerators. Solve.

   $$\frac{1 \text{ mL}}{0.5 \text{ units}} \quad \bigg| \quad \frac{2 \text{ units}}{} \quad \bigg| \quad \frac{1 \times 2}{0.5} = 4 \text{ mL}$$

   To calculate the rate to infuse the bolus dose, Literature states to give over 5 minutes. Use the conversion factor 60 min/1 hr to convert minutes to hours.

   $$\frac{4 \text{ mL}}{5 \text{ min}} \quad \bigg| \quad \frac{60 \text{ min}}{1 \text{ hr}}$$

   Cancel "min." Multiple the numerators. Solve.

   $$\frac{4 \text{ mL}}{5 \text{ min}} \quad \bigg| \quad \frac{60 \text{ min}}{1 \text{ hr}} \quad \bigg| \quad \frac{4 \times 12}{1 \times 1} = 48 \text{ mL/hr}$$

2. Calculate the infusion rate

   Supply: Humulin R 50 units in 100 mL 0.9% sodium chloride (concentration 0.5 units/mL)

   Order: blood glucose 12.1 mmol/L. Start infusion at 2 units/hr

   Set up the equation. The answer will be in mL/hr on an infusion pump.

   $$\frac{2 \text{ units}}{1 \text{ hr}} \quad \bigg| \quad \frac{1 \text{ mL}}{0.5 \text{ units}}$$

   Cancel "units." Multiply numerators. Solve.

   $$\frac{2 \text{ units}}{1 \text{ hr}} \quad \bigg| \quad \frac{1 \text{ mL}}{0.5 \text{ units}} \quad \bigg| \quad \frac{2 \times 2}{1 \times 1} = 4 \text{ mL/hr}$$

   Set the infusion pump at 4 mL/hr. 4 mL to be absorbed. Recheck the blood glucose in 1 hour and titrate according to the insulin protocol.

SELF TEST 6   Advanced IV Calculations

Solve these problems using dimensional analysis. Answers are given at the end of the chapter. The answers show how to set up the problem and how to solve it.

1. Order: infuse heparin at 1000 units/hr via infusion pump
   Supply: heparin 25,000 units in 250 mL D5W IV
   How many mL/hr?

2. Order: infuse insulin at 20 units/hr via infusion pump
   Supply: insulin 125 units in 250 mL NS IV
   How many mL/hr?

3. Order: infuse aminophylline at 50 mg/hr via infusion pump
   Supply: aminophylline 250 mg in 250 mL D5W
   How many mL/hr?

4. Order: infuse heparin at 40 mL/hr
   Supply: heparin 25,000 units in 500 mL D5W
   How many units are infusing per hour?

5. Order: infuse aminophylline at 60 mL/hr
   Supply: aminophylline 500 mg/250 mL D5W
   How many mg are infusing per hour?

6. Order: infuse Bretylol (bretylium) 2 mg/min via infusion pump
   Supply: Bretylol (bretylium) 1 g/500 mL D5W
   How many mL/hr?

7. Order: lidocaine 3 mg/min via infusion pump
   Supply: lidocaine 2 g/500 mL D5W
   How many mL/hr?

8. Order: nitroglycerine 20 mcg/min via infusion pump
   Supply: nitroglycerin 50 mg/250 mL D5W
   How many mL/hr?

9. Order: Isuprel (isoproterenol) 5 mcg/min via infusion pump
   Supply: Isuprel (isoproterenol) 2 mg/250 mL D5W
   How many mL/hr?

10. Order: Intropin (dopamine) 5 mcg/kg/min via infusion pump
    Supply: Intropin (dopamine) 200 mg/250 mL D5W; weight, 70 kg
    How many mL/hr?

11. Order: Pitocin (oxytocin) 5 milliunits/min via infusion pump
    Supply: Pitocin (oxytocin) 15 units/250 mL NS
    Solve using the same equation used for questions 8 and 9. Use the equivalency
    1 unit = 1000 milliunits.
    How many mL/hr?

12. Order: Nipride (nitroprusside) 2 mcg/kg/min via infusion pump
    Supply: Nipride (nitroprusside) 50 mg/250 mL D5W; weight, 50 kg
    How many mL/hr?

Solve these problems using the dimensional analysis method. Set up the equation first, then cancel out any like measurement systems, reduce the fraction, and solve. Answers are given in Appendix A.

1. Order: Augmentin (amoxicillin) 500 mg q8h
   Supply: 125 mg/5 mL

2. Order: heparin 5000 units subcutaneous bid
   Supply: heparin 10,000 units/mL

3. Order: Lasix (furosemide) 20 mg IV bid
   Supply: Lasix (furosemide) 40 mg/4 mL

4. Order: Halcion (triazolam) 0.25 mg po at bedtime
   Supply: Halcion (triazolam) 0.125 mg/tablet

5. Order: Tylenol (acetaminophen) elixir 650 mg po q4h
   Supply: Tylenol (acetaminophen) elixir 325 mg/5 mL

6. Order: calcium gluconate 0.5 g IV × 1
   Supply: calcium gluconate 10%

7. Order: Lanoxin (digoxin) 125 mcg IV every day
   Supply: Lanoxin (digoxin) 0.25 mg/mL

8. Order: Amoxil (amoxicillin) 375 mg q6h
   Supply: Amoxil (amoxicillin) 125 mg/5 mL

9. Order: Deltasone (prednisone) 40 mg/m^2 × 1 dose; BSA, 0.44 m^2
   What is the calculated dose?

10. Order: morphine 0.1 to 0.2 mg/kg IM; weight, 15 kg
    Supply: 10 mg/mL

11. Order: Ancef (cefazolin) 0.44 g IM q12h
    Supply: Ancef (cefazolin) vial
    Follow reconstitution directions to yield solution 330 mg/1 mL

12. Order: penicillin 1 million units
    Supply: penicillin vial
    Follow reconstitution directions to yield solution 500,000 units/1 mL.

13. Order: D5W 500 mL over 6 hr
    How many mL/hr?

14. Order: NS 1000 mL over 16 hr
    How many mL/hr?

15. Order: D5W 1000 mL over 10 hr
    Drop factor is 60 gtt/mL. How many gtt/min?

16. Order: D5W 250 mL over 2 hr
    Drop factor is 15 gtt/mL. How many gtt/min?

17. Order: regular insulin 5 units/hr via infusion pump
    Supply: regular insulin 125 units/125 mL NS
    How many mL/hr?

(continued)

18. Order: heparin 1500 units/hr via infusion pump
Supply: heparin 25,000 units/500 mL D5W
How many mL/hr?

19. Order: heparin 30 mL/hr via infusion pump
Supply: heparin 25,000 units/250 mL D5W
How many units infusing per hour?

20. Order: nitroglycerine 15 mcg/min per infusion pump
Supply: nitroglycerine 50 mg/250 mL D5W
How many mL/hr?

21. Order: Pronestyl (procainamide) 2 mg/min per infusion pump
Supply: Pronestyl (procainamide) 2 g/500 mL D5W
How many mL/hr?

22. Order: Dobutrex (dobutamine) 10 mcg/kg/min per infusion pump
Supply: Dobutrex (dobutamine) 500 mg/500 mL D5W; weight, 100 kg
How many mL/hr?

23. Order: Nipride (nitroprusside) 5 mcg/kg/min per infusion pump
Supply: Nipride (nitroprusside) 50 mg/250 mL D5W; weight, 100 kg
How many mL/hr?

24. Order: starting dose heparin 16 units/kg/hr
Supply: heparin 25000 units in 500 mL
Patient's weight 50 kg.
How many mL/hr?

25. Order: heparin bolus dose 60 units/kg
Patient's weight 50 kg.
What is the bolus dose?

26. Order: increase heparin drip by 2 units/kg/hr
Supply: heparin 25000 units/500 mL NS
Current rate: 21.5 mL/hr
Patient's weight: 55 kg.
How many mL/hr?

Answers to Self Tests

Self Test 1 Calculation of Medications

1. $\dfrac{0.5 \text{ mg}}{} \left|\dfrac{1 \text{ tablet}}{0.25 \text{ mg}}\right.$

$$\dfrac{\overset{2}{\cancel{0.5}} \text{ mg}}{} \left|\dfrac{1 \text{ tablet}}{\underset{1}{\cancel{0.25}} \text{ mg}}\right| \dfrac{2 \times 1}{} = 2 \text{ tablets}$$

2. $\dfrac{800{,}000 \text{ units}}{} \left|\dfrac{1 \text{ tablet}}{400{,}000 \text{ units}}\right.$

$$\dfrac{\overset{2}{\cancel{800{,}000}} \text{ units}}{} \left|\dfrac{1 \text{ tablet}}{\underset{1}{\cancel{400{,}000}} \text{ units}}\right| \dfrac{2 \times 1}{} = 2 \text{ tablets}$$

3. $\dfrac{400 \text{ mg}}{} \left|\dfrac{5 \text{ mL}}{200 \text{ mg}}\right.$

$$\dfrac{\overset{2}{\cancel{400}} \text{ mg}}{} \left|\dfrac{5 \text{ mL}}{\underset{1}{\cancel{200}} \text{ mg}}\right| \dfrac{2 \times 5}{} = 10 \text{ mL}$$

4. $\dfrac{10 \text{ mg}}{} \left|\dfrac{1 \text{ tablet}}{2.5 \text{ mg}}\right.$

$$\dfrac{\overset{4}{\cancel{10}} \text{ mg}}{} \left|\dfrac{1 \text{ tablet}}{\underset{1}{\cancel{2.5}} \text{ mg}}\right| \dfrac{4 \times 1}{} = 4 \text{ tablets}$$

5. $\dfrac{60 \text{ mg}}{} \left|\dfrac{1 \text{ tablet}}{40 \text{ mg}}\right.$

$$\dfrac{\overset{3}{\cancel{60}} \text{ mg}}{} \left|\dfrac{1 \text{ tablet}}{\underset{2}{\cancel{40}} \text{ mg}}\right| \dfrac{3 \times 1}{2} = \dfrac{3}{2} = 1.5 \text{ or } 1\tfrac{1}{2} \text{ tablets}$$

6. $\dfrac{75 \text{ mg}}{} \left|\dfrac{1 \text{ mL}}{50 \text{ mg}}\right.$

$$\dfrac{\overset{3}{\cancel{75}} \text{ mg}}{} \left|\dfrac{1 \text{ mL}}{\underset{2}{\cancel{50}} \text{ mg}}\right| \dfrac{3 \times 1}{2} = \dfrac{3}{2} = 1.5 \text{ mL}$$

7. $\dfrac{0.5 \text{ mg}}{} \bigg| \dfrac{1 \text{ mL}}{0.25 \text{ mg}}$

$$\dfrac{\overset{2}{\cancel{0.5}} \text{ mg}}{} \bigg| \dfrac{1 \text{ mL}}{\underset{1}{\cancel{0.25}} \text{ mg}} \bigg| \dfrac{2 \times 1}{1} = 2 \text{ mL}$$

8. $\dfrac{1500 \text{ units}}{} \bigg| \dfrac{1 \text{ mL}}{5000 \text{ units}}$

$$\dfrac{\overset{3}{\cancel{1500}} \text{ units}}{} \bigg| \dfrac{1 \text{ mL}}{\underset{10}{\cancel{5000}} \text{ units}} \bigg| \dfrac{3 \times 1}{10} = \dfrac{3}{10} \text{ or } 0.3 \text{ mL}$$

9. $\dfrac{15 \text{ mg}}{} \bigg| \dfrac{1 \text{ mL}}{10 \text{ mg}}$

$$\dfrac{\overset{3}{\cancel{15}} \text{ mg}}{} \bigg| \dfrac{1 \text{ mL}}{\underset{2}{\cancel{10}} \text{ mg}} \bigg| \dfrac{3 \times 1}{2} = \dfrac{3}{2} = 1.5 \text{ mL}$$

10. $\dfrac{80 \text{ mg}}{} \bigg| \dfrac{2 \text{ mL}}{125 \text{ mg}}$

$$\dfrac{\overset{16}{\cancel{80}} \text{ mg}}{} \bigg| \dfrac{2 \text{ mL}}{\underset{25}{\cancel{125}} \text{ mg}} \bigg| \dfrac{16 \times 2}{25} = \dfrac{32}{25} = 1.28 \text{ or } 1.3 \text{ mL}$$

Self Test 2 Calculation of Medications Involving Equivalencies

1. $\dfrac{0.8 \text{ g}}{} \bigg| \dfrac{1 \text{ tablet}}{400 \text{ mg}} \bigg| \dfrac{1000 \text{ mg}}{1 \text{ g}}$

$$\dfrac{0.8 \cancel{\text{ g}}}{} \bigg| \dfrac{1 \text{ tablet}}{\cancel{400} \text{ mg}} \bigg| \dfrac{\cancel{1000} \text{ mg}}{1 \cancel{\text{ g}}} \bigg| \dfrac{0.8 \times 1 \times 10}{4 \times 1} = \dfrac{8}{4} = 2 \text{ tablets}$$

2. $\dfrac{0.3 \text{ mg}}{} \bigg| \dfrac{1 \text{ tablet}}{300 \text{ mcg}} \bigg| \dfrac{1000 \text{ mcg}}{1 \text{ mg}}$

$$\dfrac{0.3 \cancel{\text{ mg}}}{} \bigg| \dfrac{1 \text{ tablet}}{\cancel{300} \text{ mcg}} \bigg| \dfrac{\cancel{1000} \text{ mcg}}{1 \cancel{\text{ mg}}} \bigg| \dfrac{0.3 \times 1 \times 10}{3 \times 1} = \dfrac{3}{3} = 1 \text{ tablet}$$

3. $\dfrac{1 \text{ mg}}{} \bigg| \dfrac{1 \text{ mL}}{1000 \text{ mcg}} \bigg| \dfrac{1000 \text{ mcg}}{1 \text{ mg}}$

$$\dfrac{1 \cancel{\text{ mg}}}{} \bigg| \dfrac{1 \text{ mL}}{\underset{1}{\cancel{1000}} \text{ mcg}} \bigg| \dfrac{\overset{1}{\cancel{1000}} \text{ mcg}}{1 \cancel{\text{ mg}}} = 1 \text{ mL}$$

4. $\dfrac{500 \text{ mg}}{} \left| \dfrac{1 \text{ mL}}{1 \text{ g}} \right| \dfrac{1 \text{ g}}{1000 \text{ mg}}$

$\dfrac{\overset{1}{\cancel{500}} \cancel{\text{mg}}}{} \left| \dfrac{1 \, \cancel{\text{mL}}}{\cancel{1} \cancel{\text{g}}} \right| \dfrac{\cancel{1} \cancel{\text{g}}}{\underset{2}{\cancel{1000}} \cancel{\text{mg}}} = \dfrac{1}{2}$ or 0.5 mL

5. $1:1000 = 1 \text{ g in } 1000 \text{ mL}$

$\dfrac{0.4 \text{ mg}}{} \left| \dfrac{1000 \text{ mL}}{1 \text{ g}} \right| \dfrac{1 \text{ g}}{1000 \text{ mg}}$

$\dfrac{0.4 \, \cancel{\text{mg}}}{} \left| \dfrac{\overset{1}{\cancel{1000}} \, \cancel{\text{mL}}}{\cancel{1} \cancel{\text{g}}} \right| \dfrac{\cancel{1} \cancel{\text{g}}}{\underset{1}{\cancel{1000}} \cancel{\text{mg}}} = 0.4 \text{ mL}$

6. $2\% = 2 \text{ g in } 100 \text{ mL}$

$\dfrac{30 \text{ mg}}{} \left| \dfrac{100 \text{ mL}}{2 \text{ g}} \right| \dfrac{1 \text{ g}}{1000 \text{ mg}}$

$\dfrac{30 \, \cancel{\text{mg}}}{} \left| \dfrac{\overset{1}{\cancel{100}} \, \cancel{\text{mL}}}{\underset{2}{\cancel{2}} \, \cancel{\text{g}}} \right| \dfrac{\overset{1}{\cancel{1}} \cancel{\text{g}}}{\underset{10}{\cancel{1000}} \cancel{\text{mg}}} = \dfrac{30}{10 \times 2} = \dfrac{30}{20} = 1.5 \text{ mL}$

Self Test 3 Calculation of Medications Using Weight or BSA

1. $\dfrac{1 \text{ mg}}{\text{kg}} \left| \dfrac{1 \text{ mL}}{10 \text{ mg}} \right| \dfrac{70 \text{ kg}}{}$

$\dfrac{1 \, \cancel{\text{mg}}}{\cancel{\text{kg}}} \left| \dfrac{1 \, \cancel{\text{mL}}}{\underset{1}{\cancel{10}} \, \cancel{\text{mg}}} \right| \dfrac{\overset{7}{\cancel{70}} \, \cancel{\text{kg}}}{} = 7 \text{ mL}$

2. $\dfrac{10 \text{ mg}}{\text{kg}} \left| \dfrac{5 \text{ mL}}{125 \text{ mg}} \right| \dfrac{30 \text{ kg}}{}$

$\dfrac{10 \, \cancel{\text{mg}}}{\cancel{\text{kg}}} \left| \dfrac{\overset{1}{\cancel{5}} \, \cancel{\text{mL}}}{\underset{25}{\cancel{125}} \, \cancel{\text{mg}}} \right| \dfrac{30 \, \cancel{\text{kg}}}{} \left| \dfrac{10 \times 30}{25} = 12 \text{ mL} \right.$

3. $\dfrac{25 \text{ mg}}{\text{kg/day}} \left| \dfrac{5 \text{ mL}}{250 \text{ mg}} \right| \dfrac{22.7 \text{ kg}}{} \left| \dfrac{\text{day}}{4 \text{ doses}} \right.$

$\dfrac{\overset{1}{\cancel{25}} \, \cancel{\text{mg}}}{\cancel{\text{kg}} / \text{day}} \left| \dfrac{5 \, \cancel{\text{mL}}}{\underset{10}{\cancel{250}} \, \cancel{\text{mg}}} \right| \dfrac{22.7 \, \cancel{\text{kg}}}{} \left| \dfrac{\cancel{\text{day}}}{4 \, \cancel{\text{doses}}} \right| \dfrac{5 \times 22.7}{10 \times 4} = \dfrac{113.5}{40} = 2.84$

$= 2.8 \text{ mL per dose}$

4. $\dfrac{0.4 \text{ mg}}{\text{kg/day}} \left| \dfrac{1 \text{ mL}}{4 \text{ mg}} \right| \dfrac{11.4 \text{ kg}}{} \left| \dfrac{\text{day}}{4 \text{ doses}} \right.$

$\dfrac{\overset{0.1}{\cancel{0.4}} \, \cancel{\text{mg}}}{\cancel{\text{kg/day}}} \left| \dfrac{1 \, \cancel{\text{mL}}}{\underset{1}{\cancel{4}} \, \cancel{\text{mg}}} \right| \dfrac{11.4 \, \cancel{\text{kg}}}{} \left| \dfrac{\cancel{\text{day}}}{4 \, \cancel{\text{doses}}} \right| \dfrac{0.1 \times 11.4}{4} \left| \dfrac{1.14}{4} \right.$

$= 0.29 \text{ mL per dose}$

5. $\dfrac{10\ \text{mg}}{\text{m}^2}\ \Big|\ \dfrac{1\ \text{tablet}}{2.5\ \text{mg}}\ \Big|\ 1.29\ \text{m}^2$

$\dfrac{\overset{4}{\cancel{10}}\ \cancel{\text{mg}}}{\cancel{\text{m}^2}}\ \Big|\ \dfrac{1\ \cancel{\text{tablet}}}{\underset{1}{\cancel{2.5}}\ \cancel{\text{mg}}}\ \Big|\ 1.29\ \cancel{\text{m}^2}\ \Big|\ 4 \times 1 \times 1.29 = 5.16$ or 5 tablets

Self Test 4 Reconstitution

1. $\dfrac{0.5\ \text{g}}{}\ \Big|\ \dfrac{1\ \text{mL}}{250\ \text{mg}}\ \Big|\ \dfrac{1000\ \text{mg}}{1\ \text{g}}$

$\dfrac{0.5\ \cancel{\text{g}}}{}\ \Big|\ \dfrac{1\ \cancel{\text{mL}}}{\underset{1}{\cancel{250}}\ \cancel{\text{mg}}}\ \Big|\ \dfrac{\overset{4}{\cancel{1000}}\ \cancel{\text{mg}}}{1\ \cancel{\text{g}}}\ \Big|\ \dfrac{0.5 \times 4}{1 \times 1} = 2\ \text{mL}$

2. $\dfrac{1{,}000{,}000\ \text{units}}{}\ \Big|\ \dfrac{1\ \text{mL}}{1{,}000{,}000\ \text{units}}$

$\dfrac{\cancel{1{,}000{,}000}\ \cancel{\text{units}}}{}\ \Big|\ \dfrac{1\ \cancel{\text{mL}}}{5{,}000{,}000\ \cancel{\text{units}}} = 1\ \text{mL}$

3. $\dfrac{0.3\ \text{g}}{}\ \Big|\ \dfrac{1\ \text{mL}}{225\ \text{mg}}\ \Big|\ \dfrac{1000\ \text{mg}}{1\ \text{g}}$

$\dfrac{0.3\ \cancel{\text{g}}}{}\ \Big|\ \dfrac{1\ \cancel{\text{mL}}}{\underset{45}{\cancel{225}}\ \cancel{\text{mg}}}\ \Big|\ \dfrac{\overset{200}{\cancel{1000}}\ \cancel{\text{mg}}}{1\ \cancel{\text{g}}}\ \Big|\ \dfrac{0.3 \times 1 \times 200}{45 \times 1} = \dfrac{60}{45} = 1.33\ \text{mL}$ or 1.3 mL

4. $\dfrac{1500\ \text{mg}}{}\ \Big|\ \dfrac{5\ \text{mL}}{1.5\ \text{g}}\ \Big|\ \dfrac{1\ \text{g}}{1000\ \text{mg}}$

$\dfrac{\cancel{1500}\ \cancel{\text{mg}}}{}\ \Big|\ \dfrac{\overset{1}{\cancel{5}}\ \cancel{\text{mL}}}{1.5\ \cancel{\text{g}}}\ \Big|\ \dfrac{1\ \cancel{\text{g}}}{\underset{2}{\cancel{1000}}\ \cancel{\text{mg}}}\ \Big|\ \dfrac{15 \times 1 \times 1}{1.5 \times 2}\ \Big|\ \dfrac{15}{3} = 5\ \text{mL}$

5. $\dfrac{0.25\ \text{g}}{}\ \Big|\ \dfrac{1\ \text{mL}}{500\ \text{mg}}\ \Big|\ \dfrac{1000\ \text{mg}}{1\ \text{g}}$

$\dfrac{0.25\ \cancel{\text{g}}}{}\ \Big|\ \dfrac{1\ \cancel{\text{mL}}}{\underset{1}{\cancel{500}}\ \cancel{\text{mg}}}\ \Big|\ \dfrac{\overset{2}{\cancel{1000}}\ \cancel{\text{mg}}}{1\ \cancel{\text{g}}}\ \Big|\ 0.25 \times 2 = 0.5\ \text{mL}$

Self Test 5 Basic IV Calculations and Drop Factors

1. $\dfrac{1000 \text{ mL}}{8 \text{ hr}}$

$$\dfrac{\overset{250}{\cancel{1000}} \,\cancel{(\text{mL})}}{\underset{2}{\cancel{8}} \,\cancel{(\text{hr})}} \; \Big| \; \dfrac{250}{2} = 125 \text{ mL/hr}$$

2. $\dfrac{500 \text{ mL}}{5 \text{ hr}}$

$$\dfrac{\overset{100}{\cancel{500}} \,\cancel{(\text{mL})}}{\underset{1}{\cancel{5}} \,\cancel{(\text{hr})}} \; \Big| \; \dfrac{100}{1} = 100 \text{ mL/hr}$$

3. $\dfrac{250 \text{ mL}}{5 \text{ hr}}$

$$\dfrac{\overset{50}{\cancel{250}} \,\cancel{(\text{mL})}}{\underset{1}{\cancel{5}} \,\cancel{(\text{hr})}} \; \Big| \; \dfrac{50}{1} = 50 \text{ mL/hr}$$

4. $\dfrac{500 \text{ mL}}{4 \text{ hr}}$

$$\dfrac{\overset{125}{\cancel{500}} \,\cancel{(\text{mL})}}{\underset{1}{\cancel{4}} \,\cancel{(\text{hr})}} \; \Big| \; \dfrac{125}{1} = 125 \text{ mL/hr}$$

5. $\dfrac{250 \text{ mL}}{2 \text{ hr}} \; \Big| \; \dfrac{20 \text{ gtt}}{\text{mL}} \; \Big| \; \dfrac{1 \text{ hr}}{60 \text{ min}}$

$$\dfrac{\overset{125}{\cancel{250}} \,\cancel{\text{mL}}}{\underset{1}{\cancel{2}} \,\cancel{\text{hr}}} \; \Big| \; \dfrac{\overset{1}{\cancel{20}} \,\cancel{(\text{gtt})}}{\cancel{\text{mL}}} \; \Big| \; \dfrac{1 \,\cancel{\text{hr}}}{\underset{3}{\cancel{60}} \,\cancel{(\text{min})}} \; \Big| \; \dfrac{125 \times 1 \times 1}{1 \times 3} = \dfrac{125}{3} = 41.6 \text{ or } 42 \text{ gtt/min}$$

6. $\dfrac{100 \text{ mL}}{30 \text{ min}} \; \Big| \; \dfrac{15 \text{ gtt}}{\text{mL}}$

$$\dfrac{100 \,\cancel{\text{mL}}}{\underset{2}{\cancel{30}} \,\cancel{(\text{min})}} \; \Big| \; \dfrac{\overset{1}{\cancel{15}} \,\cancel{(\text{gtt})}}{\cancel{\text{mL}}} \; \Big| \; \dfrac{100}{2} = 50 \text{ gtt/min}$$

7. $\dfrac{500 \text{ mL}}{4 \text{ hr}} \; \Big| \; \dfrac{60 \text{ gtt}}{\text{mL}} \; \Big| \; \dfrac{1 \text{ hr}}{60 \text{ min}}$

$$\dfrac{500 \,\cancel{\text{mL}}}{4 \,\cancel{\text{hr}}} \; \Big| \; \dfrac{\overset{1}{\cancel{60}} \, \text{gtt}}{\cancel{\text{mL}}} \; \Big| \; \dfrac{1 \,\cancel{\text{hr}}}{\underset{1}{\cancel{60}} \,\cancel{(\text{min})}} \; \Big| \; \dfrac{500 \times 1 \times 1}{4 \times 1} = \dfrac{500}{4} = 125 \text{ gtt/min}$$

8. $\dfrac{300\ \text{mL}}{90\ \text{min}}\ \Big|\ \dfrac{60\ \text{gtt}}{\text{mL}}$

$$\dfrac{300\ \cancel{\text{mL}}}{\underset{3}{\cancel{90}}\ \cancel{(\text{min})}}\ \Big|\ \dfrac{\overset{2}{\cancel{60}}\ \cancel{(\text{gtt})}}{\cancel{\text{mL}}}\ \Big|\ \dfrac{600}{3} = 200\ \text{gtt/min}$$

9. $\dfrac{1000\ \text{mL}}{8\ \text{hr}}\ \Big|\ \dfrac{20\ \text{gtt}}{\text{mL}}\ \Big|\ \dfrac{1\ \text{hr}}{60\ \text{min}}$

$$\dfrac{1000\ \cancel{\text{mL}}}{8\ \cancel{\text{hr}}}\ \Big|\ \dfrac{\overset{1}{\cancel{20}}\ \cancel{(\text{gtt})}}{\cancel{\text{mL}}}\ \Big|\ \dfrac{1\ \cancel{\text{hr}}}{\underset{3}{\cancel{60}}\ \cancel{(\text{min})}}\ \Big|\ \dfrac{1000\times1\times1}{8\times3} = \dfrac{1000}{24} = 41.6\ \text{or}\ 42\ \text{gtt/min}$$

10. $\dfrac{500\ \text{mL}}{4\ \text{hr}}\ \Big|\ \dfrac{10\ \text{gtt}}{\text{mL}}\ \Big|\ \dfrac{1\ \text{hr}}{60\ \text{min}}$

$$\dfrac{500\ \cancel{\text{mL}}}{4\ \cancel{\text{hr}}}\ \Big|\ \dfrac{\overset{1}{\cancel{10}}\ \cancel{(\text{gtt})}}{\cancel{\text{mL}}}\ \Big|\ \dfrac{1\ \cancel{\text{hr}}}{\underset{6}{\cancel{60}}\ \cancel{(\text{min})}}\ \Big|\ \dfrac{500\times1\times1}{4\times6} = \dfrac{500}{24} = 20.8\ \text{or}\ 21\ \text{gtt/min}$$

Self Test 6 Advanced IV Calculations

1. $\dfrac{1000\ \text{units}}{\text{hr}}\ \Big|\ \dfrac{250\ \text{mL}}{25{,}000\ \text{units}}$

$$\dfrac{1000\ \cancel{\text{units}}}{\cancel{(\text{hr})}}\ \Big|\ \dfrac{\overset{1}{\cancel{250}}\ \cancel{(\text{mL})}}{\underset{100}{\cancel{25{,}000}}\ \cancel{\text{units}}}\ \Big|\ \dfrac{1000}{100} = 10\ \text{mL/hr}$$

2. $\dfrac{20\ \text{units}}{\text{hr}}\ \Big|\ \dfrac{250\ \text{mL}}{125\ \text{units}}$

$$\dfrac{20\ \cancel{\text{units}}}{\cancel{(\text{hr})}}\ \Big|\ \dfrac{\overset{2}{\cancel{250}}\ \cancel{(\text{mL})}}{\underset{1}{\cancel{125}}\ \cancel{\text{units}}}\ \Big|\ 2\times20 = 40\ \text{units/hr} = 40\ \text{mL/hr}$$

3. $\dfrac{50\ \text{mg}}{\text{hr}}\ \Big|\ \dfrac{250\ \text{mL}}{250\ \text{mg}}$

$$\dfrac{50\ \cancel{\text{mg}}}{\cancel{(\text{hr})}}\ \Big|\ \dfrac{\overset{1}{\cancel{250}}\ \cancel{(\text{mL})}}{\underset{1}{\cancel{250}}\ \cancel{\text{mg}}} = 50\ \text{mL/hr}$$

4. $\dfrac{40\ \text{mL}}{\text{hr}}\ \Big|\ \dfrac{25{,}000\ \text{units}}{500\ \text{mL}}$

$$\dfrac{40\ \cancel{\text{mL}}}{\cancel{(\text{hr})}}\ \Big|\ \dfrac{\overset{50}{\cancel{25{,}000}}\ \cancel{(\text{units})}}{\underset{1}{\cancel{500}}\ \cancel{\text{mL}}}\ \Big|\ 40\times50 = 2000\ \text{units/hr}$$

5. $\dfrac{60\ mL}{hr}\ \Big|\ \dfrac{500\ mg}{250\ mL}$

$\dfrac{60\ \cancel{mL}}{\cancel{hr}}\ \Big|\ \dfrac{500\ \overset{2}{\cancel{mg}}\ \textcircled{mg}}{250\ \cancel{mL}_{\ 1}}\ \Big|\ \dfrac{60\times 2}{} = 120\ mg/hr$

6. $\dfrac{2\ mg}{min}\ \Big|\ \dfrac{500\ mL}{1\ g}\ \Big|\ \dfrac{1\ g}{1000\ mg}\ \Big|\ \dfrac{60\ min}{1\ hr}$

$\dfrac{2\ \cancel{mg}}{\cancel{min}}\ \Big|\ \dfrac{\overset{1}{\cancel{500}}\ \textcircled{mL}}{1\ \cancel{g}}\ \Big|\ \dfrac{1\ \cancel{g}}{\underset{2}{\cancel{1000}}\ \cancel{mg}}\ \Big|\ \dfrac{60\ \cancel{min}}{1\ \textcircled{hr}}\ \Big|\ \dfrac{2\times 60}{2} = \dfrac{120}{2} = 60\ mL/hr$

7. $\dfrac{3\ mg}{min}\ \Big|\ \dfrac{500\ mL}{2\ g}\ \Big|\ \dfrac{1\ g}{1000\ mg}\ \Big|\ \dfrac{60\ min}{1\ hr}$

$\dfrac{3\ \cancel{mg}}{\cancel{min}}\ \Big|\ \dfrac{\overset{1}{\cancel{500}}\ \textcircled{mL}}{2\ \cancel{g}}\ \Big|\ \dfrac{1\ \cancel{g}}{\underset{2}{\cancel{1000}}\ \cancel{mg}}\ \Big|\ \dfrac{60\ \cancel{min}}{1\ \textcircled{hr}}\ \Big|\ \dfrac{3\times 1\times 1\times 60}{2\times 2\times 1} = \dfrac{180}{4} = 45\ mL/hr$

8. $\dfrac{20\ mcg}{min}\ \Big|\ \dfrac{250\ mL}{50\ mg}\ \Big|\ \dfrac{1\ mg}{1000\ mcg}\ \Big|\ \dfrac{60\ min}{1\ hr}$

$\dfrac{20\ \cancel{mcg}}{\cancel{min}}\ \Big|\ \dfrac{\overset{5}{\cancel{250}}\ \textcircled{mL}}{\underset{1}{\cancel{50}}\ \cancel{mg}}\ \Big|\ \dfrac{1\ \cancel{mg}}{1000\ \cancel{mcg}}\ \Big|\ \dfrac{60\ \cancel{min}}{1\ \textcircled{hr}}\ \Big|\ \dfrac{20\times 5\times 60}{1000} = \dfrac{6000}{1000} = 6\ mL/hr$

9. $\dfrac{5\ mcg}{min}\ \Big|\ \dfrac{250\ mL}{2\ mg}\ \Big|\ \dfrac{1\ mg}{1000\ mcg}\ \Big|\ \dfrac{60\ min}{1\ hr}$

$\dfrac{5\ \cancel{mcg}}{\cancel{min}}\ \Big|\ \dfrac{\overset{1}{\cancel{250}}\ \textcircled{mL}}{2\ \cancel{mg}}\ \Big|\ \dfrac{1\ \cancel{mg}}{\underset{4}{\cancel{1000}}\ \cancel{mcg}}\ \Big|\ \dfrac{60\ \cancel{min}}{1\ \textcircled{hr}}\ \Big|\ \dfrac{5\times 60}{2\times 4} = \dfrac{300}{8} = 37.5\ or\ 38\ mL/hr$

10. $\dfrac{5\ mcg}{kg/min}\ \Big|\ \dfrac{250\ mL}{200\ mg}\ \Big|\ \dfrac{1\ mg}{1000\ mcg}\ \Big|\ \dfrac{70\ kg}{}\ \Big|\ \dfrac{60\ min}{1\ hr}$

$\dfrac{\overset{1}{\cancel{5}}\ \cancel{mcg}}{kg/min}\ \Big|\ \dfrac{\overset{1}{\cancel{250}}\ \textcircled{mL}}{\underset{40}{\cancel{200}}\ \cancel{mg}}\ \Big|\ \dfrac{1\ \cancel{mg}}{\underset{4}{\cancel{1000}}\ \cancel{mcg}}\ \Big|\ \dfrac{70\ \cancel{kg}}{}\ \Big|\ \dfrac{60\ \cancel{min}}{1\ \textcircled{hr}}\ \Big|\ \dfrac{1\times 1\times 1\times 70\times 60}{40\times 4\times 1} = \dfrac{4200}{160} = 26.2\ or\ 26\ mL/hr$

11.

$$\frac{5 \text{ milliunits}}{\text{min}} \left| \frac{250 \text{ mL}}{15 \text{ units}} \right| \frac{1 \text{ unit}}{1000 \text{ milliunits}} \left| \frac{60 \text{ min}}{1 \text{ hr}} \right.$$

$$\frac{\overset{1}{\cancel{5}} \text{ milliunits}}{\text{min}} \left| \frac{\overset{1}{\cancel{250}} \cancel{\text{mL}}}{\underset{3}{\cancel{15}} \text{ units}} \right| \frac{1 \text{ unit}}{\underset{4}{\cancel{1000}} \text{ milliunits}} \left| \frac{60 \cancel{\text{min}}}{1 \cancel{\text{hr}}} \right| \frac{1 \times 1 \times 1 \times 60}{3 \times 4 \times 1} = \frac{60}{12} = 5 \text{ mL/hr}$$

12.

$$\frac{2 \text{ mcg}}{\text{kg/min}} \left| \frac{250 \text{ mL}}{50 \text{ mg}} \right| \frac{1 \text{ mg}}{1000 \text{ mcg}} \left| 50 \text{ kg} \right| \frac{1 \text{ kg}}{1 \text{ kg}} \left| \frac{60 \text{ min}}{1 \text{ hr}} \right.$$

$$\frac{\overset{1}{\cancel{2}} \cancel{\text{mcg}}}{\text{kg / min}} \left| \frac{\overset{1}{\cancel{250}} \cancel{\text{mL}}}{\underset{25}{\cancel{50}} \cancel{\text{mg}}} \right| \frac{1 \cancel{\text{mg}}}{\underset{4}{\cancel{1000}} \cancel{\text{mcg}}} \left| 50 \text{ kg} \right| \frac{1 \cancel{\text{kg}}}{1 \cancel{\text{kg}}} \left| \frac{60 \cancel{\text{min}}}{1 \cancel{\text{hr}}} \right| \frac{1 \times 1 \times 1 \times 50 \times 1 \times 60}{25 \times 4 \times 1 \times 1} = \frac{300}{100} = 30 \text{ mL/hr}$$

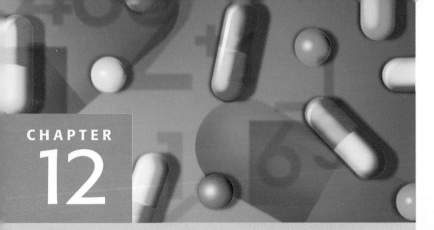

CHAPTER 12

Information Basic to Administering Drugs

LEARNING OBJECTIVES

1. Generic names and trade names

2. Drug classification and drug categories

3. Side effects and adverse effects

4. Basic knowledge essential for safe drug administration

5. Pharmacokinetics

6. Legal considerations: criminal and civil

7. Ethical values in drug administration

8. Information on preparation and administration of medications

In previous chapters, you learned drug forms and preparations, how to read prescriptions, and how to calculate dosages. This chapter provides the opportunity to focus on some of the nurse's responsibilities for drug therapy—drug knowledge, legal and ethical considerations, and finally, specific points that may prove helpful in giving medications.

Drug Knowledge

Nursing drug handbooks are the best references for the nurse who needs a variety of information specifically designed to help assess, manage, evaluate, and teach the patient. The following headings represent the kind of information found in a nursing handbook.

- Generic and trade names
- Classification and category
- Side and adverse effects
- Pregnancy category
- Dosage and route
- Action

- Indications
- Contraindications and precautions
- Interactions and incompatibilities
- Nursing implications
- Signs of effectiveness
- Patient teaching

Two long-standing web sites that include drug information are Health Canada (www.hc.sc.gc.ca) and Rx Med (www.rxmed.com). Nursing publishing companies include drug information on their web sites. Lippincott's is www.nursingcenter.com.

Generic and Trade Names

The generic name, which is not capitalized, is the official name given to a drug. In Canada, a drug can have only one generic name. The letters USP (United States Pharmacopeia) following a generic name indicate that the drug meets government standards for purity and assay.

A trade name is the brand name under which a company manufactures a generic drug. While a drug has only one generic name, it may have several trade names. The trade name is capitalized and is sometimes followed by the symbol ®.

The generic name of MS Contin is morphine sulfate sustained release.

Consumer groups have advocated that drugs be prescribed by generic name only so that the pharmacist may dispense the least expensive drug available on the market. The nurse should understand that generic drugs, because they are manufactured by different companies, are not exactly the same. Although the active ingredient in the drug meets standards of uniformity and purity, manufacturers use different fillers and dyes. These substances can cause adverse effects (e.g., severe nausea caused by the dye used in colouring).

Also, when a pharmacist dispenses the same drug with a different trade name, the patient may become confused and distressed about medication that appears unlike previous doses. While the active ingredient is the same, the medication size, shape, or colour may vary according to trade name and manufacturer.

Drug Classification and Drug Category

Drug classification is a way to categorize drugs by the way they act against diseases or disorders, especially by their effect on a particular area of the body or on a particular condition. A diuretic, for instance, acts on the kidneys; an anticonvulsant prevents seizures. Because drug classifications are a quick reference to a drug's therapeutic actions, uses, and adverse effects, they provide the administering nurse with a drug's general indications, precautions, and nursing implications.

Category (in this text) refers to the way a drug works at the molecular, tissue, or body system level (e.g., beta blocker, SSRI).

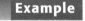 The classification of **morphine sulfate (MS Contin)** is an opioid analgesic, and the category is narcotic antagonist/agonist. This drug's main action and use are to relieve pain; its adverse effects are sedation and respiratory depression. Sometimes it will decrease the effect of other opioids.

Side Effects and Adverse Effects

Side effects are non-therapeutic reactions to a drug. Because these reactions are transient, they may not require any nursing intervention. Side effects occur as a consequence of drug administration; often they are unrelated to the desired action of the drug.

Adverse effects are non-therapeutic effects that may be harmful to the patient and thus require lowering the dosage or discontinuing the drug. Because these effects can be life-threatening, they may require medical intervention.

Drowsiness is a **side effect** that occurs with some antihistamines. A serious decrease in white blood cells (WBCs) is an **adverse effect,** resulting in lowered resistance to infection. The nurse must watch for these effects, know how to manage them, and if necessary, teach the patient about them.

Example **Morphine sulfate (MS Contin)** can cause these side effects: sedation headache, dizziness, nausea, vomiting, dry mouth, and sweating. **Morphine sulfate,** in high doses, can cause these adverse effects: hypotension and drug addiction.

Pregnancy Category

Product monographs may refer to risk factors for drug use during pregnancy (A, B, C, D, or X). They are an indication of the level of risk that the drug poses to the fetus and are the definitions used by the Food and Drug Administration in the US. A brief summary of each category is presented.

A: No risk to the fetus in any trimester

B: No adverse effect demonstrated in animals; no human studies available

C: Studies with animals have shown adverse reactions; no human studies are available; given only after risks to the fetus have been considered

D: Definite fetal risk exists; may be given despite risk to the fetus if needed for a life-threatening condition

X: Absolute fetal abnormality; not to be used anytime during pregnancy

A nurse administering a drug to any woman of child-bearing age should know the pregnancy categories. If the drug has a category of D or X, the nurse should inform the woman of that category's significance and determine whether there is any possibility of the woman being pregnant. If a woman has a confirmed pregnancy, the nurse should find out the pregnancy's current gestational week. The nurse also should use this circumstance as an opportunity to educate the client about the risks of *any* current medication (whether prescribed, over-the-counter, herbal, or nutritional supplement) and its known or potential effects on a fetus.

Example   **MS Contin (morphine sulfate sustained release)** is pregnancy category C, which indicates possible fetal risk.

Dosage and Route

Information about the dosage and route of administration is crucial to protect against medication error. Most handbooks include, for each drug, appropriate dosage ranges for adults, the elderly, and children.

Example   MS Contin (morphine sulfate sustained release)
Adult: Usual initial dose is 30 mg every 12 hours.
Elderly or debilitated: 15 mg every 12 hours.
Those patients already taking oral morphine: divide total daily dosage into two 12 hourly doses.
Dosage in children not determined.
Do not break, chew, or crush tablets. Swallow whole.

Action

Action explains how the drug works—that is, what medical experts know or believe about how the drug acts to produce a therapeutic effect. This knowledge helps the nurse understand whether a drug should be taken with food or between meals, with other drugs or alone, orally, or parenterally.

The nurse who knows drug action can better assess, manage, and evaluate drug therapy. For example, if a particular drug is metabolized in the liver and kidney, then the nurse can apply this knowledge. Because patients with liver or kidney disease may not be able to metabolize or excrete certain drugs, this particular drug could accumulate in the body and possibly cause adverse effects.

Example   **MS Contin (morphine sulfate sustained release)** binds to opiate receptors in the central nervous system (CNS), alters the perception of and response to painful stimuli, and produces generalized CNS depression.

Indications

Indications give the reasons for using the drug. This information helps the nurse watch not only for expected effects and therapeutic response but also for any side effects and adverse effects. One of the most common questions patients ask nurses is "Why am I getting this drug?" With a good understanding of indications, the nurse can answer the patient's question, describing the drug's expected effects.

Often a drug can be used for an indication "off label"—that is, for an indication other than the one(s) "labelled," or approved. The drug may be widely known to be effective in "off-label" conditions because of its side effects (e.g., Benadryl—generic diphenhydramine—causes sleep); or research studies may have proven the drug effective for that particular indication, but the drug hasn't yet been licensed as a treatment for it (e.g., Wellbutrin—generic bupropion—helps a patient stop smoking).

The nurse should become familiar with the typical off-label uses of particular drugs. If a medication order requests a drug for an indication other than the one for which it is labelled and approved, or other than off-label uses with which the nurse is familiar, the nurse should question the medication order.

Example | **MS Contin (morphine sulfate sustained release)** is used to alleviate moderate to severe chronic pain.

Contraindications and Precautions

These terms refer to conditions in which a drug should be either given with caution or not given at all. For instance, patients who have exhibited a previous reaction to penicillin should be cautioned against taking that drug again; if a patient has poor kidney function, certain antibiotics must be administered with caution. Because the nurse has a responsibility to safeguard the patient and carry out effective nursing care, a knowledge of contraindications and precautions is important—especially in relation to patients with glaucoma, renal disease, or liver disease, and patients who are very young or very old.

Example | **MS Contin (morphine sulfate sustained release)** is contraindicated if hypersensitivity to the drug exists or if the patient has a dependency on other opioids. Use this drug cautiously in head trauma, increased intracranial pressure (ICP), severe respiratory disease, undiagnosed abdominal pain, and pregnancy (depressed respirations in newborn). The drug's safety is not established in children.

Interactions and Incompatibilities

When more than one drug is administered at a time, unexpected or non-therapeutic responses may occur. Some interactions are desirable: for example, naloxone (Narcan) is a narcotic antagonist that reverses the effects of a morphine overdose. Other interactions, however, are undesirable: aspirin, for instance, should not be taken with an oral anticoagulant because that combination increases the possibility of an adverse effect (e.g., increased bleeding). The nurse must carefully consider some drug-herbal interactions as well.

Some drugs are incompatible and thus should not be mixed. Knowledge of incompatibilities is especially important when medications are combined for injection in IV administration. *Chemical incompatibility* usually produces a visible sign such as precipitation or colour change. *Physical incompatibility*, however, may not give a visible sign, so the nurse should never combine drugs without checking a suitable reference.

A good rule of thumb: *When in doubt, do not mix.*

COMMON DRUGS AND DRUG CLASSIFICATIONS THAT CAUSE UNEXPECTED OR NON-THERAPEUTIC RESPONSES

Refer to a drug handbook for specific interactions:

- MAO inhibitors–anticonvulsants–lithium
- Tricyclic antidepressants–antifungals–methotrexate
- Alcohol–barbiturates–NSAIDs
- Aluminum–beta blockers–oral contraceptives
- Aminoglycosides–cimetidine–phenothiazines
- Antacids–clonidine–phenytoin
- Anticoagulants–cyclosporine–probenecid
- Heparin–digoxin–rifampin
- Coumadin–erythromycin–theophylline
- ASA–isoniazid

Interactions also may occur between drugs and certain foods. Here are some common examples. The calcium present in dairy products interferes with the absorption of tetracycline. Foods high in vitamin B6 can decrease the effect of an antiparkinsonian drug. Foods high in tyramine, such as wine and cheese, can precipitate a hypertensive crisis in patients taking monoamine oxidase (MAO) inhibitors. Grapefruit juice interferes with the absorption of multiple drugs.

Additionally, cigarette smoke—which can increase the liver's metabolism of drugs—may decrease drug effectiveness. People exposed even to secondhand cigarette smoke may require higher doses of medication.

> **Example** **MS Contin (morphine sulfate sustained release)** produces additive CNS depression with alcohol, antihistamines, and sedative/hypnotics. It can produce withdrawal in patients dependent on opioids and can diminish the analgesic effect. Exercise care when giving to patients receiving MAO inhibitors, because severe reactions are possible. Some manufacturer's recommend avoiding use within 14 days of MAO inhibitors.

Nursing Implications

To administer a drug safely and to assess, manage, and teach the patient, the nurse needs a knowledge of implications: whether the drug should be taken with or without food; what specific vital signs to monitor; and what lab values may be affected by the drug or may need to be ordered to check the drug's effectiveness or toxicity.

> **Example** Some nursing implications related to **MS Contin (morphine sulfate sustained release)** include the following: assess pain both before the dose and after the dose; assess BP, pulse, and respiration both before the dose and periodically after the dose; assess for dependency and for tolerance. It may cause GI upset; take with food if GI upset occurs. It is not to be used to manage acute pain.

Signs of Effectiveness

Few drug references actually list this heading, yet the nurse is expected to evaluate the drug regimen and to record and report observations. Knowledge of the drug's class, its action, and its use helps the nurse understand the expected therapeutic outcomes.

Ampicillin sodium, for instance, is a broad-spectrum antibiotic that is used for urinary, respiratory, and other infections. Signs of effectiveness might include these: normal temperature; the lab report of the WBC count, indicating a normal result; clear urine, no pain on urination, and no WBC in urine; decreased pus in an infected wound; wound healing; a patient showing alertness, interest in surroundings, and improved appetite.

> **Example** For **MS Contin (morphine sulfate sustained release),** signs of effectiveness are relief of pain and sedation.

Teaching the Patient

The patient has a right to know the drug's name and dose, why the drug is ordered, and what effects to expect or watch for. A patient who will be taking a drug at home also needs specific information. Making sure that patients are knowledgeable about their drugs is a professional responsibility shared by three people: the physician or healthcare provider, the nurse, and the pharmacist.

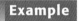 Pharmacokinetics

When a drug is taken *orally,* the villi of the small intestine absorb it, and the bloodstream distributes it to the cells. The body metabolizes the drug to a greater or lesser extent and then excretes it. When a drug is given *parenterally,* it bypasses the gastrointestinal system, entering the circulation more quickly—or, in the case of the intravenous route, immediately. The general term **pharmacokinetics** includes these drug activities: absorption, distribution, biotransformation, and excretion.

Absorption

Effective absorption of an oral drug depends on several conditions: the degree of stomach acidity, the time required for the stomach to empty, whether food is present, the amount of contact with villi in the small intestine, and the flow of blood to the villi.

Other circumstances may affect a drug's absorption too. Enteric-coated (EC) tablets, for instance, are not meant to dissolve in the acidic stomach; they ordinarily pass through the stomach to the duodenum. When a patient receives an antacid along with an EC tablet, the pH of the stomach rises, perhaps causing the tablet to dissolve prematurely—which either can make the drug less potent or can irritate the gastric lining. Timed-release EC capsules that dissolve prematurely can deliver a huge dose of the drug, producing adverse effects.

Here's another example: laxatives increase GI movement and decrease the time a drug is in contact with the villi of the small intestine, where most absorption occurs. The presence of food in the stomach, however, can impair absorption. In particular, foods that contain calcium, such as milk and cheese, form a complex with some drugs and inhibit absorption. Penicillin is a good example of a drug that should be taken on an empty stomach.

Distribution

Distribution describes the drug's movement through body fluids—chiefly the bloodstream—to the cells. Drugs do not travel freely in the blood; instead, most travel attached to plasma proteins, especially albumin. If a drug is not attached to a plasma protein, it can attach to cells and can affect them in various ways.

When the bloodstream contains more than one drug, the drugs may compete for binding with protein sites. One drug may displace another, leaving the displaced drug free to interact with the cells, and its effect on the cells will be more pronounced. Aspirin is a common drug that displaces others; it should not be given with oral anticoagulants, which are 99% bound to albumin. Because aspirin displaces the anticoagulant, it leaves the anticoagulant free to act at the cellular level, sometimes causing the toxic effect of bleeding.

Biotransformation

Biotransformation refers to the chemical change of a drug into a form that can be excreted. Most biotransformation occurs in the liver, because that's where oral drugs go first. The process, called the first-pass effect, begins when the drug is absorbed. Here, too, one drug can interfere with the effects of another Barbiturates increase the liver's enzyme activity. Since this activity makes the body metabolize the drugs more rapidly, it reduces their effect. Conversely, acetaminophen (Tylenol) blocks the breakdown of penicillin in the liver, thereby increasing the effect of the drug.

Excretion

The major organ of excretion—the process by which the body removes a drug—is the kidney. Drug interactions may also occur at this point. The drug probenecid, for example, inhibits the excretion of penicillin and increases its length of action. Furosemide (Lasix), a diuretic, blocks the excretion of aspirin and can cause aspirin to produce adverse effects.

Drug interactions at the excretion stage are not necessarily harmful. For instance, narcotic antagonists are used intentionally to reverse the adverse effects of general anesthetics. This reversal action is termed *antagonism*. The term *synergism*, on the other hand, describes what happens when a second drug increases the intensity or prolongs the effect of a first drug. A narcotic and a minor tranquilizer together, for example, produce more pain relief than the narcotic alone. The nurse administering medications needs to be aware of possible drug interactions and must carefully evaluate the patient's response.

To minimize adverse interactions, the nurse should closely review the patient's drug profile, administer as low a dose as possible, know the actions, the side and adverse effects of the drugs administered, and monitor the patient. Continued monitoring is important, because some drug interactions may take several weeks to develop.

Tolerance

When a medication for pain or sleeping is administered frequently, the liver enzymes become skilled at rapid biotransforming. Thus less of the drug is available, and the drug is less effective in relieving pain or aiding sleep. This reaction may be labelled "addiction" because the patient complains that the drug is not working and asks for more; but in fact, it is a physiologic response rather than an addictive one. The patient requires more of the drug, or a drug with a different molecular structure.

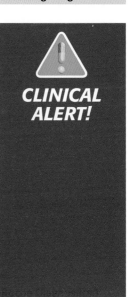

Cultural Considerations

- Drug metabolism and side effects can vary among different cultures, races, and ethnic groups.

- *Pharmacoanthropology* deals with differences in drug responses among racial and ethnic groups. *Ethnocultural perception* deals with various cultural perceptions and beliefs related to illness, disease, and drug therapy.

- Assessing the personal beliefs of the patient and the family is an essential step in drug administration.

- The nurse's communication about drugs must meet the cultural needs of the patient and family and must respect their culture and cultural practices.

CLINICAL ALERT!

Cumulation

When a condition—such as liver or kidney disease—inhibits biotransformation or excretion, the drug accumulates in the body. The same thing can happen when a patient receives too much of a drug or takes a drug too frequently. This activity, called cumulation, can produce an adverse effect. Other factors that affect drug action include these:

- Weight: Larger individuals need a higher dose.

- Age: People at either extreme of life respond more strongly. The liver and kidneys of infants are not well developed; in the elderly, systems are less efficient.

- Pathologic conditions, especially of liver and kidneys.

- Hypersensitivity to a drug, which causes an allergic reaction.

- Psychological and emotional state: Depression or anxiety can decrease or increase body metabolism and thus affect drug action.

Side effects and adverse reactions can occur in any system or organ. Drug knowledge will enhance the nurse's skill in observation and will lead to responsible and appropriate intervention.

Half-Life

The half-life of a drug, which correlates roughly with its duration of action, indicates how often the drug may be given to continue therapeutic effect. Literally, the half-life is the time required for half of the drug to be excreted and therefore no longer available for therapeutic use. For example, penicillin's half-life is 30 minutes: after 30 minutes, only half of the dose is still therapeutic. After 30 more minutes, only half of *that* dose is therapeutic, and so on, until most of the drug is eliminated. Then the patient needs another dose. In this case, the patient receives oral penicillin every 6 to 8 hours. Another example is piroxicam (Feldene), which has a half-life of 48 to 72 hours and is given by mouth as a single dose once a day. Carisoprodol (Soma) has a half-life of 4 to 6 hours and is administered three to four times daily.

Therapeutic Range

To evaluate the effects of drug therapy, the drug concentration in the patient's blood or serum can be monitored through the use of lab tests that measure the therapeutic level. The International System of Units (Système International d'Unités—SI) is a standard measurement system adopted by most countries. One of the units in SI is used to quantify the amount of drug in the blood or serum. (More details on SI can be found at http://www.bipm.org/en/si/) Some drugs, such as Theo-Dur (theophylline), Dilantin (pheny-toin), Lanoxin (digoxin), and others, require periodic measurements of the drug in order to ensure that the patient is receiving the right amount, or not receiving too much of the drug. Antibiotics often are measured with peak and trough therapeutic levels; the trough level is drawn from the blood before the next dose of antibiotic is due to see if there is too much drug left in the body. The peak level is drawn from the blood after a dose of antibiotic to see if there is enough drug in the body to have a therapeutic effect.

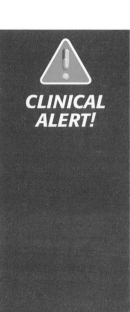

Herbs, Herbs, Herbs

- Herbal therapy is one of the oldest forms of medication. Today its use is worldwide, with more and more people taking herbal remedies.

- Clients should consult with their healthcare provider before beginning herbal therapy, while taking herbal therapy, whenever they experience any side effects from the products, and before discontinuing herbal medications.

- Refer to Health Canada's website for details on Natural Health Products Regulations (www.hc-sc.gc.ca).

- Healthcare providers need to be aware of potential drug interactions between herbal therapy and conventional drugs (both prescription and over-the-counter).

CLINICAL ALERT!

Legal Considerations

Nurses must know the scope of nursing practice in the province in which they function. They should be familiar not only with government regulations – federal and provincial – that affect nursing but also with the policies and procedures of the agency where they practice, which also have legal status. Failure to follow guidelines, or even just a lack of knowledge, can lead to liability. The web site for the Canadian Nurses Association (www.can.aiic.ca) gives information on nurse regulation and licensure in each province and up-to-date information on legal issues. The Institute for Safe Medication Practices (www.ismp-canada.org) is devoted entirely to medication error prevention and safe medication use. The Canadian Nurses Protective Society (www.cnps.ca) is a non-profit society, owned and operated by nurses for nurses, that offers legal liability protection related to nursing practice to *eligible* Registered Nurses, by providing information, education, and financial and legal assistance.

The Health Protection Branch of the Department of National Health and Welfare (www.hc-sc.gc.ca/ahc-asc/index_e.html) maintains the quality and safety of drug development. Details regarding the Canadian Food and Drugs Act appear on the same site. For information about narcotics control, see the web page for the Canadian Narcotics Control act: laws.justice.gc.ca/en/C-38.8/index.html

Nursing practice is also affected by two other types of law: criminal and civil.

Criminal Law

Criminal law relates to offenses against the general public that are detrimental to society as a whole. Actions considered criminal are prosecuted by governmental authorities. If the defendant is judged guilty, the penalty may be a fine, imprisonment, or both.

Nurses in Canada cannot prescribe medications. Nurse Practitioners, however, are licensed to prescribe medications. Criminal charges include unlawful use, possession, or administration of a controlled substance. In Canada, prescription (Schedule F) drug labels are clearly marked with the Pr symbol. Controlled Substance (Schedule G – CDSI III, IV) labels are marked with the C symbol and Narcotics (CDSI

I, II) are labelled with the N symbol. An order for a narcotic is usually valid only for 3 days, after which a new order is required. A nurse who administers a controlled drug after its order has expired commits a mediation error.

In the hospital setting, all controlled and narcotic medications are stored in a locked cupboard or cabinet and a record is kept for each medication administered. Controlled drugs and narcotics are counted for each shift and discrepancies are reported. Government and institutional policies specify how these drugs are stored and protected.

Nurses who become impaired (unable to function) because of alcohol or drug abuse leave themselves open to criminal action, as well as to disciplinary action by their provincial licensing body. Provincial practice standards require mandatory reporting of impaired nurses.

Civil Law

Civil law is concerned with the legal rights and duties of private persons. When an individual believes that a wrong was committed against him or her personally, he or she can sue for damages in the form of money.

The legal wrong is called a tort. *Malpractice,* or negligence on the part of the nurse, involves four elements:

1. A claim that the nurse owed the patient a special duty of care—i.e., that a nurse-patient relationship existed.

2. A claim that the nurse failed to meet the required standard. To prove or disprove this element, both sides bring in expert witnesses to testify.

3. A claim that harm or injury resulted because the nurse did not meet the required standard.

4. A claim of damages for which compensation is sought.

The nurse-patient relationship is a legal status that begins the moment a nurse actually provides nursing care to another person.

For administration of medications, a nurse is required by law to exercise the degree of skill and care that a reasonably prudent nurse with similar training and experience, practicing in the same community, would exercise under the same or similar circumstances. When a nursing student performs duties that are customarily performed by a registered nurse, the courts have held the nursing student to the higher standard of care, that of the registered nurse.

Mistakes in administering medications are among the most common causes of malpractice. Liability may result from administering the wrong dose, giving a medication to the wrong patient, giving a drug at the wrong time, or failing to administer a drug at the right time or in the proper manner.

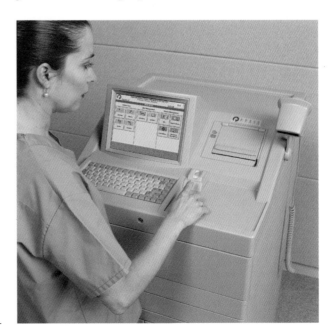

FIGURE 12-1

Pyxis Controlled Medication System. (With permission from Roach, S. [2004]. *Introductory clinical pharmacology* [7th ed.]. Philadelphia: Lippincott Williams & Wilkins, p. 18.)

A frequent cause of medication errors is either misreading the order of the physician or healthcare provider or failing to check with the physician or healthcare provider when the order is questionable. Faulty technique in administering medications, especially injections that result in injury to the patient, is another common medication error.

Not all malpractice is a result of negligence. Malpractice claims are also founded on the daily interaction between the nurse and the patient; consequently, the nurse's personality plays a major role in fostering or preventing malpractice claims. All nurses should be familiar with the principles of psychology. The surest way to prevent claims is to recognize the patient as a human being who has emotional as well as physical needs and to respond to these needs in a humane and competent manner.

If an error does occur, primary consideration must be given to the patient. Assessment of the patient is done first. The nurse notifies the physician and the immediate nursing supervisor; students notify the instructor. Error-in-medication forms are filled out, and appropriate action is taken under the direction of the physician or healthcare provider.

To prevent malpractice claims, the nurse must render, as consistently as possible, the best possible care to patients. Every nurse involved in direct care should regard prevention of malpractice claims as an integral part of daily nursing responsibilities, for two fundamental reasons:

1. Such measures result in higher-quality care.

2. All affirmative measures taken to minimize malpractice will minimize the nurse's exposure to liability.

How can a nurse avoid medication errors? First and foremost are the three checks and 5 + 2 rights (see p. 351). Accurate dosage calculation is also a safeguard against medication errors and potential liability claims.

OTHER SAFEGUARDS INCLUDE

- Know and follow institutional policies and procedures.
- Look up what you do not know.
- Avoid interruptions when preparing medications.
- Do not leave medicines at the bedside.
- Chart carefully.
- Listen to the patient: "I never took that before," and the like.
- Check and double-check when a dose seems high. Most oral tablet doses range from ½ to 2 tablets. Most intramuscular, intradermal, and subcutaneous injections are less than 3 mL.
- Label any powder you dilute. Label any IV bag you use.
- When necessary, seek advice from competent professionals.
- Do not administer drugs prepared by another nurse.
- Report near-misses to prevent future errors.
- Keep drug knowledge up to date. Attend continuing education programs and update your nursing skills.

It is possible to render high-quality nursing care and never commit a medication error. Safe effective drug therapy is a combination of knowledge, skill, carefulness, and caring.

Ethical Values in Drug Administration

Complex issues in nursing practice, such as medication administration, have both legal and ethical dimensions. The Canadian Nurses Association *Code of Ethics for Registered Nurses* sets out the ethical behaviour expected of nurses in Canada. The code delineates what nurses must know about their ethical responsibilities. The *Code of Ethics for Registered Nurses* is structured around eight primary values that are grounded in the professional nursing relationship with individuals and indicate what nurses care about in that relationship. These eight primary values are central to ethical nursing practice.

Safe, competent, and ethical care

Nurses value the ability to provide safe, competent and ethical care that allows them to fulfill their ethical and professional obligations to the people they serve.

Health and well-being

Nurses value health promotion and well-being and assisting persons to achieve their optimum level of health in situations of normal health, illness, injury, disability, or at the end of life.

Choice

Nurses respect and promote the autonomy of persons and help them to express their health needs and values and also to obtain desired information and services so they can make informed decisions.

Dignity

Nurses recognize and respect the inherent worth of each person and advocate for respectful treatment of all persons

Confidentiality

Nurses safeguard information learned in the context of a professional relationship and ensure it is shared outside the healthcare team only with the person's informed consent, or as may be legally required, or where the failure to disclose would cause significant harm.

Justice

Nurses uphold principles of equity and fairness to assist persons in receiving a share of health services and resources proportionate to their needs and in promoting social justice.

Accountability

Nurses are answerable for their practice, and they act in a manner consistent with their professional responsibilities and standards of practice.

Quality practice environments

Nurses value and advocate for practice environments that have the organizational structures and resources necessary to ensure safety, support, and respect for all persons in the work setting (Canadian Nurses Association, Code of Ethics, 2002).

Specific Points in Giving Medications Safely

The 5 + 2 Rights and Three Checks

The nurse observes the three checks and 5+2 rights of medication administration.

The 5+2 rights of medication administration are:

1. The right drug
2. To the right patient
3. At the right time
4. By the right route
5. In the right amount

Plus:

1. Using the right approach (safety, comfort, allergy check, position, etc.)

2. Completing the right documentation

The Three Checks of the Five Rights when Preparing Medications:

1. Check the drug label against the medication administration record (MAR) when removing the drug from where it is stored (e.g., narcotic cupboard, drug cart, ward stock). Do you have the right drug for the right patient in the right amount and route at the right time?

2. Check the drug label against the MAR as you open, prepare, and/or pour the medication. Ensure the five rights match *exactly*.

3. Check the drug label against the MAR one last time before throwing out the wrapper, or discarding your waste into the sharps container, or replacing the ward stock back into the cupboard. Ensure you have the right drug in the right amount to be given by the right route at the right time to the right patient. This is the "Oh my!!" check and will save your patient from harm. Do not miss this check—even if you are in a hurry. Ensure you check your patient's ID bracelet prior to administering any medication.

N.B.—You cannot check the five rights *after* you have given the drug to your patient. All three of these checks must occur Prior to administration. You must know that the each of the five rights has been verified.

Medication Orders

A correct medication order bears the patient's name and room number, the date, the name of the drug (generic or trade), the dose of the drug, the route of administration, and the times to administer the drug. It ends with the signature of the physician or healthcare provider.

Types of orders:

1. Standing order with termination

> **Example**   Keflex (cephalexin) 500 mg po every 6 hours × 7 days

2. Standing order without termination

> **Example**   Digoxin (Lanoxin) 0.5 mg po every day

3. A prn order

> **Example**   Demerol (meperidine) 50 mg IM q4h prn pain

4. Single-dose order

> **Example**   atropine 0.3 mg subcutaneous 0730h on call to OR

5. Stat order

> **Example**   morphine sulfate 4 mg IV stat

Hospital guidelines provide for an automatic stop time on some classes of drugs; narcotic orders may be valid for only 3 days, antibiotics for 10 days. When first reading the order and transferring the order, the nurse must take care to note the expiration time, thus alerting all staff who pour medications. Hospital policies vary.

6. Range dose order

> **Example**   Tylenol #3 1–2 tabs po of q4–6h prn

Following are general guidelines in regards to several areas of medication administration:

Medication Orders for Physicians and Healthcare Providers

- Medical students may write orders on charts, but orders must be countersigned by a house physician before they are legal. Medical students are not licensed.

- Do not carry out an order that is not clear or that is illegible. Check with the physician or healthcare provider who wrote the order. Do not assume anything.

- Do not carry out an order if a conflict exists with nursing knowledge. For example, Demerol (meperidine) 500 mg IM is above the average dose. Check with the physician or healthcare provider who wrote the order.

- Nursing students should not accept oral or telephone orders. The student should refer the physician to the instructor or staff nurse.

- Professional nurses may take oral or telephone orders in accord with institutional policy. Orders should be restated verbally to the prescriber to confirm the accuracy of the order. The nurse must write these orders on the chart, and the physician or healthcare provider must sign them within 24 hours.

Knowledge Base

- Nurses should know the generic and trade names of drugs to be administered, as well as their class, average dose, routes of administration, use, side effects and adverse effects, contraindications, and nursing implications in administration. Nurses should also know what signs of effectiveness to look for and what drug interactions are possible. New or unfamiliar drugs require research.

- The nurse should be aware of the patient's diagnosis and medical history, especially relative to drugs taken. Be especially alert to OTC drugs, which patients often do not consider important. Check for allergies.

- Assess the patient's need for drug information. Be prepared to implement and evaluate a nursing care plan in drug therapy.

Medication Safety

- The patient has a right to considerate and respectful care and the right to refuse a medication. The patient also has a right to know the name of the medication, what it is supposed to do, any side effects that may occur, and what to do should they occur.

- It is a fallacy that the nurse is no longer required to calculate or prepare drugs dispensed as unit dose. In some instances, the pharmacy may not have the exact dose on hand, or the nurse may need to administer a partial dose. The label must still be read three times.

- Labels must be clear. If not, return them to the pharmacy.

- In the unit-dose mobile cart system, the nurse has the medication sheets of each patient together in a folder or on a computer printout. If unsure of an order, take the sheet to the patient's chart and check from the date ordered to the current date.

- In the ticket system, the Kardex is the main check against the medication ticket. If the medication ticket does not match the Kardex, further checking is necessary. First go to the chart and find the original order; then check through every order up until the current date to verify when the order changed. (The ticket system is rarely used.)

- If any doubt about a drug exists, do not administer it. Check further with the physician, the healthcare provider, the pharmacist, or a supervising nurse.

- PRN medications must be administered only for the purpose they were ordered.

- Keys to a locked system or a Pyxis system are needed to obtain controlled drugs (e.g., narcotics) and to prevent others' access to medications. Student nurses cannot access controlled drugs unless supervised by a registered nurse.

- Pour oral medications first, then injections. For oral administration, use medical asepsis (clean technique). Injections require aseptic technique.

- Orders issued as "stat" take precedence and must be carried out immediately.

- Perform indicated nursing actions before administering certain medications. Example: Digitalis preparations require an apical heart rate, whereas antihypertensives require a blood pressure reading.

- Administer medications within 30 minutes of the time scheduled.

- Keep medications within sight at all times. Never leave medications unattended.

- Do not administer a medication if assessment shows that the drug is contraindicated or that an adverse effect may have occurred as a result of a previous dose. If you withhold a drug, notify the physician or healthcare provider who wrote the order.

Oral Medications—Tablets and Capsules

- Administer irritating oral drugs along with meals or a snack (unless contraindicated), to decrease gastric irritation.

- If the patient is nauseated or vomiting, withhold oral medications and notify the physician or the healthcare provider. Be sure to chart this action.

- Break a tablet only if it is scored.

- Never open capsules or break EC tablets. If the patient cannot swallow capsules or tablets, either ask the physician or healthcare provider to order a liquid or check with the pharmacist.

- Check the tablets in a stock container. Are they the same size? Same colour? If not, return them to the pharmacy.

- Hydrophilic capsules are not medications. They are labelled DO NOT EAT and are placed in stock containers of tablets and capsules to absorb dampness and to maintain the drug in a solid state.

Liquid Medications

- Read labels three times: (1) when removing the drug from storage, (2) when calculating the dose, and (3) after pouring the drug.

- Quiet and concentration are needed to pour drugs. Follow a routine in pouring. Methodology is the best safeguard in preventing error.

- Never return any poured drug to a stock bottle once the drug has been taken from the preparation room.

- Never combine medications from two stock bottles. Return both bottles to the pharmacy. It is the responsibility of the pharmacists to combine drugs.

- Some liquid medications require dilution. Check references for directions.

- Some liquids may have to be administered through a straw. Liquid iron preparations, for example, cause discolouring and should not come in contact with teeth.

- Pour liquids at eye level, using a medicine cup. Measure at the centre of the meniscus. To keep from spilling the medication onto the label (which could make it unreadable), pour with the label up.

- After the patient has taken a liquid antacid, add 5 to 10 mL water to the cup, mix, and have the patient drink it as well. Because antacids are thick, some medication often remains in the cup.

- The nurse who pours medications is responsible for administering and charting.

- Do not give drugs that another nurse has poured.

- Aqueous or water-based solutions do not need to be shaken before pouring.

Giving Medications

- Follow the universal safeguards in administration of medication (see Chapter 13).

- **Always check the patient's ID band before administering medications (Fig. 12-2). If the patient does not have an ID band, have a responsible person identify the patient for you and obtain an ID band for the patient.**

- Listen to the patient's comments and act on them. If a patient says something like "That's not mine" or "I never took this before," check carefully, then return to the patient with the result of your investigation. Failure to do this will cause you to lose the patient's trust and confidence and may result in a medication error.

- If a patient refuses a drug, find out why. First check the chart, to see if the drug was in fact ordered; then talk to the patient to understand his or her reasons. After charting the reason for refusal, notify the physician or healthcare provider who wrote the order.

- Watch to make sure the patient takes the drugs. Stay until oral drugs are swallowed.

- Keep drugs within view at all times.

- Never leave any drug at the bedside stand unless hospital policy permits this. If a medication is left with the patient, inform the patient why the drug is ordered, how to take it, and what to expect. Later, check to determine whether the drug was taken and record the findings.

Charting

Documentation is the "seventh right" of medication administration. The always quoted axiom is still true: "If it's not charted, it's not done."

- Chart all medications after administration.

- Chart single doses, stat doses, and prn medications immediately, and note the exact time when they were administered.

- When a range dose has been ordered, clearly document the amount of dosage given.

- Chart any nursing actions done before administering drugs (e.g., apical heart rate [with digoxin], or blood pressure [with antihypertensives]). The safest place to chart these actions is on the medication administration record where the drug is documented.

- If the drug was refused or was withheld (not given), write the reason on the nurse's notes and/or on the medication administration record, and notify the healthcare provider who ordered the medication. Also note the time you notified the healthcare provider, and any response.

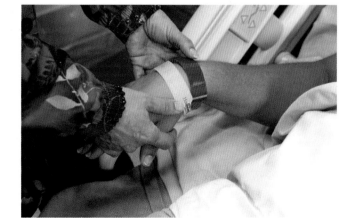

FIGURE 12-2

Checking the patient's armband. (With permission from Evans-Smith, P. [2005] *Lippincott's atlas of medication administration* [2nd ed.] Philadelphia: Lippincott Williams and Wilkins, p. 8.)

Evaluation

- Check for the expected effect of the drug. Did side effects or adverse effects occur? Perform indicated nursing actions. Record your observations.

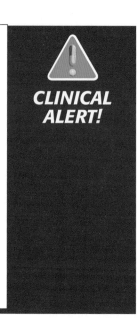

Age-Specific Considerations

- Neonatal clients—The nurse needs to consider the immaturity of organ function, the importance of weight, and the precision of dosage calculation (rounding to the nearest one hundredth).

- Pediatric clients—The nurse needs to remember the principles of atraumatic care and to consider developmental stages.

- Geriatric clients—The nurse needs to take into account decreasing organ function (especially liver and kidney), circulatory changes leading to decreased perfusion, and physical limitations (poor eyesight, decreased coordination, decreased ability to chew and/or swallow).

CLINICAL ALERT!

Error in Medication Administration

- Report any error immediately to the charge nurse and the physician or healthcare provider.

- Always give primary concern to the patient.

- Fill out an error-in-medication form. Follow the physician's or healthcare provider's directions in caring for the patient.

CRITICAL THINKING: TEST YOUR CLINICAL SAVVY

Mr. T is a patient receiving a drug that is in a drug study.

A. As a nurse administering this drug, what is your ethical responsibility?

B. If the patient asks "Is it safe to take this drug?" what is an appropriate response? If the patient refuses to take the drug, what should you do?

C. You agree with the patient that he should not take the experimental drug. What are your ethical responsibilities? What are your legal responsibilities?

Mr. T discovers from the Internet that the drug he is taking is an experimental drug and that another drug with similar actions has been released by Health Canada and is available by prescription.

D. How do you respond to the information that he has acquired? What are some questions that the patient should ask regarding information acquired over the Internet?

E. If the patient asks you whether he should continue to take the experimental drug, or whether he should discontinue his participation in the drug study and obtain a prescription for the similar drug, what is an appropriate response?

F. What reasons can you give Mr. T regarding the benefits of participating in a drug study?

SELF TEST 1   Basic Information

Give the information requested. (Answers appear at the end of the chapter.)

1. List at least 10 kinds of information the nurse needs to know in order to administer drugs safely.

   _____   _____

   _____   _____

   _____   _____

   _____   _____

   _____   _____

2. List the five pregnancy categories used to identify the safety of drugs for the fetus and briefly define each.

   _____

   _____

   _____

   _____

   _____

3. Name the major organ for the following drug activities.

   a. Absorption _____   **c.** Biotransformation _____

   b. Distribution _____   **d.** Excretion _____

4. Define these terms:

   a. Tolerance _____

   _____

   _____

   b. Cumulation _____

   _____

   _____

5. List the four elements of negligence.

   _____ ,

   _____ ,

   _____ , and

   _____

6. What is the standard by which a tort is judged?

   _____

   _____

   _____

(continued)

7. List at least five positive actions to avoid liability.

_____

_____

_____

_____

_____

8. List and briefly describe five ethical values in drug therapy.

_____

_____

_____

_____

_____

9. What are the seven elements of a correct medication order?

_____

_____

_____

_____

_____

_____

_____

10. When an order is not clear, what action should a nurse take?

_____

PROFICIENCY TEST 1   Basic Drug Information

Name: _____

Choose the correct answer. Answers are given in Appendix A.

1. Two drugs are given for different reasons, but drug Y interferes with the excretion of drug X. The effect of drug X would be

   a. increased
   b. decreased
   c. unchanged
   d. stopped

2. Major biotransformation of drugs occurs in the

   a. lungs
   b. kidney
   c. liver
   d. urine

3. Toxicity to a drug is more likely to occur when

   a. elimination of the drug is rapid
   b. the drug is bound to the plasma protein albumin
   c. the drug will not dissolve in the lipid layer of the cell
   d. the drug is free in the blood circulation

4. The term USP after a drug name indicates that the drug

   a. is made only in the United States
   b. meets official standards in the United States
   c. cannot be made by any other pharmaceutical company
   d. is registered by the US Public Health Service

5. When an order is written to be administered "as needed" it is called a

   a. standing order
   b. prn order
   c. single order
   d. stat order

6. Signs of effectiveness of a drug are based on what information?

   a. action and use
   b. untoward effects
   c. generic and trade names
   d. drug interaction

7. Drug classification is an aid in understanding

   a. use of the drug
   b. drug idiosyncrasy
   c. the trade name
   d. the generic name

(continued)

8. Names of many drugs include

   a. several generic, several trade names
   b. several generic, one trade name
   c. one generic, one trade name
   d. one generic, several trade names

9. Which pregnancy category is considered safe for the fetus?

   a. A
   b. B
   c. C
   d. D

10. What is the primary purpose of EC medications?

    a. improve taste
    b. delay absorption
    c. code the drug for identification
    d. make the drug easier to swallow

11. Which of the following drug preparations does *not* have to be shaken before pouring?

    a. magma
    b. gel
    c. suspension
    d. aqueous solution

12. Most oral drugs are absorbed in the

    a. mouth
    b. stomach
    c. small intestine
    d. large intestine

13. Nursing legal responsibilities associated with controlled substances include

    a. storage in a locked place
    b. assessing vital signs
    c. evaluating psychological response
    d. establishing automatic 24-hour stop orders

14. The responsibilities of the nurse regarding medication in the hospital include all except

    a. prescribing drugs
    b. teaching patients
    c. regulating automatic expiration times of drugs
    d. preparing solutions

15. Under what condition does a nurse have a right to refuse to administer a drug?

    a. The pharmacist ordered the drug.
    b. The drug is manufactured by two different companies.
    c. The drug is prescribed by a licensed physician.
    d. The dose is within the range given in the physician's desk reference.

(continued)

16. When administering medication in the hospital, the nurse should

 a. chart medications before administering them
 b. chart only those drugs that she or he personally gave the patient
 c. chart all medications given for the day at one time
 d. determine the best method for giving the drugs

17. Which of the following illustrates a medication error?

 a. administering a 1000h dose at 1020h
 b. giving 2 tablets of gantrisin (sufisoxazole) 500 mg when 1 g is ordered
 c. holding a medication when client refuses to take it
 d. giving digoxin (Lanoxin) IM when digoxin po 0.25 mg is ordered

18. A nurse reads a medication order that is not clear. What action is indicated?

 a. Ask the charge nurse to explain the order.
 b. Ask a doctor at the nurses' station for help.
 c. Check the drug reference on the unit.
 d. Check with the doctor who wrote the order.

19. Which nursing action is illegal?

 a. Pouring medication from one stock bottle into another.
 b. Counting control drugs in the narcotic cabinet or Pyxis each shift.
 c. Labelling a vial of powder after dissolving it.
 d. Refusing to carry out an order that is confusing.

Answers to Self Tests

Self Test I Basic Information

1. Generic/trade name, drug class and drug classification, pregnancy category, dose and route, action, use, side/adverse effects, contraindications/ precautions, interactions/incompatibilities, nursing implications, evaluation of effectiveness, patient teaching

2. **A.** No risk to fetus
   B. No adverse effects in animals, but no human studies
   C. Animals show adverse effects; calculated risk to fetus
   D. Fetal risk exists
   X. Absolute fetal abnormality

3. **a.** Small intestines
   b. Blood
   c. Liver
   d. Kidney

4. **a.** Repeated administration of a drug increases microsomal enzyme activity in the liver. The drug is broken down more quickly and its effectiveness is decreased.
   b. Biotransformation is inhibited and the drug level remains high. Adverse effects are more likely to occur.

5. A claim that a nurse-patient relationship existed
   The nurse was required to meet a standard of care
   A claim that harm or injury occurred because the standard was not met
   A claim of damages for which compensation is sought

6. Whether the nurse exercised the degree of skill and care that a reasonably prudent nurse with similar training and experience, practicing in the same community, would exercise under the same or similar circumstances

7. Know policies and practices of the institution.
   Research unfamiliar drugs.
   Do not leave medicines at the bedside.
   Chart carefully.
   Listen to the patient's complaints.
   Check yourself (e.g., read labels three times).
   Label anything you dilute.
   Keep up to date.

8. Safe, competent and ethical care—professional practice
   Health and well-being—health promotion and optimal level of health
   Choice—freedom to decide based on knowledge with no constraint
   Dignity—respect
   Confidentiality—keep secrets
   Justice—ensure all are treated fairly and equally
   Accountability—nurses are responsible for their actions
   Quality practice environments—safe work settings

9. Patient's name and room, date, name of drug, dose, route, times of administration, doctor's or healthcare provider's signature

10. The nurse does not administer the drug and checks with the physician or healthcare provider who wrote the order.

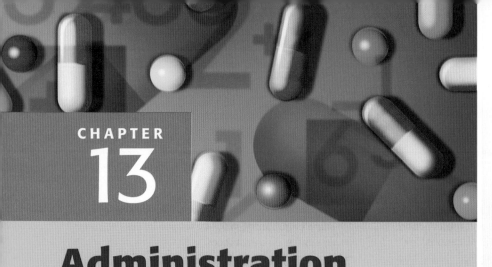

LEARNING OBJECTIVES

1. Standard precautions

2. Systems of administration

3. Guidelines for administration of drugs:

   Oral

   Parenteral—IM, subcutaneous, IV, IVPB, ID

4. Administering injections:

   Topical—skin, mucous membran⬤

5. Special considerations

CHAPTER
13

Administration Procedures

Throughout this text, we have calculated dosages and studied information related to drug therapy. This chapter is the "how to" chapter—describing the actual methods of administering drugs orally, parenterally, and topically. The adages "practice makes perfect" and "one picture is worth a thousand words" apply. Administering medications is a skilled activity that requires practice—with supervision—to ensure correct technique. Because this chapter covers only the basics, you will want to work with a medication administration skill book and a pharmacology textbook as well.

Every institution has a standard procedure for administering medications, which depends on the way its drugs are dispensed: by unit-dose, in multidose containers, or a combination of the two. Institutional procedure may call for the use of a mobile cart with medication administration records, a locked medication dispensing system, or the use of a computer printout or a bar code device.

Whatever the procedure's specifications, follow them carefully. Step-by-step attention to detail is the best safeguard to ensure the patient's 5 + 2 rights.

⬤▬ Standard Precautions Applied to Administration of Medications

When you are administering drugs, there's a chance that the patient's blood, body fluids, or tissues can come into contact with your skin or mucous membranes. So you always risk potential exposure to a long list of viruses, including these: hepatitis A (HAV), hepatitis B (HBV), hepatitis C (HCV), hepatitis D (HDV), hepatitis E (HEV), and the human immunodeficiency virus (HIV).

The Centers for Disease Control and Prevention (CDC) in Atlanta recommends standard precautions in caring for all patients and when handling equipment that's contaminated with blood or blood-streaked body fluids. In 1996, the term *standard precautions* replaced "universal precautions." *Transmission-based precautions* are those used with patients who have a suspected infection. For more information on these procedures, see the CDC web site: http://www.cdc.gov/ ncidod/dhqp/index.html

The following points, based on CDC guidelines, can help you determine appropriate safeguards in giving medications. The safeguards you need to follow depend on the type of contact you have with patients.

General Safeguards in Administering Medications

- Oral medications: Hand washing is adequate. If there's a possibility of exposure to blood or body secretions, wear gloves.

- Injections: Both hand washing and gloves are required. Do not recap needles. Use a needleguard device if provided. Carefully dispose of used sharps in an appropriate, labelled, puncture-proof container.

- Intermittent infusion plugs, IV catheters, and IV needles: Wash your hands and wear gloves when inserting or removing IV needles and catheters. Dispose of used sharps in a puncture-proof container or use a needleguard device.

- Secondary administration sets or IVPB (IV piggyback) sets: Before removing this equipment from the main IV tubing, wash your hands and put on gloves. Either use a needleless device or place used needles in a puncture-proof container.

- Application of medication to mucous membranes: Wash your hands and wear gloves (see the following guidelines for using gowns, masks, and protective eyewear).

- Applications to skin: Before applying such drug forms as transdermal patches or applying lotions, ointments, or creams, wash your hands and wear gloves.

Hand Washing

- When washing with soap and water, rub hands together vigorously for 15 seconds, covering all surfaces of hands and fingers.

- With each patient, always wash your hands twice: before preparing medications and after administering medications.

- Wash your hands after removing your gloves.

- If your hands have come into contact with a patient's blood or body fluids, wash them *immediately*.

- Wash your hands after handling any equipment soiled with blood or body fluids.

- If hands are not visibly soiled, use an alcohol-based hand rub for routine hand cleaning.

Protective Equipment

Gloves

- While administering medications, wear gloves for any direct ("hands-on") contact with a patient's blood, bodily fluids, or secretions.

- Wear gloves when handling materials or equipment contaminated with blood or body fluids.

- Whenever you use gloves, you must change them after completing procedures for each patient and between patients.

Gowns

- When administering medications, you need to wear a gown if there's a risk that your clothing may become contaminated with a patient's blood or body fluids.

Masks, Protective Eyewear, and Face Shields

- A mask is required when you are caring for a patient on strict or respiratory isolation procedures.

- Masks and protective eyewear or face shields are required when a medication procedure may cause blood or body fluids to splash directly onto your face, eyes, or mucous membranes.

- You must wear masks and protective eyewear during any medication procedure known to cause aerosolization of fluids that contain chemicals or body fluids.

Management of Used Needles and Sharps

- All used needles, syringes, sharps, stylets, butterfly needles, and IV catheters must be discarded in appropriate, labelled, puncture-proof containers.

- Do not break, bend, or recap needles after using them. Immediately place needles in a puncture-proof container.

- Wear gloves and exercise caution when removing an intermittent infusion plug, IV catheters, and IV needles. Place them in a puncture-proof container. Never remove the IV needle from the IV tubing by hand. Instead, use either a clamp or the needle unlocking device on the sharps container. It's best to use needleless systems or needleguard devices.

- As you dispose of a sharp, keep your eyes on the sharps (puncture-proof) container.

Needleless Systems and Needleguard Devices

- Needleless systems, used to reduce the risk of needle-sticks and blood-borne pathogens, work in several ways.
- Some syringes have a needleguard device that retracts the needle into the syringe or a cap after it is used.
- Needleless adapters for syringes to withdraw medication from vials (Fig. 13-1).

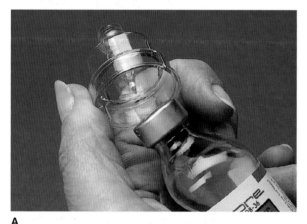

A

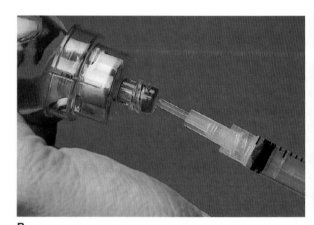

B

FIGURE 13-1

(**A**) Needleless system adapter for vial. (**B**) Use syringe (without needle) to withdraw medication.

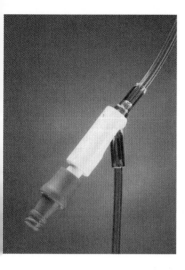

FIGURE 13-2

Needleless system for IV tubing

- Needleless systems are also available for IV tubing (Fig. 13-2) and for use at the patient's IV site. All needleless equipment must be discarded into sharp containers.

Management of Materials Other Than Needles and Sharps

- Paper cups, plastic cups, and other equipment not contaminated with blood or body fluids may be discarded according to routine hospital procedures.
- In situations that require strict or respiratory isolation precautions, follow the institution's established protocol.

Management of Nurse Exposed to Blood or Body Fluids

If a personal needle-stick, an injury, or a skin laceration causes contact with the blood or blood-streaked body fluids of any patient, *act immediately*. Wash the area with soap and copious amounts of water, and apply an acceptable antiseptic. If mucous membrane exposure occurs, flush the exposed areas with copious amounts of warm water. Follow the protocol established by the healthcare institution for management of needle-stick injury or accidental exposure to blood or body fluids.

Systems of Administration

Institutions establish their own systems for administering medication. You might need to use tickets, the mobile cart, a locked medication cabinet near the patient's bedside, and/or computer printouts.

Unit-dose packaging is the most widely used system. Drugs are dispensed by the pharmacy and placed in individual patient drawers, either on a mobile cart or in a locked cabinet at the patient's bedside. The mobile cart can be wheeled into the patient's room so that you can prepare medications at the bedside for administration.

A newer system uses a scanner device, scanning the patient's ID band, the nurse's ID, the medication administration record, and the medication in unit-dose packaging. If the scan reveals any discrepancy, the device alerts the nurse.

The ticket system, rarely used, works with drugs that are dispensed in multidose containers. The nurse prepares the drugs in a medication room and then carries them on a tray to the patient.

Computer Order Entry

Some institutions have computerized medication procedures, which enable doctors or prescribing healthcare providers to input medication orders directly onto the computer. The nurse can immediately see the new order on the computer screen and plan care accordingly. This system presents several advantages: Neither the nurse nor the pharmacist has to interpret the handwriting of the doctor or healthcare provider.

The nurse does not have to transfer the written orders to a Medication Administration Record (MAR)—lessening the chance for error while also saving time. Moreover, a computer check identifies possible interactions among the patient's medications and alerts the nurse and the pharmacist. The nurse marks details of administration on the patient's computer record.

Medication Administration Record

The MAR, a daily (24-hour) record of what medications are ordered for the patient, also documents the medications given by the nurse. Most MARs consist of a computerized printout (Fig. 13-3), with key identifying information—the patient's name, ID number, room, date of admission, age, diagnosis,

MCFARLAND MEDICAL CENTRE
Medication Administration Record

Patient Name	Room Number	Hospital Number	Diagnosis
Velder, Chelsea	1401	204452896	CHF

Allergies	Admitted	Age	Sex	Physician
PCN	6/25/07	50	F	Richardson

DOSAGE ADMINISTRATION PERIOD: 6/26/07 0600-6/27/07 0600

	0601-1400	1401-2200	2201-0600
Digoxin 0.25 mg PO every day Hold if HR <60	0900		
Aspirin 325 mg PO daily	0900		
Protonix 40 mg PO every day	0900		
Ampicillin 250 mg PO q 6h	1400	1800	0200 0600
Lopressor 50 mg PO BID Hold if SBP <100	0900	2100	
Coumadin 5 mg PO once a day		1700	
Morphine Sulfate 4-6 mg IV every 2-3h prn pain			
Tylenol gr X q4h prn temp >101			

Signature _____ Initials __( )__   Signature _____ Initials __( )__   Signature _____ Initials __( )__

FIGURE 13-3

A sample 24-hour computerized medication record. Scheduled drugs are listed at the top of the sheet and prn orders at the bottom. Military time is used. The nurse draws a line through the time administered, initials to indicate that the drug was administered, then signs at the bottom of the sheet.

gender, and attending physician—printed at the top. Orders written during the shift have to be added to the printout by hand, a procedure that can lead to medication errors. Therefore, hospitals require that every shift, the nurse must check the MAR against the original orders in the chart to make sure that the orders are correct.

Each healthcare setting will have different guidelines on charting medications. Generally, routine medications are assigned a scheduled time on the MAR. After the nurse gives the medication, a line is drawn through the time and initialed. If the medication is refused or held, the time is circled and initialed and then a reason given why the medication was not given. PRN meds are not assigned a scheduled time on the MAR, rather, after the medication is given, the time is then written on the MAR, a line crossed through that time, and then initialed. Different medications may be given at different scheduled times throughout the day, for example, Coumadin is given at 1700 or 1800 in the evening so that the therapeutic effect is maximized. Follow institutional guidelines for medication administration times.

Computer Scanner

This system uses a portable computer scanning device, which stores information about the patient and the medication. The unit-dose packaging used with this system shows bar codes. The nurse's process is simple: Prepare the medications and check each one against the MAR. Use the scanning device to scan the patient's ID band, your own ID, the medication package, and the MAR. If the computer detects no discrepancy, you can continue to administer the medications as described in the previous paragraph.

Mobile Cart System

In this system, pharmacy dispenses unit-dose medications directly to the patient's drawer in the mobile cart, which is labelled with the patient's name. The cart contains all the equipment the nurse might require to administer medications.

When a drug is ordered, the nurse transcribes the order to only one place: the patient's MAR, either in a medication book on the cart or in the patient's chart.

Here's the appropriate procedure: When it's time to administer medications, wash your hands and roll the cart to the bedside of the first patient. Identify the patient verbally by name, unlock the cart, and open the medication book to that patient's medication sheet.

Before giving the medication, check the sheet for special nursing actions required, such as obtaining a blood pressure or heart rate. Carry out the orders, record the results, and decide whether to withhold the medication or to administer it.

First check: Place the patient's drawer on the top of the cart. Read each medication order, starting with the first medication listed. If you're giving a dose, choose the unit-dose from the drawer and compare the label with the order (Fig. 13-4).

Second check: After comparing the order with the unit measure, compute the dose. Then open or prepare the unit-dose, and pour the amount.

Third check: Label the unit dose, read the order again, and verify the dose. After preparing all the patient's medications, read the name and ID number on the medicine sheet, check the patient's ID band, ensuring hospital number matches the MAR, and administer the drugs. Remain with the patient until he or

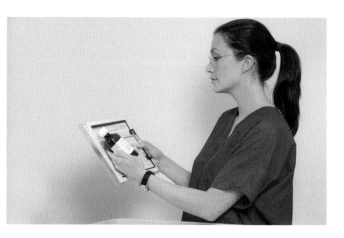

FIGURE 13-4

The nurse compares the medication with the order.

she has taken the medications; then provide any comfort measures, wash your hands, and return to the cart to chart the drugs administered. Replace the patient's drawer and roll the cart to the next patient. When all the medications have been administered, return the mobile cart to its designated area.

This system has several advantages. Two professionals—the pharmacist and the nurse—check the medication in the drawer. All the MARs are together on the cart, which saves time. The nurse can carry out assessment and can chart the results before pouring any medication. Immediately after administering the drugs, the nurse can sign for them.

Note that with any type of medication system, you must *check the label three times:* when choosing the drug, when pouring the dose or opening the medication, and before replacing the container or giving the unit-dose to the patient.

In a variation of the mobile cart system, the medications are locked in a cabinet at or near the patient's bedside. As with the original mobile cart system, the pharmacy fills the cabinet with the unit-dose medications. MARs are in the patient chart, which is in the cabinet; and the nurse prepares the medications in the same manner, using the three checks and the 5 + 2 rights. Having the medications and the patient's chart closer to the patient's bedside saves time for both the patient and the nurse.

Many hospitals are using the computerized narcotic cart or cabinet (Pyxis system) to dispense all medications (controlled substances and noncontrolled medications). The computer in the cart or cabinet stores a record of each medication, when it is due, and lists this information for each patient. The nurse simply goes to the Pyxis with the MAR and removes the unit-doses for each patient by accessing the computer. This system provides yet another check to make sure that the right patient receives the right medication, the right dose, at the right time, by the right route.

Ticket System

This system transfers a medication order to three places: a medication ticket, the patient's medication sheet, and the patient's Kardex file, which contains the nursing care plan. Tickets for all patients are kept in a central location. The nurse sorts them according to time of administration and compares them with the Kardex entry. If there is a discrepancy, the nurse checks the original order on the patient's chart, using three-check system:

First check: Separate the first patient's tickets and place them together in a pile; read each ticket, locate the medication in the medication cart or medication room, and verify that the label matches the ticket.

Second check: Compare the dose on the ticket with the label, then calculate and pour the amount of the drug.

Third check: Before discarding the unit-dose packet or returning the container to the shelf, read the order and the label again, verifying the poured dose.

Having finished these checks, place each medication on a tray with the ticket in front to identify it. Then dispense the medication to the patient, identifying the patient by ID band, ensuring hospital number matches the MAR, and keeping the medications in sight. Complete any required nursing assessment (e.g., obtain a blood pressure or heart rate). Administer the drugs, then take the medication tray to the next patient and follow the same procedure. After giving all the medications, chart them on each patient's chart. If you give a stat medication, chart it and destroy the ticket.

This system has a number of disadvantages: Because every order must be transcribed to three different places, that opens three opportunities for error. Also, tickets can be lost or misplaced; an error may occur while the nurse is choosing the stock medication; and if the tickets become mixed, a medication may go to the wrong patient. Medications requiring assessment need some kind of tag for identification and locating the chart of each patient takes a lot of time.

◼◻ Routes of Administration

Oral Route

Regardless of which system you use to prepare the medications, the procedure for administering drugs requires specific steps. The oral route is the least expensive, the safest, and also the easiest to administer.

For oral administration, you first identify the patient verbally by name, check the ID band, ensuring hospital number matches the MAR, and make sure the patient is alert and able to swallow. If so, assist the patient to a sitting position. Give oral solids first, along with a full glass of water whenever possible (unless contraindicated). Then give oral liquid medications. Watch to be sure that the patient has swallowed all the drugs. Discard the paper and/or plastic cups according to routine hospital procedure, unless the patient is on strict or respiratory isolation. For this condition, use special isolation bags. Finally, make the patient comfortable, wash your hands, and chart the medications given.

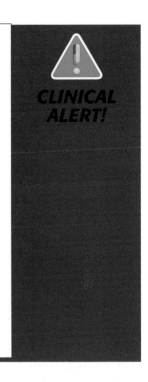

Medication Errors

- Medication errors can cause unnecessary side effects, adverse effects, illnesses, and sometimes death.

- Medication errors are among the most common medical errors, harming at least 1.5 million people every year, according to the Institute of Medicine of the National Academies.

- The three most common errors are administering an improper dose, administering the wrong drug, and using the wrong route of administration.

- Medication errors are preventable. As a nurse, you can prevent medication errors by following the 5 +2 rights of medication administration and the three checks of medication identification. For information on medication errors, visit the ISMP-Canada web site (www.ismp-canada.org).

CLINICAL ALERT!

Special Considerations for Oral Administration

- Check patients for allergies to drugs. This should be a routine procedure.

- Some drugs are best taken on an empty stomach; others may be taken with food.

- Check expiration dates on all labels. Never administer expired drugs.

- Be aware of foods or fluids that are safe for ingesting with the drug and those that are contraindicated.

- Even if the patient is NPO (nothing by mouth), the patient may need to receive certain drugs (e.g., an anticonvulsant for a patient with epilepsy). Check with the doctor or healthcare provider to determine whether you can administer oral medication with a small amount of water.

- When administering solid stock medications, pour them first into the container lid and then into a paper cup, using medical asepsis. *Do not touch the medication.* You can combine several solids in the cup, but you should first pour each medication into a separate cup. Check all unit-dose medications three times before you discard the package container.

- To break a scored tablet, use medical asepsis: clean (not sterile) technique. One method is to place the tablet in a paper towel, fold the towel over and, with your thumbs and index fingers in apposition, break the tablet along the score line. You can also use commercial pill splitters. *Don't break any tablets that are not scored.*

- If the patient has difficulty swallowing solids, first determine whether the medication is available in a liquid form. Don't crush enteric-coated and film-coated tablets and don't open capsules; instead, check with the pharmacist for alternative forms. If opening a capsule won't compromise the medication inside it, you can open the capsule and mix the drug with a small amount of applesauce, custard, or other soft food that will make the medication more palatable and easy to swallow.

- If crushing a pill won't compromise its medication, you can crush it, preferably using a commercial pill crusher. You can also crush a pill using a mortar and pestle; just make sure to clean both implements before and after crushing so no residue remains. To help a patient swallow the medication, you can mix a crushed drug with water or semisolids, such as applesauce or custard.

- Be knowledgeable about food-drug, drug-drug, and herb-drug interactions and always act to safeguard the patient.

- Patients with decreased tongue mobility and/or a decreased gag reflex may have difficulty swallowing medication. To promote swallowing, you may have to place the tablet or capsule in the patient's mouth, toward the pharynx and on the unaffected side. Afterwards, thoroughly inspect the patient's mouth to determine whether the tablet or capsule has been swallowed.

Liquid Medications

Special considerations for liquid medications include:

- Shake liquid medications (magmas, gels, suspensions) thoroughly before pouring; otherwise, the drug in the liquid may settle to the bottom.

- Pour liquids at eye level and then place them on a flat surface to accurately measure the dose. When pouring liquids, keep the label face up so it will not become stained. Before recapping, wipe the lip of the bottle with a paper towel.

- Note any unusual colour change or precipitate in a liquid. If such a change occurs, do not use the medication. Send the container to the pharmacy with a note describing what you've observed.

- Check references to determine how to disguise liquids that are distasteful or irritating. Two possibilities are to mix them with juice or to administer them through a straw after diluting well. Because liquid iron preparations stain the teeth, have the patient take them through a straw placed in the back of the mouth. Always dilute tinctures.

- Don't dilute liquid cough mixtures. Besides their antitussive action, they have a secondary soothing (demulcent) effect on the mucous membranes.

Parenteral Route

The term parenteral refers to drugs that are given via the intradermal (ID), subcutaneous, intramuscular (IM), or intravenous (IV) routes. Drugs are given via these routes because

- The patient is unable to take the drug orally
- A rapid systemic effect is required, or
- The oral route would destroy a drug or render it ineffective (e.g., insulin)

Parenteral drugs must be prepared and administered using aseptic technique. For ID, subcutaneous, and IM injections choose an injection site that is free from large blood vessels, nerves, sensitivity, bruises, hardened areas, abrasions and inflammation. Avoid areas not viable due to previous medical procedures, e.g. mastectomy, renal shunts, or grafts.

For each route there are considerations the nurse must make when choosing the site, equipment, and technique.

ID Injections

ID injections are used for diagnostic purposes such as allergy and tuberculin testing.

SITES

Suitable sites for ID testing are similar to those used for subcutaneous injections but also include the inner forearm.

EQUIPMENT

Use a 25-gauge ⅝ needle and a tuberculin syringe.

TECHNIQUE

1. Perform all necessary assessments prior to preparing the medication.

2. Wash hands and don gloves.

3. Identify patient verbally by name.

4. Check patient's ID band, ensuring hospital number matches the MAR.

5. Cleanse skin with an alcohol pad for 30 seconds and allow to dry for at least 30 seconds.

6. Place your nondominant hand around the arm from below and pull the skin tightly to make the forearm tissue taut.

7. Holding the syringe parallel to the skin with your four fingers and thumb, keep the bevel facing up.

8. Insert needle 3 mm into the intradermal space at a 10°–15° angle (Fig. 13-5).

9. Inject up to 0.5 mL until a wheal appears on the skin (Fig. 13-6).

10. If there is bleeding from the site, apply gentle pressure using gauze or alcohol swab. Do not massage the site.

11. Do not recap needle. Dispose of needle and syringe in a sharps container. Make the patient comfortable, wash your hands, and chart the medication, documenting the site of the injection.

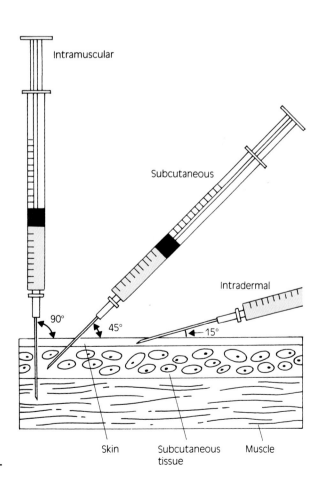

FIGURE 13-5

Comparison of angles of intersection for IM, subcutaneous, and ID injections.

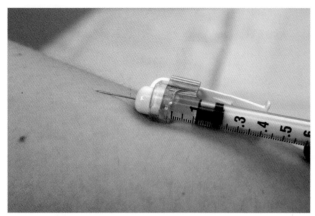
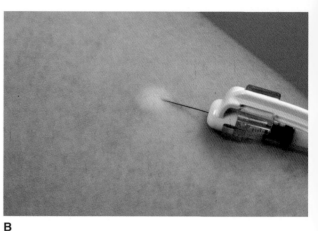

A   B

FIGURE 13-6

(**A**) Inserting the needle almost level with the skin. (**B**) Observing for wheal while injecting medication. (Used with permission from Evans-Smith, P. [2005]. *Taylor's clinical nursing skills.* Philadelphia: Lippincott Williams & Wilkins, p. 132.)

Subcutaneous Injection

The subcutaneous route is used for slow, sustained absorption of medications. Up to 1 mL can be injected safely. This route is used for immunizations, insulin, anticoagulants, and narcotics. This route is ideal for insulin because a slow and steady release is required. It is relatively painless and can tolerate frequent injections, making this route ideal for insulin therapy.

SITE

Figure 13-7 shows acceptable subcutaneous sites. A good layer of subcutaneous tissue is required in order for the steady release to be achieved and the medication not be given directly into the muscle.

EQUIPMENT

Use a short, small-gauge needle: 25–28 gauge, 9 mm, 13 mm, or 16 mm (⅜, ½, ⅝). Syringes may be pre-filled, insulin, or 1 or 3 mL. Insulin MUST be administered using equipment that measures in units in order to avoid errors in dosage.

TECHNIQUE

1. Perform all necessary assessments prior to preparing the medication.

2. Wash hands and don gloves.

3. Identify patient verbally by name

4. Check patient's ID band, ensuring hospital number matches the MAR

5. Skin should be pinched up with nondominant hand to lift the adipose tissue away from the underlying muscle, especially in thin patients.

6. Inject at an angle between 45° and 90° (as close to 90° as possible) (see Fig. 13-5).

7. Do not aspirate for subcutaneous injections.

8. Administer the medication slowly, ensuring the medication is deposited within the subcutaneous layer.

9. Do not massage the site.

10. Do not recap needle. Dispose of needle and syringe in a sharps container. Make the patient comfortable, wash your hands, and chart the medication, documenting the site of the injection.

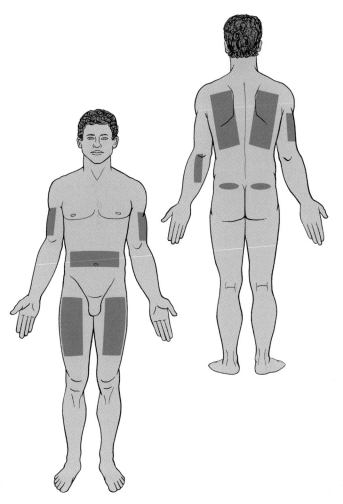

FIGURE 13-7

Sites for subcutaneous injection.

SPECIAL CONSIDERATIONS

Skin Preparation. Studies show that swabbing with alcohol before subcutaneous insulin injections predisposes the skin to be hardened and that such cleansing is not always necessary and the lack of skin prep has not been shown to result in higher infection rates. Aspirating is not necessary because piercing a blood vessel during an subcutaneous injection is very rare. Ensure injection sites are systematically rotated to avoid damage to the underlying tissue (lipohypertrophy, lipoatrophy, or lipodystrophy).

Insulin. Insulin can also be administered via a prefilled pen. The pen has a needle attached for each injection and a dial on the pen to measure the correct insulin dose. The technique matches the one described above, but you must hold the device for 5 seconds before removing it from the skin.

Heparin. Aspiration during heparin injections increases the likelihood of a haematoma forming. Heparin must be injected deep into subcutaneous tissue to minimize bruising. Most anticoagulant manufacturers recommend injecting into the lower abdomen.

IM Injection

IM injections deliver medication into well-perfused muscle, providing rapid systemic action. If frequent injections are required, sites must be clearly documented in the patient's chart to ensure an even rotation. This reduces patient discomfort from overuse of any one area and lessens the likelihood of the development of complications, such as muscle atrophy or abscesses.

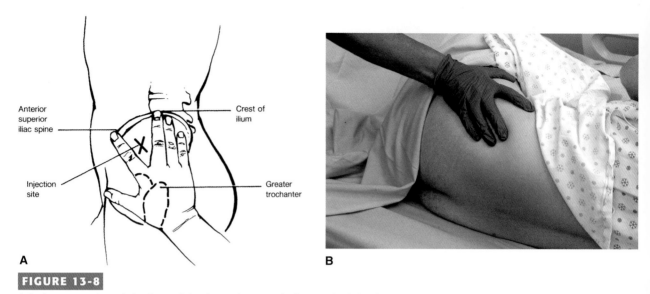

A   **B**

FIGURE 13-8

(**A**) The ventrogluteal site for IM injections; the cross indicates the injection site. (**B**) Locating the exact site. (Used with permission from Evans-Smith, P. [2005]. *Lippincott's atlas of medication administration* [2nd ed.]. Philadelphia: Lippincott Williams & Wilkins, p. 31.)

SITES

There are four sites used for IM injections (ventrogluteal, deltoid, vastus lateralis, and rectus fermoris). Consideration of patient's general physical status, age, and amount of drug will help to determine the safest site.

Ventrogluteal. The ventral part of the gluteal muscle (Fig 13-8). No large nerves or blood vessels and less adipose tissue over it. This is the optimal choice for IM injections in both children over 2 years and adults. Usual adult volume is 1–3 mL; the volume for children is 1 mL.

- Patient's position: supine, side lying, sitting, or standing.
- Landmark: Place the palm of your right hand on the greater trochanter of the patient's left hip (or your left hand to patient's right hip – "thumb towards pubis"). Extend your index finger up to the anterior superior iliac crest and stretch the middle finger to form a V as far along the iliac crest as you can reach. If you have small hands, you may have difficulty reaching the iliac crest, so slide the palm of your hand up from the greater trochanter until you can reach the anterior superior iliac crest with your index finger. The injection site is between the second joint of your index and middle fingers in the middle of the V over the body of the ventrogluteal muscle.

Deltoid. The deltoid muscle of the upper arm (Fig. 13-9). Use this site for IM injections only if specifically ordered. It is commonly used for vaccines. Usual adult volume is less than 2 mL; volume for children is up to 1 mL.

- Patient's position: Sitting with hand resting in lap.
- Landmark: Identify the acromion process and the point on the lateral arm in line with the axilla. Give the injection about 2.5 cm below the acromion process at a 90° angle into the densest part of the muscle.

Vastus lateralis. The quadriceps muscle located on the outer edge of the thigh (Fig. 13-10). This muscle is used most often when giving injections to infants because it's usually the best developed. It is recommended that this site be used only up to the age of 2 years to avoid accidental injury to the femoral nerve and muscle atrophy through overuse.

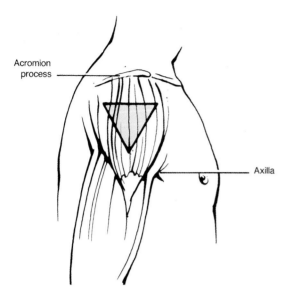

FIGURE 13-9

The deltoid muscle site for IM injections. The triangle indicates the injection site.

- Patient's position: Supine with foot inverted or side lying.

- Landmark: A handbreadth below the greater trochanter to a handbreadth above the knee. Insert the needle into the middle third of the muscle. You may have to bunch up the muscle before insertion.

Rectus femoris. The anterior quadriceps muscle. This site is rarely used by nurses except in infants (Fig. 13-11), but it is easily accessible for adults who must self-administer injections. Usual adult volume is 1–3 mL; volume for children 1 mL, infants 0.5 mL.

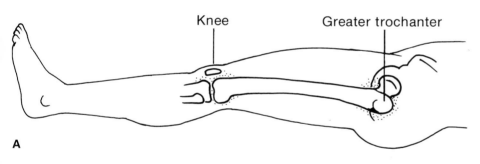

A

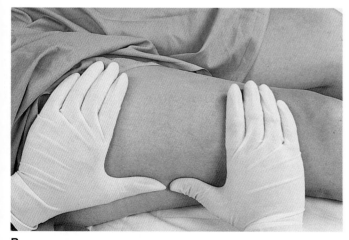

B

FIGURE 13-10

(**A**) Vastus lateralis injection site. (**B**) Locating the site.

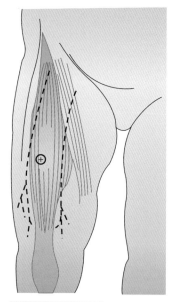

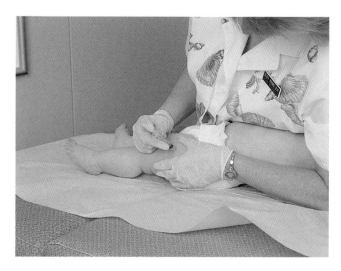

FIGURE 13-11

For infants under walking age, use the rectus femoris muscle for IM injections. (With permission from Pillitteri, A. [2002]. *Maternal and child health nursing* [4th ed.]. Philadelphia: Lippincott Williams & Wilkins, p. 1102.)

- Patient's position: Supine, sitting,

- Landmark: Middle third of anterior thigh. In children and very thin adults, may need to be bunched up in a handful to provide sufficient depth for injection.

Note: Although the dorsogluteal site was once a commonly used site for IM injections, frequent complications are associated with this site. Damage to the sciatic nerve or the superior gluteal artery can occur. Additionally, due to the increased amount of adipose tissue over this site, medications are more likely to be injected into adipose tissue than muscle, resulting in poor absorption and increased discomfort to the patient. For these reasons, this site is not recommended for use.

EQUIPMENT

Adults: 21 gauge/25–50 mm (1–2 inch) needle.
Children: 21–23 gauge/25–38 mm (1–1½ inch) needle.
Infants (less than 2 years): 23 gauge/25 mm (1 inch)
Newborn–2 months: 25 gauge/16–25 mm (⅝–1 inch)
Syringe: 1 or 3 mL

TECHNIQUE

1. Perform all necessary assessments prior to preparing the medication (vital signs, apical pulse, site integrity, pain).

2. Wash hands and don gloves.

3. Identify patient verbally by name

4. Check patient's ID band, ensuring hospital number matches the MAR

5. If previous injection site not documented in patient's chart, ask patient to ensure sites are rotated. Choose a site that is free from large blood vessels, nerves, sensitivity, bruises, hardened areas, abrasions, and inflammation.

6. Landmark carefully to ensure injection is given into body of muscle.

7. Cleanse the injection site for 30 seconds, and allow to dry for at least 30 seconds.

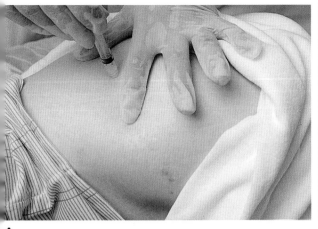

A

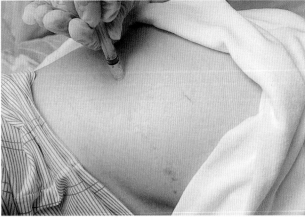

B

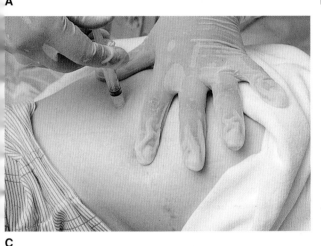

C

FIGURE 13-12

(**A**) Dart the needle into the skin; (**B**) aspirate slowly; (**C**) inject medication slowly.

8. Children should be restrained by a parent or another nurse or wrapped securely to prevent harm to themselves.

9. With nondominant hand, stretch the skin over the site or bunch the muscle up in order to ensure medication will be given in muscle not adipose tissue.

10. With dominant hand, insert the needle directly at a 90° angle with a *quick*, dart-like motion to ensure the needle goes well into the muscle (Fig. 13-12). Medication must reach muscle in order to achieve desired effect and to reduce pain.

11. Aspirate by steadying the barrel with the thumb and forefinger of your nondominant hand and gently pull the plunger back (with dominant hand) approximate 3 mm, checking for blood.

12. If blood is present, withdraw needle, discard needle and syringe, and prepare a new injection.

13. If no blood is present, inject slowly at a rate of approximately 1 mL every 10 seconds. Hold the syringe steady so needle does not move within the patient's muscle, causing discomfort.

14. Wait 10 seconds prior to withdrawing the needle to allow the medication to diffuse into the muscle. Withdraw the needle quickly.

15. If there is bleeding from the site, apply gentle pressure using gauze or alcohol swab. Do not massage the site.

16. Do not recap needle. Dispose of needle and syringe in a sharps container. Make the patient comfortable, wash your hands, and chart the medication, documenting the site of the injection.

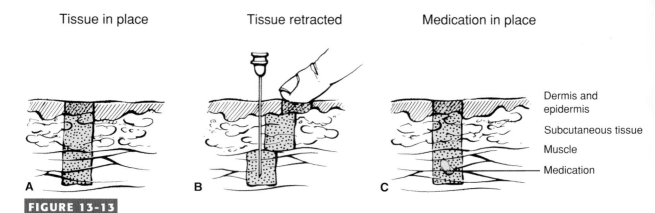

Tissue in place	Tissue retracted	Medication in place	Dermis and epidermis
			Subcutaneous tissue
			Muscle
A	B	C	Medication

FIGURE 13-13

Z-track technique. The tissue is retracted to one side and held there until the injection is given. When the hand is removed, the tissue closes over the injection tract, preventing medication from rising to the surface.

Z-TRACK TECHNIQUE FOR IM INJECTIONS

Some medications, such as iron dextran (Imferon) and hydroxyzine (Vistazine), are irritating to the tissues and can stain the skin. The Z-track method, used at the ventrogluteal site, can prevent medication from seeping into the needle tract and onto the skin.

1. After preparing the medication, change the needle to prevent leakage along the tract.

2. Prepare the patient and the site in the usual manner.

3. Use the heel on your nondominant hand to retract the tissue to the side. Hold this position during the injection (Fig. 13-13). Spread the skin taut over the injection site.

4. Inject at a 90° angle, as usual. Before giving this injection, be sure to aspirate.

5. After giving the injection, count 10 seconds.

6. Then remove the needle quickly.

7. Remove the hand that has been retracting the tissue.

8. Do not massage the site.

9. Using an alcohol pad or dry gauze pad, press down on the site to inhibit bleeding.

IV Route

IV drugs may be given in a number of ways: continuous IV infusion; secondary or IVPB (IV piggyback) infusion; IV push (slow or fast); and flushing of an intermittent infusion plug. Because IV medications introduce the drug directly into the bloodstream—thus having an immediate effect—you must follow strict asepsis technique.

Several types of IV needles are appropriate for inserting into a vein. The most common is the cathlon or "over the needle," in which a plastic catheter covers the needle. After inserting the needle in the vein, you withdraw the needle and the plastic catheter stays in place for a specified amount of time.

Usually, IV needles are inserted peripherally in the hand or forearm (Fig. 13-14). For long-term IV therapy, a central venous catheter (Fig. 13-15) or peripherally inserted central catheter (PICC) (Fig. 13-16) may be inserted by a specially trained health professional. Information on IV calculations is found in Chapters 8 and 9.

Basic guidelines for peripheral IV therapy include:

- Use aseptic technique for insertion of IV needle.

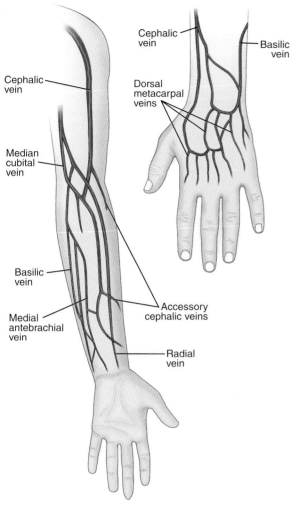

Cephalic vein
Basilic vein
Dorsal metacarpal veins
Cephalic vein
Median cubital vein
Basilic vein
Medial antebrachial vein
Accessory cephalic veins
Radial vein

FIGURE 13-14

Infusion sites available in the hand or forearm. (Used with permission from Taylor, C. [2008]. *Fundamentals of nursing* [6th ed.]. Philadelphia: Lippincott Williams & Wilkins, p. 1709.)

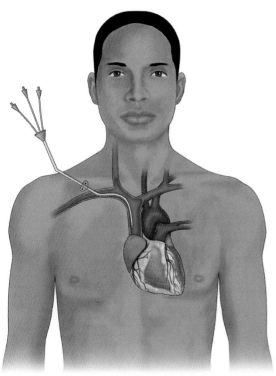

FIGURE 13-15

Triple-lumen central venous catheter (TLC or CVC). (Used with permission from Taylor, C. [2008]. *Fundamentals of nursing* [6th ed.]. Philadelphia: Lippincott Williams & Wilkins, p. 1708.)

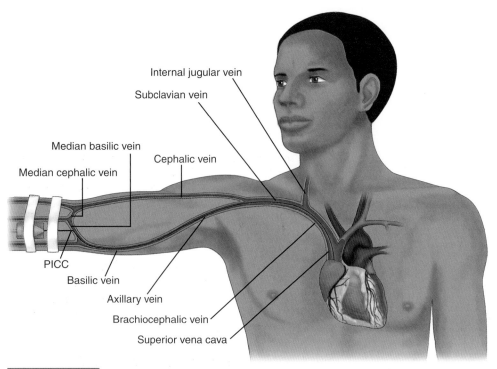

Internal jugular vein

Subclavian vein

Median basilic vein

Cephalic vein

Median cephalic vein

PICC

Basilic vein

Axillary vein

Brachiocephalic vein

Superior vena cava

FIGURE 13-16

Peripherally inserted central catheter (PICC). (Used with permission from Taylor, C. [2008]. *Fundamentals of nursing* [6th ed.]. Philadelphia: Lippincott Williams & Wilkins, p. 1708.)

- Use an occlusive dressing to secure IV needle. Most healthcare settings use a clear plastic dressing over the IV needle site so that constant monitoring of the site can occur.

- Verify IV fluids and IV medications orders before administration. Calculate the correct dose. Check an approved compatibility guide to determine the compatibility of IV fluids and IV medications.

- Infuse IV fluids and IV medications according to policy and procedures of the institution. Use an infusion pump if available.

- Monitor and assess the IV site frequently and according to institutional guidelines. Monitor the IV site for: swelling, colour, temperature, and pain.

- Follow institutional guidelines for changing the IV site, changing the IV fluids, and changing the IV tubing. Generally, a peripheral IV site is changed every 72 hours; IV fluids every 24 hours; and IV tubing every 72 hours.

For further information about IV insertion and IV medication administration, consult a nursing pharmacology or a nursing fundamentals textbook.

Buccal Tablet

Use standard precautions: hand washing and gloves. Identify the patient verbally by name. Check the ID band, ensuring hospital number matches the MAR, explain the procedure, and then give the tablet to the patient. The patient should place the tablet between the gum and the cheek. Withhold food and liquids until the tablet is dissolved, (approximately 14 – 25 minutes) and warn the patient not to disturb the tablet. Medication applied across mucous membranes causes rapid systemic absorption. To minimize irritation, alternate doses between cheeks.

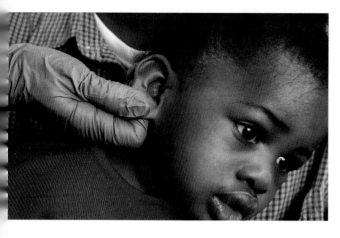

FIGURE 13-17

Technique for administering ear drops in children under 3 years old. (Used with permission from Evans-Smith, P. [2005]. *Taylor's clinical nursing skills.* Philadelphia: Lippincott Williams & Wilkins, p. 173.)

Ear Drops

Use standard precautions: hand washing and gloves. The ear drops, labelled either "otic" or "auric," should be warmed to body temperature or fainting can occur. Identify the patient verbally by name, check the patient's ID band, ensuring hospital number matches the MAR, and explain the procedure. Help the patient into a comfortable position; lying on side with the affected ear up is recommended. With a dropper, draw the medication into the dropper. Straighten the ear canal by pulling the pinna up and back (for an adult) or down and back (for a child 3 years or younger) (Fig. 13-17).

Placing the tip of the dropper at the opening of the canal, instill the medication into the canal (Fig. 13-18). The patient should then rest on the unaffected side for 10 to 15 minutes. If the patient wishes, place a cotton ball in the canal. Make sure the patient is comfortable, and then wash your hands and chart the medication.

Ear Drop Administration

- Should the ear pinna be pulled up or down with adults?
- Should the ear pinna be pulled up or down with children?
- Adults are usually taller than children, so the ear pinna is pulled "up" and back for ear drops.
- Children younger than 3 years old are smaller than adults, so the ear pinna is pulled "down" and back for ear drops.

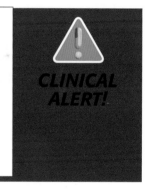

CLINICAL ALERT!

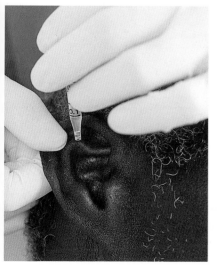

FIGURE 13-18

In adults, pull the pinna up and back to straighten the ear canal and instill the medication.

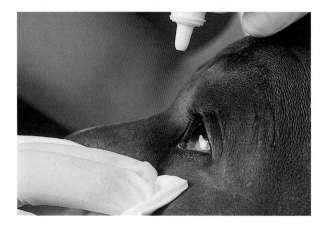

FIGURE 13-19

Applying eye drops: Gently draw the lower eyelid down to create a pocket. Insert the medication into this pocket.

Eye Drops or Ointment

Use standard precautions: hand washing and gloves. Identify the patient by name, check the patient's ID band, ensuring hospital number matches the MAR, and explain the procedure. Hand the patient a tissue. The patient may sit or lie down. If exudate is present, you may need to cleanse the eyelid with cotton or gauze and either normal saline or distilled water for the eye. Eye medications—which must be labelled "ophthalmic" or "for the eye"—come in either a monodrop container (a container with a drop-like lid); in a bottle with a dropper; or as an ophthalmic ointment. Gently draw the patient's lower eyelid down to create a sac (Fig. 13-19). Instruct the patient to look up. Then instill the liquid medication into the lower conjunctival sac, taking care not to touch the membrane. If you're administering ophthalmic ointment, spread a small amount from the inner to the outer canthus of the eye. Advise the patient that some ophthalmic medications may cause stinging when first administered to the eye surface.

After either of these procedures, instruct the patient to close her or his eyelids gently and rotate her or his eyes. The patient may use a tissue to wipe away excess medication. Also, after instilling eye drops, have the patient apply gentle pressure with the index finger to the inner canthus for a minute. This action keeps the medication from entering the tear duct.

To prevent cross-contamination, each patient should have individual medication containers. If the medication impairs the patient's vision, provide a safe environment. Make the patient comfortable. Then dispose of the gloves according to institutional procedure, wash your hands, and chart the medication.

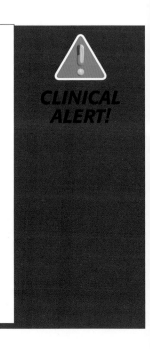

Eye and Ear Abbreviations

The use of abbreviations—including those for eye and ear medications—can cause confusion. The Institute for Safe Medication Practices recommends *avoiding using these abbreviations:*

- AS (left ear), AD (right ear), AU (both ears). These are often confused with the terms for eyes: OS (left eye), OD (right eye), OU (both eyes).

- Recommendations: Write out the phrases "left ear," "right ear," or "both ears," as appropriate. As well as "left eye," "right eye," "both eyes."

- Be sure to write out "every day" or "daily" rather than using the abbreviation "qd," which is easily confused with "OD."

CLINICAL ALERT!

Nasogastric (N/G) Route

PRECAUTIONS

Use standard precautions: hand washing and gloves. Medications given via the N/G route are not routinely to be mixed together in a syringe for administration. Each medication is to be administered separately and the tube flushed between each medication (usually with 10–30 mL of sterile water). If patient is severely fluid restricted (e.g., neonates), some medications may be mixed together if compatible. Medications are to be instilled using clean technique.

EQUIPMENT

Sterile water for flush (clean water is used in community settings)
Syringe (50–60 mL) (5–30 mL for infant/child) with appropriate tip attached to connect to N/G tube
30 mL plastic med cup

TECHNIQUE

1. Check patient's ID band, ensuring hospital number matches the MAR.

2. Elevate head of bed 30°–45° (if not contraindicated).

3. Don gloves.

4. Prior to instilling any medications into tube, ensure you follow institutional or hospital policy regarding checking N/G tube placement. Checking gastric aspirate for acidity using pH paper is more accurate and considered more reliable than injecting air and listening for "swoosh."

5. Flush N/G tube prior to administration of medications and again after administration of medications with a minimum of 10 mL sterile water (2–3 mL for infants; 5–10 mL for children). Flush tube using gravity flow method (Fig. 13-20).

6. Prepare medications to instill into N/G tube:

   • Use liquid medications whenever possible. Dilute liquids with two to three times their volume to prevent tube from clogging.

   • Crush oral tablets (immediate release) into a fine powder and mix in sterile water (10–30 mL) and administer immediately.

   • Open hard gelatin capsules (immediate release), crush, and mix contents with sterile water (10–30 mL) and administer immediately.

   • Dissolve soft gel capsules (immediate release) in warm sterile water (15–30 mL). NOTE: Complete dilution may take up to 1 hour.

   • DO NOT CRUSH

      • Enteric-coated tablets

      • Sustained-release or long-acting tablets

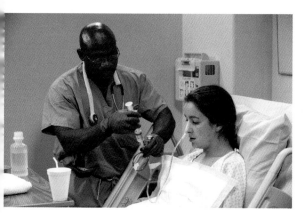

FIGURE 13-20

Flush the tube with at least 10–30 mL water. (Used with permission from Taylor, C. [2008]. *Fundamentals of nursing* [6th ed.]. Philadelphia: Lippincott Williams & Wilkins, p. 1473.)

- Cytotoxics or hormones
- Draw up each medication in syringe separately and administer via N/G tube.

7. Flush tube with a minimum of 10 mL (0.5 mL for infants) sterile water.

8. Wash syringe well between incompatible medications or use a different syringe.

9. Ensure N/G tube is closed or reattached to continuous feeds if ordered.

10. Ensure patient is comfortable. Leave head of bed elevated for 30 minutes if possible. Wash hands.

11. Document medications given and amount of water given with flushes.

Nose Drops

Use standard precautions: hand washing and gloves. Identify the patient verbally by name, check the patient's ID band, ensuring hospital number matches the MAR, and explain the procedure. The patient, either sitting or lying down, may have to blow his or their nose gently to clear the nasal passageway. Have the patient tilt their head back. If the patient is lying in bed, place a pillow under their shoulders to hyperextend the neck (unless contraindicated). Insert the dropper about one-third of the way into first one nostril, then the other. Do not touch the nostril. Instill the nose drops (Fig. 13-21), and then instruct the patient to maintain the position for 1 to 2 minutes. If the patient feels the medication flowing down their throat, assist the patient to sit up and bend their head down so the medication will flow into the sinuses instead.

To prevent cross-contamination, each patient should have their own medication container. After making the patient comfortable, wash your hands and chart the medication.

If a nasal spray is ordered, push the tip of patient's nose up and then place the nozzle tip just inside the nares, so when you give the medication, the spray is aiming toward the back of the nose.

Rectal Suppository

Use standard precautions: hand washing and gloves. Identify the patient verbally by name, then check the patient's ID band, ensuring hospital number matches the MAR, and explain the procedure. Encourage the patient to defecate (unless the suppository is ordered for this purpose). Position the patient in the left lateral recumbent position (Fig. 13-22). After moistening the suppository with a water-soluble lubricant, instruct the patient to breathe slowly and deeply through the mouth. To open the anal sphincter, ask the patient to "bear down" as if having a bowel movement. Using a gloved finger, insert the suppository past the sphincter. You will feel the suppository move into the canal. Wipe away excess lubricant, and encourage the patient to retain the suppository as long as possible (up to 30 minutes if possible). Make the patient comfortable. Then dispose of gloves according to institutional procedure, wash your hands, and chart the medication.

The patient may insert her or his own suppository if she or he is able and wishes to do so. Provide a glove, lubricant, and suppository. After insertion, check to make sure that the suppository is in place and is not in the bed.

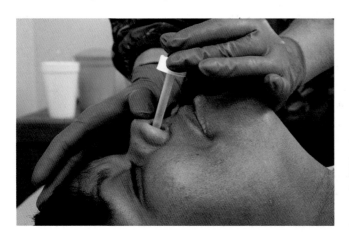

FIGURE 13-21

Administering nose drops. (Used with permission from Evans-Smith, P. [2005]. *Taylor's clinical nursing skills.* Philadelphia: Lippincott Williams & Wilkins, p. 178.)

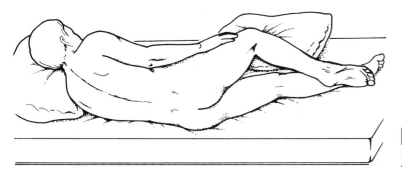

FIGURE 13-22

Left lateral recumbent position.

Respiratory Inhaler

Use standard precautions: hand washing and gloves. An inhaler delivers medication directly to the airway as the patient inhales. Inhalers come in several forms, including metered-dose inhaler (MDI) with a spacer and mouthpiece (Fig. 13-23) and dry powder inhalers such as Discus, Turbuhaler, and Handihaler.

METERED DOSE INHALER TECHNIQUE

Using an inhaler without a spacer is NOT recommended.

1. Identify the patient verbally by name, check the patient's ID band, ensuring hospital number matches the MAR, and explain the procedure.

2. Instruct the patient to:

   - Open mouthpiece.
   - Shake the MDI inhaler 10 times.
   - Insert MDI into spacer.
   - Breathe out.
   - Place mouthpiece between lips and form a seal.
   - Press down on MDI.
   - Slowly breathe in and hold breath for 10 seconds (if whistle sounds, it is a warning to slow breathing).
   - If another puff is needed, wait 30 seconds then repeat.
   - Rinse and spit to remove medication from mucous membranes and teeth

3. If institutional policy permits, the inhaler can be left at the patient's bedside.

4. Make the patient comfortable, wash your hands, and chart the medication.

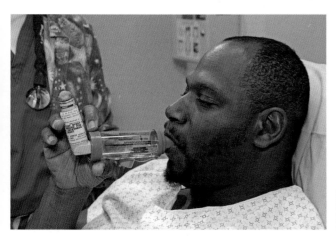

FIGURE 13-23

Example of a metered-dose inhaler (MDI) with spacer.

5. Clean spacer once a week by soaking spacer in warm soapy water. Rinse gently in warm water. Drip dry.

DRY POWDER INHALER TECHNIQUE

1. Identify the patient verbally by name, check the patient's ID band, ensuring hospital number matches the MAR, and explain the procedure.

2. Instruct patient to:

   - Open device and load medication (slide and click, twist, or insert capsule).
   - Breathe out (do not blow breath directly into device due to contamination risk).
   - Place device between lips and form seal.
   - Breathe in quickly and hold breath for 10 seconds.
   - Rinse and spit to remove medication from mucous membranes and teeth.
   - Remove capsule (if applicable) and close device. Keep device dry.

3. If institutional policy permits, the inhaler can be left at the patient's bedside.

4. Make the patient comfortable, wash your hands, and chart the medication.

Topical Route

Topical drug preparations have two purposes: to cause a local effect or to act systematically. To create a systemic effect, the drug must be absorbed into the circulation.

Skin Applications

Use standard precautions: hand washing and gloves. Identify the patient verbally by name, check the patient's ID band, ensuring hospital number matches the MAR, and explain the procedure. Avoid personal contact with the medication so that you don't absorb any of the drug. Apply the medication with a tongue blade, a glove, a gauze pad, or a cotton-tipped applicator. Cleanse the area as appropriate before beginning a new application.

Many kinds of medications are applied topically. Before you proceed, obtain the following information:

- How to prepare the skin
- How to apply the medication
- Whether to cover the skin or leave skin uncovered following application

The following are some typical drug preparations:

- Powders: The patient's skin should be dry. Sprinkle the medication on your gloved hands, then apply it. Use sparingly to avoid caking.
- Lotions: Using a gloved hand or gauze pad, pat the medication on lightly.
- Creams: Using gloves, rub the medication into the patient's skin.
- Ointments: Using a gloved hand or an applicator, apply an even coat and then place a dressing on the patient's skin.

After any of these procedures, make the patient comfortable and dispose of gloves according to institutional policy. Then wash your hands and chart the medication.

Transdermal Disks, Patches, and Pads

Use standard precautions: hand washing and gloves. All of these products are unit-dose adhesive bandages, consisting of a semipermeable membrane that allows medication to be released continuously over time. Some patches are effective for 24 hours, some for 72 hours, and some last as long as 1 week.

The skin at the site should be free of hair and not subject to excessive movement; therefore, avoid distal extremities. At each administration, change the site. If the patch loosens with bathing, contact doctor or ordering health professional to decide if new patch should be applied.

Medications appropriate for this route include hormones, nitroglycerin, narcotics for chronic, severe pain, antihypertensive drugs such as clonidine (Catapres), and anti–motion sickness drugs such as scopolamine.

Identify the patient verbally by name, check the patient's ID band, ensuring hospital number matches the MAR, and explain the procedure Don gloves. Select a site where the skin is clear and dry, with no signs of irritation. Ensure previous patch has been removed before administering a new one. Open the packet and remove the cover from the adhesive transdermal drug. Don't touch the inside of the pad. Apply the pad to the skin, pressing firmly to be certain all edges adhere. Chart on the pad the date, time, and your initials. Then make the patient comfortable, wash your hands, and chart the medication.

Sublingual Tablets

Use standard precautions: hand washing and gloves. The most common sublingual medication is nitroglycerin, which is prescribed to alleviate symptoms of angina pectoris. If a patient does not feel relief within 5 minutes, a second and then a third dose at 5-minute intervals is commonly ordered. If the pain continues after 15 minutes, notify the physician.

To administer a sublingual tablet, first identify the patient by name, check the patient's ID band, ensuring hospital number matches the MAR, and explain the procedure. Instruct the patient to sit down and to place the tablet under his or her tongue. If the patient is unable to place the tablet under the tongue, the nurse should do it, and should wear a glove. The patient should not swallow or chew the tablet, but allow it to dissolve. Make sure the patient does not eat or drink anything with the tablet, because that will interfere with the effectiveness of the medication. Stay with the patient until the pain has stopped. For more information, consult an appropriate text. To conclude, wash your hands and chart the medication.

Vaginal Suppository or Tablet

Use standard precautions: hand washing and gloves. Identify the patient by name, check the patient's ID band, ensuring hospital number matches the MAR, and explain the procedure. Ask her to void in a bedpan. (If the perineal area has excessive secretions, you may need to perform perineal care after the patient voids.) Insert the suppository or tablet into the applicator. Then assist the patient into a lithotomy position (lying on her back, with knees flexed and legs apart) and drape her, leaving the perineal area exposed. Put on gloves.

Separate the labia majora and identify the vaginal opening. Then insert the applicator down and back (Fig. 13-24), and eject the suppository or tablet into the vagina. (If the patient wishes, she can do this procedure herself.) You may also insert the suppository—using gloved fingers—into the vagina. Place a pad at the vaginal opening to collect secretions, and make the patient comfortable before you leave.

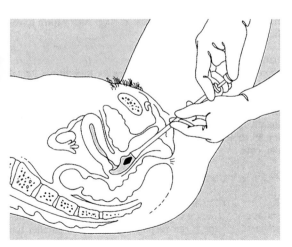

FIGURE 13-24

Vaginal applicator should be inserted down and back. (From Taylor, C., Lillis, C., and LeMone, P. [2001]. *Fundamentals of nursing* [4th ed.]. Philadelphia: Lippincott Williams & Wilkins, p. 627.)

Wash the applicator with soap and water, wrap it in a paper towel, and leave it at the bedside. Dispose of gloves and equipment according to institutional procedure wash your hands, and chart the medication.

Vaginal Cream or Vaginal Tablet

Use standard precautions: hand washing and gloves. Vaginal cream is packaged either in a prefilled disposable syringe or in a tube with its own applicator. To fill the applicator, remove the cap from the tube and screw the top of the tube into the applicator's barrel. Squeeze the tube and fill the barrel to the prescribed dose. Then unscrew the tube from the applicator and cap it.

Prepare the patient as described in the previous section. Insert the applicator down and back, and press the plunger to empty the barrel of medication. The patient may do this herself if she wishes. After removing the applicator, place a pad at the vaginal opening to collect secretions. Before you leave, make sure the patient is comfortable. She should remain in bed for a minimum of 20 minutes.

If the applicator is a prefilled unit dose, dispose of it according to institutional policy. If it is reusable, wash it with soap and water, and place it in a clean paper towel on the bedside stand. Dispose of your gloves wash your hands, and chart the medication.

◖▭ Special Considerations

The basics of medication administration apply to all age groups. However, administering drugs to pediatric and geriatric patients requires special considerations.

Neonatal and Pediatric Considerations

Dosages of medications for neonatal and pediatric administration are covered in Chapter 10.

Differences in medication administration are mainly developmental; consult a nursing pediatric textbook for specifics and for special skills needed.

Suggestions for administering oral medication to children include:

- Before you administer an oral medication, offer the child a popsicle, which will numb the taste buds.

- Mix the drug with a teaspoon of puréed fruit, ice cream, or syrup. Using essential foodstuffs is not a good idea, because the child may refuse those foods later.

- Have older children pinch their nostrils closed and drink the medication through a straw. Because this technique interferes with their ability to smell, it keeps them from tasting the medication.

- For infants, use a specially manufactured medication nipple or pacifier.

Suggestions for IM administration in children include:

• Explain the procedure to the child, using terms she or he can easily understand.

• Predetermine the injection site to make sure the muscle is large enough to accommodate the amount and type of medication.

• A topical anesthetic (if ordered) can help reduce the pain of a needle-stick.

• A child's behaviour and movements are unpredictable, so have someone help you hold the child securely.

• Distract the child with conversation or a toy.

• Insert the needle quickly and inject the medication slowly.

• Use a decorative adhesive bandage to cover the injection site.

CRITICAL THINKING: TEST YOUR CLINICAL SAVVY

A client in your outpatient clinic is to receive an IM injection. The drug literature states that the preferred site is the ventrogluteal.

A. When would the deltoid muscle be preferable over this site? What are the contraindications for using the deltoid muscle?

B. The client requests the injection in the deltoid. What is your response in light of the recommended site in the drug literature?

C. If a patient is bedridden, which site would you choose for an IM injection, and why?

D. Even though you are not actually touching the injection site, why are gloves necessary when giving IM injections?

SELF TEST 1   Standard Precautions

Complete the statements about standard precautions in medication administration. Answers appear at the end of the chapter.

1. Standard precautions should be applied when administering medications

    a. to all patients

    b. only to patients with HIV or hepatitis B virus

2. The type of precaution to be used by the nurse depends on _____

    _____.

3. Administering medications, the nurse must wear gloves when _____

    _____

    and _____.

4. After the nurse administers an injection, the syringe should be placed

    _____

    _____.

5. Five precautions stressed by the CDC are _____, _____,

    _____, _____,

    and _____.

6. If you're administering medications, you should wash your hands:

    a. _____

    b. _____

    c. _____

    d. _____

7. Standard precautions while administering ear drops or eye drops medications are:

    _____

8. A nurse should wear a gown to protect his or her uniform whenever

    _____

    _____

9. The nurse should wear protective eyewear whenever _____

    _____

    _____.

10. Wear a mask when _____

    _____ or _____

    _____.

SELF TEST 2   **Medication Administration**

Complete the statements about medication administration. Answers appear at the end of the chapter.

1. The primary reason patients should have individual eye medication is to _____

    _____ .

2. The best method of checking the positioning of an N/G tube is

    _____ .

3. For administration of a rectal suppository, the patient should lie

    _____

    _____ .

4. How should each of the following be applied to a patient's skin?

    a. powders _____

    b. lotions _____

    c. creams _____

    d. ointments _____

5. How many sublingual nitroglycerin tablets may a patient take to relieve pain? _____

    At what time interval? _____

6. Identify these administration procedures as parenteral or nonparenteral.

    a. subcutaneous injection _____   **f.** nitroglycerin ointment _____

    b. sublingual tablet _____   **g.** respiratory inhaler _____

    c. vaginal suppository _____   **h.** N/G route _____

    d. nose drops _____   **i.** ID _____

    e. IM injection _____   **j.** rectal suppository _____

7. How should the nurse insert a vaginal applicator? _____

    _____

    _____

8. How should the nurse prepare the patient's skin for an injection? _____

    _____

    _____

9. List three reasons for administering medication by injection. _____

    _____

10. What is the difference in administering ear drops to an adult and to a 2-year-old child?

    _____

    _____

PROFICIENCY TEST 1 PART A Administration Procedures

Name: _____

Choose the correct answer for each of these questions. Answers appear in Appendix A.

1. A nurse's first check when preparing medication is:

   a. checking the patient's armband before administration
   b. checking the MAR while pouring the liquid medication
   c. checking the unit-dose label with the order
   d. checking the unit-dose packaging after it is disposed

2. Which actions of the medication computer scanning device help prevent medication errors?

   a. verifying patient's identity by scanning the patient's armband
   b. verifying the correct medication by scanning the bar code on the unit-dose packaging
   c. verifying the correct time by scanning the medication administration record (MAR)
   d. all of the above

3. Checking the medication administration record (MAR) before administering medication enables the nurse to determine

   a. the name of the pharmacist who ordered the medication
   b. the correct administration time of the medication
   c. any previous medication errors
   d. orders for intake and output

4. When pouring an oral liquid medication, the nurse should

   a. place the cup on the tabletop and bend over to get the right level
   b. hold the cup in the hand and pour to the top of the meniscus
   c. hold the cup at eye level and pour to the center of the meniscus
   d. rest the cup on a flat surface and pour to the meniscus line

5. Which of these statements regarding injections from powders is *false?*

   a. Read the label twice before drawing up and once after.
   b. Draw up one medication at a time.
   c. Always use sterile water as a diluent.
   d. Pull back on the plunger before injecting the medication.

6. Injecting a specific amount of air into the vial beforehand helps in withdrawing medication from a vial. Which of these statements explains this action?

   a. It creates a partial vacuum in the vial.
   b. It makes the pressure in the vial greater than atmospheric pressure.
   c. It makes the pressure in the vial the same as atmospheric pressure.
   d. It makes the pressure in the vial less than atmospheric pressure.

7. If a patient has difficulty swallowing medications, which oral form of drug may be crushed?

   a. sugar-coated tablet
   b. enteric-coated tablet
   c. buccal tablet
   d. capsule

(continued)

8. A major advantage in the unit-dose system of drug administration is that

   a. the drug supply is always available
   b. no error is possible
   c. the drugs are less expensive than stock distribution
   d. the pharmacist provides a second professional check

9. When a drug is to be administered sublingually, the patient should be instructed to

   a. drink a full glass of water when swallowing
   b. rinse the mouth with water after taking the drug
   c. chew the tablet and allow saliva to collect under the tongue
   d. hold the medication under the tongue until it dissolves

10. Ampoules differ from vials in that ampoules

    a. are always glass containers
    b. contain only one dose
    c. contain solids as well as liquids
    d. are not used for injections

11. The Z-track technique for injections can be used to

    a. administer more than one drug at a single site
    b. inhibit hematoma formation by promoting drug absorption
    c. prevent skin discoloration by inhibiting drug seepage
    d. reduce allergic reactions at the injection site

12. Which action is correct when giving a Z-track injection?

    a. Retract the skin and hold it to one side while giving the medication.
    b. Massage the skin after giving the injection.
    c. After the needle has been inserted, do not pull back the plunger.
    d. Inject the medication quickly.

13. Which angle of injection is correctly matched with the route of administration?

    a. ID—45° angle
    b. IM—90° angle
    c. Subcutaneous—30° angle
    d. Z-track—45° angle

14. A patient asks how to put in eye drops. The nurse instructs the patient to place the drops

    a. into the lower conjunctival sac
    b. under the upper lid
    c. directly on the cornea
    d. in the inner canthus

15. When administering a vaginal suppository, which statement is false?

    a. Use standard precautions.
    b. The patient may insert the medication.
    c. The patient should be lying on her back.
    d. The applicator must be kept sterile.

(continued)

16. When applying the next dose of a transdermal medication, the nurse should

    a. shave the new area and prepare with povidone-iodine
    b. use a different site
    c. rotate the use of arms and legs as sites
    d. allow the previous patch to remain on the skin

17. Discomfort of an injection is reduced when the needle is inserted

    a. slowly into loose tissue
    b. slowly into firm tissue
    c. rapidly into loose tissue
    d. rapidly into firm tissue

18. After administering an injection, the nurse should

    a. immediately recap the needle
    b. break the needle off the syringe for safety
    c. place the used syringe in a nearby sharps container
    d. put on gloves to carry the syringe to the utility room

19. Which statement is incorrect for administering drugs to mucous membranes?

    a. Eye medications must be labelled ophthalmic.
    b. Patients may insert their own rectal suppositories.
    c. Apply sublingual medications to the space between the teeth and the cheek.
    d. The nurse may leave eye medications on the patient's bedside stand.

PROFICIENCY TEST 1   **PART B Administration Procedures**

Decide whether the following actions are correct or incorrect, according to the precautions to follow when administering medications. Explain your choice. Answers appear in Appendix A.

1. A nurse wears gloves to remove an IV intermittent infusion plug from a patient's arm. This action is

   _____

   _____

2. A nurse who has just removed a gown and gloves puts them into the disposal container in the patient's room and leaves the room. This action is

   _____

   _____

3. In the medication room, a nurse puts on gloves to prepare an IV for administration. This action is

   _____

   _____

4. A nurse puts on a mask to administer an oral medication to a patient on respiratory isolation precautions. This action is

   _____

   _____

5. A nurse applies standard precautions in caring for all patients on the unit. This action is

   _____

   _____

6. A nurse wears gloves to place a transdermal pad behind a patient's ear. This action is

   _____

   _____

7. A nurse puts on gloves and gown to administer 500 mL of a vaginal douche to a lethargic patient. This action is

   _____

   _____

(continued)

8. A nurse whose finger has been stuck with a contaminated IV needle carefully washes his/her hands with soap and water, and applies a bandage to the site. Because the patient's diagnosis is a brain tumour, the nurse decides no further action is necessary. This action is

_____

_____

9. A nurse giving an injection to a patient decides not to wear gloves. This action is

_____

_____

10. A nurse puts on gloves to administer an oral tablet to an alert patient with a positive HIV blood count. This action is

_____

_____

11. After administering an injection, the nurse carefully caps the needle. This action is

_____

_____

12. A nurse decides not to wear gloves when administering eye drops, because they are too bulky. This action is

_____

_____

Answers to Self Tests

Self Test 1 Standard Precautions

1. A. To all patients. There is a risk of potential exposure to hepatitis virus and HIV that may not have been detected by standard laboratory methods.
2. The type of contact the nurse has with the patient.
3. When there is any direct "hands-on" contact with patient's blood, bodily fluids, or secretions; when handling materials or equipment contaminated with blood or body fluids.
4. In a labelled, puncture-proof container.
5. Handwashing, gloves, gowns, masks, and protective eyewear.
6. a. Before preparing medications and after administering medicines to each patient.
   b. After removing gloves, gowns, masks, and protective eyewear and before leaving each patient.
   c. Immediately when soiled with the patient's blood or body fluids.
   d. After handling equipment soiled with blood or body fluids.
7. Hand washing and gloves.
8. The nurse's clothing may become contaminated with a patient's blood or body fluids.
9. A nurse is in extremely close contact with the patient and there is the possibility of the patient's blood or blood-tinged fluids being splashed or sprayed into the nurse's eyes or mucous membranes.
10. The patient is placed on strict or respiratory isolation precautions. Carrying out a medication procedure may cause blood or body fluids to splash directly onto the nurse's face.

Self Test 2 Medication Administration

1. Prevent cross-contamination.
2. Aspirate stomach contents and check for pH.
3. On the left side, left lateral recumbent position.
4. a. Sprinkle on gloved hands and apply, use sparingly to prevent caking.
   b. Pat on lightly with gloved hand or gauze pad.
   c. Rub into skin while wearing gloves.
   d. Use a gloved hand or applicator to apply an even coat and cover with a dressing
5. Three tablets, 5 minutes apart.
6. a. parenteral
   b. nonparenteral
   c. nonparenteral
   d. nonparenteral
   e. parenteral
   f. nonparenteral
   g. nonparenteral
   h. nonparenteral
   i. parenteral
   j. nonparenteral
7. down and back
8. Rub the skin with an alcohol pad in a circular motion from the centre of the site out.
9. The drug would be destroyed orally, a rapid effect is desired, the patient is unable to take the drug orally.
10. In the adult, pull the ear back and up. In a 2-year-old child, pull the ear back and down.

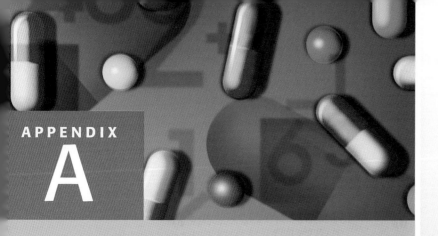

Proficiency Test Answers

Chapter 1

Test 1: Arithmetic

A. a)
$$\begin{array}{r} 647 \\ \times\ \ 38 \\ \hline 5176 \\ 1941 \\ \hline 24586 \end{array}$$

b)
$$\overset{1}{\cancel{8}}\!\!\!\!\overset{}{} \times \frac{\overset{\overset{1}{\cancel{4}}}{\cancel{12}}}{\underset{\underset{1}{\cancel{4}}}{\cancel{32}}} = \frac{1}{3}$$

$$\frac{\overset{1}{\cancel{8}}}{\underset{3}{\cancel{9}}} \times \frac{\overset{\overset{1}{\cancel{4}}}{\cancel{12}}}{\underset{\underset{1}{\cancel{4}}}{\cancel{32}}} = \frac{1}{3}$$

c)
$$\begin{array}{r} 0.56 \\ \times\ \ 0.17 \\ \hline 392 \\ 56 \\ \hline 0.0952 \end{array}$$

B. a)
$$\begin{array}{r} 9.670 = 9.67 \\ 82\overline{)793.000} \\ \underline{738} \\ 55\ 0 \\ \underline{49\ 2} \\ 5\ 80 \\ \underline{5\ 74} \\ 60 \end{array}$$

b)
$$5\frac{1}{4} \div \frac{7}{4} = \frac{\overset{3}{\cancel{21}}}{\underset{1}{\cancel{4}}} \times \frac{\overset{1}{\cancel{4}}}{\underset{1}{\cancel{7}}} = 3$$

c)
$$0.015\overset{\ \ \ 20.}{\overline{)0.300}}$$

C. a) $\dfrac{7}{15} + \dfrac{8}{15} = \dfrac{15}{15} = 1$

b) $\dfrac{3}{8} + \dfrac{2}{5} =$

$\dfrac{15}{40} + \dfrac{16}{40} = \dfrac{31}{40}$

c) $0.825 + 0.1 = 0.925$

D. a) $\dfrac{11}{15} - \dfrac{7}{10} =$

$\dfrac{44}{60} - \dfrac{42}{60} = \dfrac{2}{60} = \dfrac{1}{30}$

b) $\dfrac{8}{15} - \dfrac{4}{15} = \dfrac{4}{15}$

c) $1.56 - 0.2 =$

$$\begin{array}{r} 1.56 \\ -0.2\ \ = 1.36 \\ \hline 1.36 \end{array}$$

E. a)
$$\overset{\dfrac{1}{18}}{}\ \overset{0.055 = 0.06}{18\,\overline{)1.000}}$$
$$\begin{array}{r} \underline{90} \\ 100 \\ \underline{90} \\ 10 \end{array}$$

b)
$$\overset{\dfrac{3}{8}}{}\ \overset{0.375 = 0.38}{8\,\overline{)3.000}}$$
$$\begin{array}{r} \underline{2\ 4} \\ 60 \\ \underline{56} \\ 40 \\ \underline{40} \end{array}$$

F. a)
$$0.35 = \frac{\overset{7}{\cancel{35}}}{\underset{20}{\cancel{100}}} = \frac{7}{20}$$

b)
$$0.08 = \frac{\overset{2}{\cancel{8}}}{\underset{25}{\cancel{100}}} = \frac{2}{25}$$

G. a) 0.4

  b) 0.8

  c) 0.83

  d) 0.3

H. a)
$$\frac{\overset{5}{\cancel{20}}}{\underset{3}{\cancel{12}}} = \frac{5}{3} \quad \begin{array}{r} 1.666 = 1.67 \\ 3\overline{)5.00} \\ \underline{3} \\ 20 \\ \underline{18} \\ 20 \\ \underline{18} \\ 20 \\ \underline{18} \end{array}$$

b)
$$\frac{\overset{1}{\cancel{7}}}{\underset{12}{\cancel{84}}} = \frac{1}{12} \quad \begin{array}{r} 0.083 = 0.08 \\ 12\overline{)1.00} \\ \underline{96} \\ 40 \\ \underline{36} \\ 4 \end{array}$$

c)
$$\begin{array}{r} 6 \quad 0.461 = 0.46 \\ 13\overline{)6.00} \\ \underline{5\,2} \\ 80 \\ \underline{78} \\ 20 \\ \underline{13} \end{array}$$

I. a) 5.3

b) 0.63

c) 0.924

J. a) ratio: $\frac{1}{3}\% = 1:300$

  decimal: $\dfrac{\frac{1}{3}}{100} = \frac{1}{3} \div 100 = 0.0033$

  fraction: $\frac{1}{3} \times \frac{1}{100} = \frac{1}{300}$

  $1:300$

  0.0033

b) ratio:
$$0.8\% = \underset{\frown}{00.8} = 0.008 = 1:125$$
$$\frac{\frac{8}{1000}}{125} = \frac{1}{125} = 1:125$$

  decimal:
$$0.8\% = \frac{0.8}{100} \quad 100\overline{)0.800}^{.008} = 0.008 = 0.008$$

  fraction: $0.8\% = \dfrac{\frac{8}{10}}{100} = \frac{8}{10} \div 100 = \frac{8}{10} \times \frac{1}{100} = \dfrac{\frac{8}{1000}}{125} = \frac{1}{125}$

K. a) $\dfrac{7}{100} = \underset{\frown}{00.7} = 7\%$

b) $1:10 = \dfrac{1}{10} = \underset{\frown}{0.10} = 10\%$

c) $0.008 = \overset{\frown}{0.008} \qquad 0.8\%$

L. a) $\dfrac{32}{128} = \dfrac{4}{x}$

$$\frac{\overset{1}{\cancel{32}}x}{\underset{1}{\cancel{32}}} = \frac{\overset{4}{\cancel{128}} \times 4}{\underset{1}{\cancel{32}}}$$

  $x = 16$

b) $8:72::5:x$

$$\frac{\overset{1}{\cancel{8}}}{\underset{1}{\cancel{8}}}x = \frac{\overset{9}{\cancel{72}} \times 5}{\underset{1}{\cancel{8}}}$$

  $x = 45$

c) $\dfrac{0.4}{0.12} = \dfrac{x}{8}$

  $0.12x = 0.4 \times 8$

$$\frac{\cancel{0.12}}{\cancel{0.12}}x = \frac{0.4 \times 8}{0.12}$$

$$x = \frac{3.2}{0.12} \quad 0.12\overline{)3.2000}^{26.66 = 27}$$
$$\begin{array}{r} \underline{2\,4} \\ 80 \\ \underline{72} \\ 80 \\ \underline{72} \\ 8 \end{array}$$

  $x = 27$

Chapter 2

Test 1: Abbreviations

1. Twice a day
2. Do not use hs. Use "at bedtime."
3. When necessary
4. Write out "both eyes."
5. By mouth
6. By rectum
7. Sublingual
8. Millilitre
9. Every 4 hours
10. Do not use sc. Use "subcutaneous."
11. Do not use AU. Use "both ears."
12. Gram
13. After meals
14. Do not use qd. Use "every day."
15. Immediate
16. Every 12 hours
17. Three times a day
18. Do not use OS. Write out "left eye."
19. Kilogram
20. Every night
21. Every hour
22. Do not use OD. Write out "right eye."
23. Milliequivalent
24. Before meals
25. Four times a day
26. Milligram
27. Intramuscular
28. Do not use qod. Use "every other day."
29. Nasogastric tube
30. Every 8 hours
31. Litre
32. Microgram
33. Every 6 hours
34. Do not use μg. Use "microgram" or "mcg."
35. Do not use U. Use "unit."
36. Teaspoon (household measure)
37. Do not use AD. Use "right ear."
38. Grain (apothecary measure)
39. Intravenously
40. Suspension
41. Tablespoon (household measure)
42. Intravenous piggyback
43. Metre
44. Every 2 hours
45. Every 3 hours

Test 2: Reading Prescriptions

1. Nembutal one hundred milligrams at the hour of sleep, as needed, by mouth (e.g., 2200)
2. Propranolol hydrochloride forty milligrams by mouth twice a day (e.g., 1000, 1800)
3. Ampicillin one gram intravenous piggyback every 6 hours (e.g., 0600, 1200, 1800, 2400)
4. Demerol fifty milligrams intramuscularly every 4 hours as needed for pain
5. Tylenol three hundred twenty-five milligrams, two tablets by mouth immediately. (Give two tablets of Tylenol. Each tablet is 325 mg.) Do not use roman numerals—ii should be written as 2.
6. Pilocarpine drops two in both eyes every 3 hours (e.g., 0300, 0600, 1200, 1500, 1800, 2100, 2400). Do not use OU; write "both eyes."
7. Scopolamine eight-tenths of a milligram subcutaneously immediately. Do not use roman numerals—ii should be written as 2.
8. Elixir of digoxin twenty-five hundredths of a milligram by mouth every day (e.g., 1000). Do not use qd; write "every day."
9. Kaochlor thirty milliequivalents by mouth twice a day (e.g., 1000 and 1800)
10. Liquaemin sodium six thousand units subcutaneous every 4 hours (e.g., 0200, 0600, 1000, 1400, 1800, 2200)
11. Tobramycin seventy milligrams intramuscularly every 8 hours (e.g., 0600, 1400, 2200)
12. Prednisone ten milligrams by mouth every other day (e.g., even days of the month at 1000). You might substitute "odd days of the month."
13. Milk of magnesia one tablespoon by mouth every night (e.g., 2200). Household measurement—not acceptable. Contact physician for new order.
14. Septra one double-strength tablet every day by mouth (e.g., 1000). Do not use roman numerals—i should be written as 1.
15. Morphine sulfate fifteen milligrams subcutaneously immediately and ten milligrams every 4 hours as needed. The stat time given determines when the next dose can be administered. (Next dose must be *at least 4 hours later.*)

Test 3: Interpreting Written Prescription Orders

1. Colace one hundred milligrams by mouth three times a day (e.g., 1000, 1400, 1800).
2. Ativan one milligram intravenous push times one dose now. Do not use roman numerals—i should be written as 1.
3. Ten milliequivalents potassium chloride in one hundred cubic centimetres of normal saline over one hour, times one dose. Should be one hundred "millilitres."
4. Tylenol number three two tablets by mouth every four hours as needed for pain. Do not use roman numerals—ii should be written as 2.
5. Heparin twenty-five thousand international units in two hundred fifty cubic centimetres dextrose five percent in water at five hundred units per hour. Should write out "international unit." Should write out "500 units." Should write out "mL."
6. Ticlid two hundred fifty milligrams one tablet by mouth twice a day. Do not use roman numerals—i should be written as 1.
7. Lopressor 25 milligrams by mouth twice a day.
8. Benadryl 25 milligrams by mouth at hour of sleep; should write "at bedtime."

Chapter 3

Test 1: Exercises in Equivalents and Mixed Conversions

1. 01	**6.** 0.03	**11.** 0.6	**16.** 0.001
2. 1000	**7.** 0.5	**12.** 0.01	**17.** 125
3. 15	**8.** 1000	**13.** 0.0005 mg	**18.** 10
4. 0.01	**9.** 0.06	**14.** 0.006 g	**19.** 1
5. 200	**10.** 100	**15.** 0.25 mg	

Chapter 4

Test 1: Labels and Packaging

1. **a. 1.** Individually wrapped and labeled drugs
   2. Large stock containers of drugs
   b. 1. Glass container holding a single dose. Container must be broken to reach the drug. Any portion not used must be discarded.
   2. Glass or plastic container with a sealed top that allows medication to be kept sterile
   c. 1. Drug applied to skin or mucous membranes to achieve a local effect. May be absorbed into the circulation and cause a systemic effect.
   2. Drugs given by injection include subcutaneous, IM, IV, and IVPB
   d. 1. Brand or proprietary name of manufacturer. Identified by symbol ®.
   2. Official name of a drug as listed in the TPD
   e. 1. Liquid sterile medication ready to administer
   2. Powder or crystals diluted according to specific directions. Date and time of preparation must be written on the label and the expiration date noted.

2. a. 4   **b.** 2   **c.** 1   **d.** 1

3. 1. g   **4.** i   **7.** j   **9.** c

   2. e   **5.** d   **8.** a   **10.** b

   3. h   **6.** f

Test 2: Interpreting a Label

1. Methylprednisolone sodium succinate for injection
2. Intravenous, intramuscular
3. Anti-inflammatory, glucocorticoid
4. 1 mL
5. 40 mg/mL
6. Reconstitute with 1 mL of sterile water for injection and use solution within 24 hours or 1 mL of bacteriostatic water for injection and use solution within 48 hours.
7. Powder
8. Store powder at room temperature (15°–25°C), protected from light. Use reconstituted solution within 48 hours.
9. 06.2008 or June 30, 2008
10. None

Chapter 5

Test 1: Drug Preparations and Equipment

1. Diabetes mellitus, alcoholism
2. 10 mL or less
3. Subcutaneous, IM, IVPB, and IV
4. **a.** The date
   b. The nurse's initials
   c. The dilution made
   d. The time
5. Aseptic technique is required in preparing and administering drugs parenterally (IM, subcutaneous, IV, IVPB).
6. Milk of magnesia
7. Before an oral suspension is poured, the liquid must always be shaken.
8. Aerosol powders, creams, ointments, pastes, suppositories, transdermal medications
9. Ease in administering; prolonged action
10. An ointment is a semisolid preparation in a petroleum or lanolin base for topical use.
11. **1.** Pour to a line. Never estimate a dose.
    2. Pour liquids at eye level.
12. **a.** The natural curve of the surface of a liquid in a container
    b. Diameter or width of a needle. The higher the gauge number, the finer the needle.
13. Route of administration, size and condition of the patient, amount of adipose tissue present at the site
14. **1.** When the last number is 5 or more, add 1 to the previous number.
    2. When the last number is 4 or less, drop the number.
15. The equipment used
    3 mL syringe—nearest 10th in millilitres
    1 mL precision syringe—nearest 100th in millilitres medicine cup—metric lines

Chapter 6

Test 1: Calculation of Oral Doses

Formula Method	Proportion Expressed as Two Ratios	Proportion Expressed as Two Fractions

1. $\dfrac{\overset{10}{\cancel{20 \text{ mEq}}}}{\underset{2}{\cancel{30 \text{ mEq}}}} \times \overset{1}{\cancel{15}} \text{ mL} = 10 \text{ mL}$

$15 \text{ mL} : 30 \text{ mEq} :: x : 20 \text{ mEq}$

$\dfrac{15 \text{ mL}}{30 \text{ mEq}} \times \dfrac{x}{20 \text{ mEq}}$

$\dfrac{300}{30} = x$

$10 \text{ mL} = x$

Dimensional Analysis Method

$\dfrac{20 \cancel{\text{ mEq}} \left| \overset{1}{\cancel{15}} \cancel{\text{(mL)}} \right| 20}{\underset{2}{\cancel{30}} \cancel{\text{ mEq}} \left| 2 \right.} = 10 \text{ mL}$

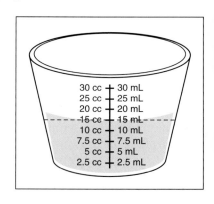

Formula Method	Proportion Expressed as Two Ratios	Proportion Expressed as Two Fractions

2. $\dfrac{\overset{2}{\cancel{150 \text{ mg}}}}{\underset{1}{\cancel{75 \text{ mg}}}} \times 7.5 \text{ mL} = 15 \text{ mL}$

$7.5 \text{ mL} : 75 \text{ mg} :: x : 150 \text{ mg}$

$\dfrac{7.5 \text{ mL}}{75 \text{ mg}} \times \dfrac{x}{150 \text{ mg}}$

$7.5 \times 150 = 75x$

$1125 = 75x$

$15 \text{ mL} = x$

Dimensional Analysis Method

$\dfrac{\overset{2}{\cancel{150}} \cancel{\text{ mg}} \left| 7.5 \cancel{\text{(mL)}} \right| 2 \times 7.5}{\underset{1}{\cancel{75}} \cancel{\text{ mg}} \left| \right.} = 15 \text{ mL}$

Formula Method

3. $\dfrac{\overset{1}{\cancel{0.125\ mg}}}{\underset{\underset{1}{2}}{\cancel{0.250\ mg}}} \times \overset{5}{\cancel{10}} = 5\ mL$

Proportion Expressed as Two Ratios

10 mL : 0.25 mg : : x : 0.125 mg

Proportion Expressed as Two Fractions

$\dfrac{10\ mL}{0.25\ mg} \bowtie \dfrac{x}{0.125\ mg}$

$$10 \times 0.125 = 0.25x$$

$$\frac{1.25}{0.25} = x$$

$$5\ mL = x$$

Dimensional Analysis Method

$\dfrac{\overset{1}{\cancel{0.125}}\ mg}{} \left|\ \dfrac{10\ \textcircled{mL}}{\underset{2}{\cancel{0.25}}\ mg}\ \right|\ \dfrac{10}{2} = 5\ mL$

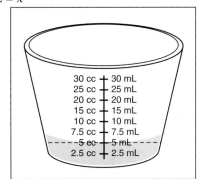

Formula Method

4. $\dfrac{\overset{3}{\cancel{375\ mg}}}{\underset{1}{\cancel{125\ mg}}} \times 5\ mL = 15\ mL$

Proportion Expressed as Two Ratios

5 mL : 125 mg : : x : 375 mg

Proportion Expressed as Two Fractions

$\dfrac{5\ mL}{125\ mg} \bowtie \dfrac{x}{375\ mg}$

$$5 \times 375 = 125x$$

$$\frac{1875}{125} = x$$

$$15\ mL = x$$

Dimensional Analysis Method

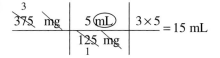

$\dfrac{\overset{3}{\cancel{375}}\ mg}{} \left|\ \dfrac{5\ \textcircled{mL}}{\underset{1}{\cancel{125}}\ mg}\ \right|\ \dfrac{3 \times 5}{} = 15\ mL$

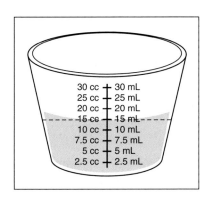

Formula Method	Proportion Expressed as Two Ratios	Proportion Expressed as Two Fractions

5. $\dfrac{\overset{2}{\cancel{40}}\ \text{mg}}{\underset{1}{\cancel{20}}\ \text{mg}} \times 2.5\ \text{mL} = 5\ \text{mL}$

$2.5\ \text{mL} : 20\ \text{mg} :: x : 40\ \text{mg}$

$\dfrac{2.5\ \text{mL}}{20\ \text{mg}} \times \dfrac{x}{40\ \text{mg}}$

$$2.5 \times 40 = 20x$$

$$\dfrac{100}{20} = x$$

$$5\ \text{mL} = x$$

Dimensional Analysis Method

$\dfrac{\overset{2}{\cancel{40}}\ \text{mg}}{\ }\ \bigg|\ \dfrac{2.5\ \cancel{\text{mL}}}{\underset{1}{\cancel{20}}\ \text{mg}}\ \bigg|\ \dfrac{2 \times 2.5}{\ } = 5\ \text{mL} = x$

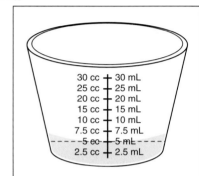

Formula Method	Proportion Expressed as Two Ratios	Proportion Expressed as Two Fractions

6. $\dfrac{0.50\ \text{mg}}{0.25\ \text{mg}} \times 1\ \text{tablet} =$

$1\ \text{tablet} : 0.25\ \text{mg} :: x : 0.5\ \text{mg}$

$\dfrac{1\ \text{tablet}}{0.25\ \text{mg}} \times \dfrac{x}{0.50}$

$0.25\overline{)0.50}\overset{2.}{} = 2\ \text{tablets}$

$$\dfrac{0.50}{0.25} = x$$

$$2\ \text{tablets} = x$$

Dimensional Analysis Method

$\dfrac{\overset{2}{\cancel{0.5}}\ \text{mg}}{\ }\ \bigg|\ \dfrac{1\ \text{tablet}}{\underset{1}{\cancel{0.25}}\ \text{mg}} = 2\ \text{tablets}$

Formula Method	Proportion Expressed as Two Ratios	Proportion Expressed as Two Fractions

7. Equivalent $0.1\ \text{mg} = 100\ \text{mcg}$

$\dfrac{\cancel{100}\ \cancel{\text{mcg}}}{\cancel{100}\ \cancel{\text{mcg}}} \times 1\ \text{capsule} = 1\ \text{capsule}$

$1\ \text{capsule} : 100\ \text{mcg} :: x : 100\ \text{mcg}$

$\dfrac{1\ \text{capsule}}{100\ \text{mcg}} \times \dfrac{x}{100\ \text{mcg}}$

$$100\ \text{mcg} = 1\ \text{capsule} = x$$

Dimensional Analysis Method

$\dfrac{\cancel{100}\ \cancel{\text{mcg}}}{\ }\ \bigg|\ \dfrac{1\ \text{capsule}}{0.1\ \text{mg}}\ \bigg|\ \dfrac{1\ \cancel{\text{mg}}}{1000\ \cancel{\text{mcg}}}\ \bigg|\ \dfrac{1}{0.1 \times 10} = \dfrac{1}{1} = 1\ \text{capsule}$

Formula Method	Proportion Expressed as Two Ratios	Proportion Expressed as Two Fractions

8. $\dfrac{\overset{5}{\cancel{250}}\ \text{mg}}{\underset{2}{\cancel{100}}\ \text{mg}} \times 1\ \text{tablet} = \dfrac{5}{2} = 2\frac{1}{2}\ \text{tablets}$

1 tablet : 100 mg : : x : 250 mg

$\dfrac{1\ \text{tablet}}{100\ \text{mg}} \times \dfrac{x}{250\ \text{mg}}$

$$\dfrac{250}{100} = x$$

$$2.5 \text{ or } 2\frac{1}{2}\ \text{tablets} = x$$

Dimensional Analysis Method

$\dfrac{\overset{2.5}{\cancel{250}}\ \text{mg}}{} \left| \dfrac{1\ \text{(tablet)}}{\underset{1}{\cancel{100}}\ \text{mg}} \right| \dfrac{2.5 \times 1}{} = 2.5\ \text{tablets or } 2\frac{1}{2}\ \text{tablets}$

Formula Method	Proportion Expressed as Two Ratios	Proportion Expressed as Two Fractions

9. Equivalent 0.5 g = 500 mg

$\dfrac{\overset{2}{\cancel{500}}\ \text{mg}}{\underset{1}{\cancel{250}}\ \text{mg}} \times 1\ \text{capsule} = 2\ \text{capsules}$

1 capsule : 250 mg : : x : 500 mg

$\dfrac{1\ \text{capsule}}{250\ \text{mg}} \times \dfrac{x}{500\ \text{mg}}$

$$\dfrac{500}{250} = x$$

$$2\ \text{capsules} = x$$

Dimensional Analysis Method

$\dfrac{0.5\ \text{g}}{} \left| \dfrac{1\ \text{(capsule)}}{\underset{1}{\cancel{250}}\ \text{mg}} \right| \dfrac{\overset{4}{\cancel{1000}}\ \text{mg}}{1\ \text{g}} \left| \dfrac{0.5 \times 4}{} \right. = 2\ \text{capsules}$

Formula Method	Proportion Expressed as Two Ratios	Proportion Expressed as Two Fractions

10. Equivalent 0.3 mg = 300 mcg

$\dfrac{\overset{1}{\cancel{300}}\ \text{mcg}}{\underset{1}{\cancel{300}}\ \text{mcg}} \times 1\ \text{tablet} = 1\ \text{tablet}$

1 tablet : 300 mcg : : x : 300 mcg

$\dfrac{1\ \text{tablet}}{300\ \text{mcg}} \times \dfrac{x}{300\ \text{mcg}}$

$$\dfrac{300}{300} = x$$

$$1\ \text{tablet} = x$$

Dimensional Analysis Method

$\dfrac{0.3\ \text{mg}}{} \left| \dfrac{1\ \text{(tablet)}}{\cancel{300}\ \text{mcg}} \right| \dfrac{\cancel{1000}\ \text{mcg}}{1\ \text{mg}} \left| \dfrac{0.3 \times 10}{3} \right. = 1\ \text{tablet}$

Test 2: Calculation of Oral Doses

Formula Method	Proportion Expressed as Two Ratios	Proportion Expressed as Two Fractions

1. Equivalent 0.8 g = 800 mg

$$\dfrac{\overset{2}{\cancel{800}}\ \text{mg}}{\underset{1}{\cancel{400}}\ \text{mg}} \times 1\ \text{tablet} = 2\ \text{tablets}$$

1 tablet : 400 mg : : x : 800 mg

$$\dfrac{1\ \text{tablet}}{400\ \text{mg}} \times \dfrac{\text{x}}{800\ \text{mg}}$$

$$\dfrac{800}{400} = \text{x}$$

2 tablets = x

Dimensional Analysis Method

$$\dfrac{0.8\ \cancel{\text{g}}}{} \ \left|\ \dfrac{1\ \text{tablet}}{400\ \cancel{\text{mg}}}\ \right|\ \dfrac{1000\ \cancel{\text{mg}}}{1\ \cancel{\text{g}}}\ \left|\ \dfrac{0.8 \times 10}{4} = 2\ \text{tablets}\right.$$

Formula Method	Proportion Expressed as Two Ratios	Proportion Expressed as Two Fractions

2. Equivalent 0.3 g = 300 mg

$$\dfrac{\overset{1}{\cancel{300}}\ \text{mg}}{\underset{1}{\cancel{300}}\ \text{mg}} \times 1\ \text{tablet} = 1\ \text{tablet}$$

1 tablet : 300 mg : : x : 300 mg

$$\dfrac{1\ \text{tablet}}{300\ \text{mg}} \times \dfrac{\text{x}}{300\ \text{mg}}$$

$$\dfrac{300}{300} = \text{x}$$

1 tablet = x

Dimensional Analysis Method

$$\dfrac{0.3\ \cancel{\text{g}}}{} \ \left|\ \dfrac{1\ \text{tablet}}{300\ \cancel{\text{mg}}}\ \right|\ \dfrac{1000\ \cancel{\text{mg}}}{1\ \cancel{\text{g}}}\ \left|\ \dfrac{0.3 \times 10}{3} = 1\ \text{tablet}\right.$$

Formula Method	Proportion Expressed as Two Ratios	Proportion Expressed as Two Fractions

3. $\dfrac{75\ \text{mg}}{50\ \text{mg}} \times 1\ \text{tablet} = 1\frac{1}{2}\ \text{tablets}$

1 tablet : 50 mg : : x : 75 mg

$$\dfrac{1\ \text{tablet}}{50\ \text{mg}} \times \dfrac{\text{x}}{75\ \text{mg}}$$

$$75 = 50\text{x}$$

$$\dfrac{75}{50} = \text{x}$$

1½ tablets = x

Dimensional Analysis Method

$$\dfrac{75\ \cancel{\text{mg}}}{} \ \left|\ \dfrac{1\ \text{tablet}}{50\ \cancel{\text{mg}}}\ \right|\ \dfrac{75}{50} = 1\frac{1}{2}\ \text{tablets}$$

Formula Method	Proportion Expressed as Two Ratios	Proportion Expressed as Two Fractions

4. 0.65 g = 650 mg

$$\dfrac{\overset{2}{\cancel{650}}\text{ mg}}{\underset{1}{\cancel{325}}\text{ mg}} \times 1 \text{ tablet} = 2 \text{ tablets}$$

1 tablet : 325 mg : : x : 650 mg

$$\dfrac{1 \text{ tablet}}{325 \text{ mg}} \diagup\!\!\!\!\diagdown \dfrac{x}{650 \text{ mg}}$$

$$\dfrac{650}{325} = x$$

$$2 \text{ tablets} = x$$

Dimensional Analysis Method

$$\dfrac{0.65 \ \cancel{g}}{} \ \bigg|\ \dfrac{1 \ \text{tablet}}{325 \ \cancel{mg}} \ \bigg|\ \dfrac{1000 \ \cancel{mg}}{1 \ \cancel{g}} \ \bigg|\ \dfrac{0.65 \times 1000}{325} = 2 \text{ tablets}$$

Formula Method	Proportion Expressed as Two Ratios	Proportion Expressed as Two Fractions

5. $\dfrac{10 \text{ mg}}{2.5 \text{ mg}} \times 1 \text{ tablet} = 4 \text{ tablets}$

1 tablet : 2.5 mg : : x : 10 mg

$$\dfrac{1 \text{ tablet}}{2.5 \text{ mg}} \diagup\!\!\!\!\diagdown \dfrac{x}{10 \text{ mg}}$$

$$10 \text{ mg} = 2.5x$$

$$\dfrac{10}{2.5} = x$$

$$4 \text{ tablets} = x$$

Dimensional Analysis Method

$$\dfrac{10 \ \cancel{mg}}{} \ \bigg|\ \dfrac{1 \ \text{tablet}}{250 \ \cancel{mg}} \ \bigg|\ \dfrac{10}{2.5} = 4 \text{ tablets}$$

Formula Method	Proportion Expressed as Two Ratios	Proportion Expressed as Two Fractions

6. $\dfrac{750,000 \text{ units}}{100,000 \text{ units}} \times 1 \text{ mL} = \dfrac{75}{10} = 7.5 \text{ mL}$

1 mL : 100,000 units : : x : 750,000 units

$$\dfrac{1 \text{ mL}}{100,000 \text{ units}} \diagup\!\!\!\!\diagdown \dfrac{x}{750,000 \text{ units}}$$

$$\dfrac{750,000}{100,000} = x$$

$$7.5 \text{ mL} = x$$

Dimensional Analysis Method

$$\frac{750,000 \text{ units}}{} \left| \frac{1 \text{ mL}}{100,000 \text{ units}} \right| \frac{75}{10} = 7.5 \text{ mL}$$

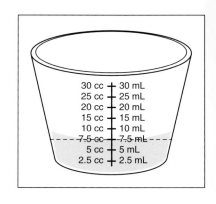

Formula Method

7. Equivalent 0.75 g = 750 mg

$$\frac{\overset{3}{\cancel{750} \text{ mg}}}{\underset{1}{\cancel{250} \text{ mg}}} \times 5 \text{ mL} = 15 \text{ mL}$$

Proportion Expressed as Two Ratios

$$5 \text{ mL} : 250 \text{ mg} :: x : 750 \text{ mg}$$

Proportion Expressed as Two Fractions

$$\frac{5 \text{ mL}}{250 \text{ mg}} \times \frac{x}{750}$$

$$5 \times 750 = 250x$$

$$\frac{3750}{250} = x$$

$$15 \text{ mL} = x$$

Dimensional Analysis Method

$$0.75 \text{ g} \left| \frac{\overset{1}{\cancel{5} \text{ mL}}}{\underset{5}{\cancel{250} \text{ mg}}} \right| \frac{1000 \text{ mg}}{1 \text{ g}} \left| \frac{0.75 \times 100}{5} \right| = 15 \text{ mL}$$

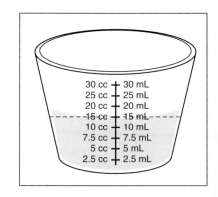

Formula Method

8. $\dfrac{\overset{2}{\cancel{500} \text{ mg}}}{\underset{1}{\cancel{250} \text{ mg}}} \times 5 \text{ mL} = 10 \text{ mL}$

Proportion Expressed as Two Ratios

$$5 \text{ mL} : 250 \text{ mg} :: x : 500 \text{ mg}$$

Proportion Expressed as Two Fractions

$$\frac{5 \text{ mL}}{250 \text{ mg}} \times \frac{x}{500 \text{ mg}}$$

$$5 \times 500 = 250x$$

$$\frac{2500}{250} = x$$

$$10 \text{ mL} = x$$

Dimensional Analysis Method

$$\frac{\overset{2}{\cancel{500}} \text{ mg}}{} \left| \frac{5 \text{ } \cancel{mL}}{\underset{1}{\cancel{250} \text{ mg}}} \right| \frac{2 \times 5}{} = 10 \text{ mL}$$

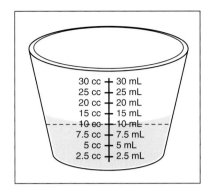

9. No arithmetic necessary. Pour 30 mL.

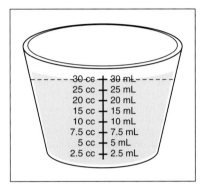

Formula Method

10. $\dfrac{\overset{2}{\cancel{160} \text{ mg}}}{\underset{1}{\cancel{80} \text{ mg}}} \times 15 \text{ mL} = 30 \text{ mL}$

Proportion Expressed as Two Ratios

$15 \text{ mL} : 80 \text{ mg} :: x : 160 \text{ mg}$

Proportion Expressed as Two Fractions

$\dfrac{15 \text{ mL}}{80 \text{ mg}} \times \dfrac{x}{160 \text{ mg}}$

$$15 \times 160 = 80x$$

$$\frac{2400}{80} = x$$

$$30 \text{ mL} = x$$

Dimensional Analysis Method

$$\frac{\overset{2}{\cancel{160} \text{ mg}}}{} \left| \frac{15 \text{ } \cancel{mL}}{\underset{1}{\cancel{80} \text{ mg}}} \right| \frac{2 \times 15}{} = 30 \text{ mL}$$

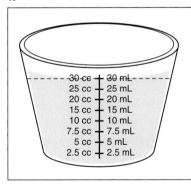

Test 3: Calculation of Oral Doses

Formula Method	Proportion Expressed as Two Ratios	Proportion Expressed as Two Fractions

1. $\dfrac{\overset{10}{\cancel{20}\ \cancel{\text{mEq}}}}{\underset{1}{\underset{2}{\cancel{30}\ \cancel{\text{mEq}}}}} \times \overset{1}{\cancel{15}}\ \text{mL} = 10\ \text{mL}$

$15\ \text{mL} : 30\ \text{mEq} :: x : 20\ \text{mEq}$

$\dfrac{15\ \text{mL}}{30\ \text{mEq}} \times \dfrac{x}{20\ \text{mEq}}$

$$15 \times 20 = 30x$$

$$\frac{300}{30} = x$$

$$10\ \text{mL} = x$$

Dimensional Analysis Method

$\dfrac{\overset{4}{\cancel{20}}\ \cancel{\text{mEq}}}{\underset{6}{\cancel{30}\ \cancel{\text{mEq}}}} \ \Bigg|\ 15\ \text{(mL)} \ \Bigg|\ \dfrac{4 \times 15}{6} = 10\ \text{mL}$

Formula Method	Proportion Expressed as Two Ratios	Proportion Expressed as Two Fractions

2. $\dfrac{\overset{16}{\cancel{80}\ \cancel{\text{mcg}}}}{\underset{25}{\cancel{125}\ \cancel{\text{mcg}}}} \times \overset{1}{\cancel{5}}\ \text{mL} = \dfrac{\overset{16}{\cancel{80}}}{\underset{5}{\cancel{25}}} =$

$5\ \text{mL} : 125\ \text{mg} :: x : 80\ \text{mg}$

$\dfrac{5\ \text{mL}}{125\ \text{mg}} \times \dfrac{x}{80\ \text{mg}}$

$$5 \times 80 = 125x$$

$$\frac{400}{125} = x$$

$$3.2\ \text{mL} = x$$

$\dfrac{16}{5}\overline{\smash{\big)}\,16.0}\ \overset{3.2}{} = 3.2\ \text{mL}$

Dimensional Analysis Method

$80\ \cancel{\text{mg}}\ \Bigg|\ \overset{1}{\cancel{5}}\ \text{(mL)}\ \Bigg|\ \dfrac{80}{25} = 3.2\ \text{mL}$, $\underset{25}{\cancel{125}}\ \cancel{\text{mg}}$

Use an oral syringe to obtain the dose.

Formula Method	Proportion Expressed as Two Ratios	Proportion Expressed as Two Fractions

3. $0.02\ \text{g} = 20\ \text{mg}$

$\dfrac{\overset{2}{\cancel{20}\ \cancel{\text{mg}}}}{\underset{1}{\cancel{10}\ \cancel{\text{mg}}}} \times 1\ \text{tablet} = 2\ \text{tablets}$

$1\ \text{tablet} : 10\ \text{mg} :: x : 20\ \text{mg}$

$\dfrac{1\ \text{tablet}}{10\ \text{mg}} \times \dfrac{x}{20\ \text{mg}}$

$$\frac{20}{10} = x$$

$$2\ \text{tablets} = x$$

Dimensional Analysis Method

$0.02\ \cancel{\text{g}}\ \Bigg|\ 1\ \text{(tablet)}\ \Bigg|\ \dfrac{\overset{100}{\cancel{1000}}\ \cancel{\text{mg}}}{1\ \cancel{\text{g}}}\ \Bigg|\ \dfrac{0.02 \times 100}{1} = 2\ \text{tablets}$, $\underset{1}{\cancel{10}}\ \cancel{\text{mg}}$

Formula Method	Proportion Expressed as Two Ratios	Proportion Expressed as Two Fractions
4. $0.5 \text{ g} = 500 \text{ mg}$		

$$\frac{\overset{2}{\cancel{500} \text{ mg}}}{\underset{1}{\cancel{250} \text{ mg}}} \times 1 \text{ capsule} = 2 \text{ capsules}$$

1 capsule : 250 mg : : x : 500 mg

$$\frac{1 \text{ capsule}}{250 \text{ mg}} \times \frac{x}{500 \text{ mg}}$$

$$\frac{500}{250} = x$$

$$2 \text{ capsules} = x$$

Dimensional Analysis Method

$$\frac{0.5 \cancel{\text{g}} \quad \Big| \quad 1 \text{ capsule} \quad \Big| \quad \overset{4}{\cancel{1000} \text{ mg}}}{\quad \Big| \quad \underset{1}{\cancel{250} \text{ mg}} \quad \Big| \quad 1 \cancel{\text{g}}} \quad \frac{0.5 \times 4}{} = 2 \text{ capsules}$$

Formula Method	Proportion Expressed as Two Ratios	Proportion Expressed as Two Fractions
5. $\dfrac{\overset{2}{\cancel{0.50} \text{ mg}}}{\underset{1}{\cancel{0.25} \text{ mg}}} \times 1 \text{ tablet} = 2 \text{ tablets}$	1 tablet : 0.25 mg : : x : 0.5 mg	$\dfrac{1 \text{ tablet}}{0.25 \text{ mg}} \times \dfrac{x}{0.5 \text{ mg}}$

$$\frac{0.5}{0.25} = x$$

$$2 \text{ tablets} = x$$

Dimensional Analysis Method

$$\frac{\overset{2}{\cancel{0.5} \text{ mg}} \quad \Big| \quad 1 \text{ tablet}}{\quad \Big| \quad \underset{1}{\cancel{0.25} \text{ mg}}} \quad \frac{2 \times 1}{} = 2 \text{ tablets}$$

Formula Method	Proportion Expressed as Two Ratios	Proportion Expressed as Two Fractions
6. $\dfrac{40 \text{ mg}}{\underset{1}{\cancel{5} \text{ mg}}} \times \overset{1}{\cancel{5}} \text{ mL} = 40 \text{ mL}$	5 mL : 5 mg : : x : 40 mg	$\dfrac{5 \text{ mL}}{5 \text{ mg}} \times \dfrac{x}{40 \text{ mg}}$

$$\frac{40 \times 5}{5} = x$$

$$\frac{200}{5} = x$$

$$40 \text{ mL} = x$$

Dimensional Analysis Method

$$\frac{40 \cancel{\text{mg}} \quad \Big| \quad 5 \text{ mL}}{\quad \Big| \quad 5 \cancel{\text{mg}}} = 40 \text{ mL}$$

Formula Method	**Proportion Expressed as Two Ratios**	**Proportion Expressed as Two Fractions**

7. $\dfrac{\overset{3}{\cancel{75}}\text{ mg}}{\underset{2}{\cancel{50}}\text{ mg}} \times 1 \text{ tablet} = \dfrac{3}{2}\,\overset{1.5}{\overline{)3.0}}$

$= 1\frac{1}{2} \text{ tablets}$

1 tablet : 50 mg : : x : 75 mg

$\dfrac{1 \text{ tablet}}{50 \text{ mg}} \times \dfrac{\text{x}}{75 \text{ mg}}$

$\dfrac{75}{50} = \text{x}$

1.5 or 1½ tablets = x

Dimensional Analysis Method

$\dfrac{\overset{15}{\cancel{75}}\text{ mg}}{} \Bigg|\ \dfrac{1\,\text{\textcircled{tablet}}}{\underset{10}{\cancel{50}}\text{ mg}}\ \Bigg|\ \dfrac{15}{10} = 1.5 \text{ tablets or } 1\frac{1}{2} \text{ tablets}$

Formula Method	**Proportion Expressed as Two Ratios**	**Proportion Expressed as Two Fractions**

8. $\dfrac{\overset{1}{\cancel{40}}\text{ mg}}{\underset{2}{\cancel{80}}\text{ mg}} \times 1 \text{ tablet} = \frac{1}{2}\,\text{tablet}$

1 tablet : 80 mg : : x : 40 mg

$\dfrac{1 \text{ tablet}}{80 \text{ mg}} \times \dfrac{\text{x}}{40 \text{ mg}}$

$\dfrac{40}{80} = \text{x}$

0.5 or ½ tablet = x

Dimensional Analysis Method

$\dfrac{\overset{1}{\cancel{40}}\text{ mg}}{} \Bigg|\ \dfrac{1\,\text{\textcircled{tablet}}}{\underset{2}{\cancel{80}}\text{ mg}}\ \Bigg|\ \dfrac{1}{2} = \frac{1}{2} \text{ tablet}$

Formula Method	**Proportion Expressed as Two Ratios**	**Proportion Expressed as Two Fractions**

9. 0.125 mg = 125 mcg

$\dfrac{\overset{1}{\cancel{125}}\text{ mcg}}{\underset{\underset{2}{4}}{\cancel{500}}\text{ mcg}} \times \overset{5}{\cancel{10}}\ \text{mL} =$

$\dfrac{5}{2}\,\overset{2.5}{\overline{)5.0}} = 2.5 \text{ mL}$

10 mL : 500 mcg : : x : 125 mcg

$\dfrac{10 \text{ mL}}{500 \text{ mcg}} \times \dfrac{\text{x}}{125}$

$10 \times 125 = 500\text{x}$

$\dfrac{1250}{500} = \text{x}$

2.5 mL = x

Dimensional Analysis Method

$\dfrac{0.125 \text{ mg}}{} \Bigg|\ \dfrac{10\,\text{\textcircled{mL}}}{\underset{1}{\cancel{500}}\text{ mcg}}\ \Bigg|\ \dfrac{\overset{2}{\cancel{1000}}\text{ mcg}}{1 \text{ mg}}\ \Bigg|\ \dfrac{0.125 \times 10 \times 2}{} = 2.5 \text{ mL}$

Formula Method

10. $\dfrac{\overset{3}{\cancel{75}} \text{ mg}}{\underset{1}{\underset{2}{\cancel{50}}} \text{ mg}} \times \overset{5}{\cancel{10}} \text{ mL} = 15 \text{ mL}$

Proportion Expressed as Two Ratios

$10 \text{ mL} : 50 \text{ mg} :: x : 75 \text{ mg}$

Proportion Expressed as Two Fractions

$\dfrac{10 \text{ mL}}{50 \text{ mg}} \times \dfrac{x}{75 \text{ mg}}$

$10 \times 75 = 50x$

$\dfrac{750}{50} = x$

$15 \text{ mL} = x$

Dimensional Analysis Method

$\dfrac{75 \text{ mg}}{} \Bigg| \dfrac{\overset{1}{\cancel{10}} \cancel{(\text{mL})}}{\underset{5}{\cancel{50}} \text{ mg}} \Bigg| \dfrac{75}{5} = 15 \text{ mL}$

Formula Method

11. $\dfrac{5 \text{ mg}}{2 \text{ mg}} \times 1 \text{ tablet} = \dfrac{5}{2} \begin{array}{r} 2.5 \\ \overline{)5.0} \end{array}$

$= 2\frac{1}{2} \text{ tablets}$

Proportion Expressed as Two Ratios

$1 \text{ tablet} : 2 \text{ mg} :: x : 5 \text{ mg}$

Proportion Expressed as Two Fractions

$\dfrac{1 \text{ tablet}}{2 \text{ mg}} \times \dfrac{x}{5 \text{ mg}}$

$\dfrac{5}{2} = x$

$2.5 \text{ or } 2\frac{1}{2} \text{ tablets} = x$

Dimensional Analysis Method

$\dfrac{5 \text{ mg}}{} \Bigg| \dfrac{1 \cancel{(\text{tablet})}}{2 \text{ mg}} \Bigg| \dfrac{5}{2} = 2.5 \text{ tablets or } 2\frac{1}{2} \text{ tablets}$

Formula Method

12. $0.15 \text{ mg} = 150 \text{ mcg}$

$\dfrac{\overset{1}{\cancel{150}} \text{ mcg}}{\underset{2}{\cancel{300}} \text{ mcg}} \times 1 \text{ tablet} = \frac{1}{2} \text{ tablets}$

Proportion Expressed as Two Ratios

$1 \text{ tablet} : 300 \text{ mcg} :: x : 150 \text{ mcg}$

Proportion Expressed as Two Fractions

$\dfrac{1 \text{ tablet}}{300 \text{ mcg}} \times \dfrac{x}{150 \text{ mcg}}$

$\dfrac{150}{300} = x$

$0.5 \text{ or } \frac{1}{2} \text{ tablet} = x$

Dimensional Analysis Method

$\dfrac{0.15 \text{ mg}}{} \Bigg| \dfrac{1 \cancel{(\text{tablet})}}{\cancel{300} \text{ mcg}} \Bigg| \dfrac{\cancel{1000} \text{ mcg}}{1 \cancel{\text{ mg}}} \Bigg| \dfrac{0.15 \times 10}{3} = 0.5 \text{ or } \frac{1}{2} \text{ tablet}$

Formula Method	Proportion Expressed as Two Ratios	Proportion Expressed as Two Fractions
13. $\dfrac{\overset{3}{\cancel{375}}\ \cancel{mg}}{\underset{2}{\cancel{250}}\ \cancel{mg}} \times 1 \text{ tablet} = \dfrac{3}{2}\overline{)\dfrac{1.5}{3.0}}$ $= 1\frac{1}{2} \text{ tablets}$	$1 \text{ tablet} : 250 \text{ mg} :: x : 375 \text{ mg}$	$\dfrac{1 \text{ tablet}}{250 \text{ mg}} \times \dfrac{x}{375 \text{ mg}}$ $\dfrac{375}{250} = x$ $1.5 \text{ or } 1\frac{1}{2} \text{ tablets} = x$

Dimensional Analysis Method

$$\dfrac{\overset{15}{\cancel{375}}\ \cancel{mg}}{\ } \left| \dfrac{1\ \cancel{tablet}}{\underset{10}{\cancel{250}}\ \cancel{mg}} \right| \dfrac{15}{10} = 1.5 \text{ or } 1\frac{1}{2} \text{ tablets}$$

Formula Method	Proportion Expressed as Two Ratios	Proportion Expressed as Two Fractions
14. $0.6 \text{ g} = 600 \text{ mg}$ $\dfrac{\overset{2}{\cancel{600}}\ \cancel{mg}}{\underset{1}{\cancel{300}}\ \cancel{mg}} \times 1 \text{ tablet} = 2 \text{ tablets}$	$1 \text{ tablet} : 300 \text{ mg} :: x : 600 \text{ mg}$	$\dfrac{1 \text{ tablet}}{300 \text{ mg}} \times \dfrac{x}{600}$ $\dfrac{600}{300} = x$ $2 \text{ tablets} = x$

Dimensional Analysis Method

$$\dfrac{0.6\ \cancel{g}}{\ } \left| \dfrac{1\ \cancel{tablet}}{300\ \cancel{mg}} \right| \dfrac{1000\ \cancel{mg}}{1\ \cancel{g}} \left| \dfrac{0.6 \times 10}{3} \right. = 2 \text{ tablets}$$

Formula Method	Proportion Expressed as Two Ratios	Proportion Expressed as Two Fractions
15. $\dfrac{\overset{3}{\cancel{1.5}}\ \cancel{mg}}{\underset{\underset{1}{2}}{\cancel{1.0}}\ \cancel{mg}} \times \overset{4}{\cancel{8}}\ mL = 12 \text{ mL}$	$8 \text{ mL} : 1 \text{ mg} :: x : 1.5 \text{ mg}$	$\dfrac{8 \text{ mL}}{1 \text{ mg}} \times \dfrac{x}{1.5 \text{ mg}}$ $8 \times 1.5 = 1x$ $\dfrac{12}{1} = x$ $12 \text{ mL} = x$

Dimensional Analysis Method

$$\dfrac{1.5\ \cancel{mg}}{\ } \left| \dfrac{8\ \cancel{mL}}{1\ \cancel{mg}} \right| \dfrac{1.5 \times 8}{\ } = 12 \text{ mL}$$

Use an oral syringe or medicine to measure the dose.

Formula Method	Proportion Expressed as Two Ratios	Proportion Expressed as Two Fractions

16. $\dfrac{\overset{2}{\cancel{25.0}}\text{ mg}}{\underset{1}{\cancel{12.5}}\text{ mg}}\times 5\text{ mL} = 10\text{ mL}$

5 mL : 12.5 mg : : x : 25 mg

$\dfrac{5\text{ mL}}{12.5\text{ mg}}\times\dfrac{x}{25\text{ mg}}$

$$5\times 25 = 12.5x$$
$$\dfrac{125}{12.5} = x$$
$$10\text{ mL} = x$$

Dimensional Analysis Method

$\dfrac{\overset{2}{\cancel{25}}\text{ mg}}{}\left|\dfrac{5\,\cancel{\text{mL}}}{\underset{1}{\cancel{12.5}}\text{ mg}}\right|\dfrac{2\times 5}{} = 10\text{ mL}$

Formula Method	Proportion Expressed as Two Ratios	Proportion Expressed as Two Fractions

17. $\dfrac{\overset{3}{\cancel{60}}\text{ mg}}{\underset{2}{\cancel{40}}\text{ mg}}\times 0.6\text{ mL} = \dfrac{1.8}{2} = 0.9\text{ mL}$

0.6 mL : 40 mg : : x : 60 mg

$\dfrac{0.6\text{ mL}}{40\text{ mg}}\times\dfrac{x}{60\text{ mg}}$

$$0.6\times 60 = 40x$$
$$\dfrac{36}{40} = x$$
$$0.9\text{ mL} = x$$

Dimensional Analysis Method

$\dfrac{\overset{3}{\cancel{60}}\text{ mg}}{}\left|\dfrac{0.6\,\cancel{\text{mL}}}{\underset{2}{\cancel{40}}\text{ mg}}\right|\dfrac{3\times 0.6}{2} = 0.9\text{ mL}$

Formula Method	Proportion Expressed as Two Ratios	Proportion Expressed as Two Fractions

18. 0.5 g = 500 mg

$\dfrac{\overset{2}{\cancel{500}}\text{ mg}}{\underset{1}{\cancel{250}}\text{ mg}}\times 5\text{ mL} = 10\text{ mL}$

5 mL : 250 mg : : x : 500 mg

$\dfrac{5\text{ mL}}{250\text{ mg}}\times\dfrac{x}{500\text{ mg}}$

$$500\times 5 = 250x$$
$$\dfrac{2500}{250} = x$$
$$10\text{ mL} = x$$

Dimensional Analysis Method

$\dfrac{0.5\,\cancel{\text{g}}}{}\left|\dfrac{5\,\cancel{\text{mL}}}{\underset{1}{\cancel{250}}\text{ mg}}\right|\dfrac{\overset{4}{\cancel{1000}}\text{ mg}}{1\,\cancel{\text{g}}}\left|\dfrac{0.5\times 5\times 4}{} = 10\text{ mL}\right.$

Formula Method	Proportion Expressed as Two Ratios	Proportion Expressed as Two Fractions
19. $\dfrac{\overset{3}{\cancel{15}}\ \text{mg}}{\underset{10}{\cancel{50}}\ \text{mg}} \times 5\ \text{mL} = 1.5\ \text{mL}$	5 mL : 50 mg : : x : 15 mg	$\dfrac{5\ \text{mL}}{50\ \text{mg}} \times \dfrac{\text{x}}{15\ \text{mg}}$

$$5 \times 15 = 50\text{x}$$
$$\frac{75}{50} = \text{x}$$
$$1.5\ \text{mL} = \text{x}$$

Dimensional Analysis Method

$$\dfrac{15\ \text{mg}}{} \ \left|\ \dfrac{\overset{1}{\cancel{5}}\ \text{mL}}{\underset{10}{\cancel{50}}\ \text{mg}}\ \right|\ \dfrac{15}{10} = 1.5\ \text{mL}$$

Formula Method	Proportion Expressed as Two Ratios	Proportion Expressed as Two Fractions
20. $\dfrac{\overset{2}{\cancel{50}}\ \text{mg}}{\underset{1}{\cancel{25}}\ \text{mg}} \times 5\ \text{mL} = 10\ \text{mL}$	5 mL : 25 mg : : x : 50 mg	$\dfrac{5\ \text{mL}}{25\ \text{mg}} \times \dfrac{\text{x}}{50\ \text{mg}}$

$$5 \times 50 = 25\text{x}$$
$$\frac{250}{25} = \text{x}$$
$$10\ \text{mL} = \text{x}$$

Dimensional Analysis Method

$$\dfrac{\overset{2}{\cancel{50}}\ \text{mg}}{}\ \left|\ \dfrac{5\ \text{mL}}{\underset{1}{\cancel{25}}\ \text{mg}}\ \right|\ \dfrac{2 \times 5}{} = 10\ \text{mL}$$

Chapter 7

Test 1: Calculations of Liquid Injections

Formula Method	Proportion Expressed as Two Ratios	Proportion Expressed as Two Fractions
1. Equivalent 0.1 g = 100 mg		
$\dfrac{\overset{1}{\cancel{100}}\ \text{mg}}{\underset{2}{\cancel{200}}\ \text{mg}} \times 3\ \text{mL} = \dfrac{3}{2}\overline{)3.0}^{\,1.5}$	3 mL : 200 mg : : x : 100 mg	$\dfrac{3\ \text{mL}}{200\ \text{mg}} \times \dfrac{\text{x}}{100\ \text{mg}}$

$$3 \times 100 = 200\text{x}$$
$$\frac{300}{200} = \text{x}$$
$$1.5\ \text{mL} = \text{x}$$

Give 1.5 mL IM.

Dimensional Analysis Method

$$\dfrac{0.1\ \text{g}}{}\ \left|\ \dfrac{3\ \text{mL}}{200\ \text{mg}}\ \right|\ \dfrac{\overset{5}{\cancel{1000}}\ \text{mg}}{1\ \text{g}}\ \right|\ \dfrac{0.1 \times 3 \times 5}{} = 1.5\ \text{mL}$$

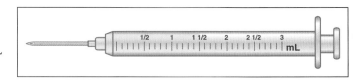

Formula Method	Proportion Expressed as Two Ratios	Proportion Expressed as Two Fractions

2. $\dfrac{\frac{1}{\cancel{5}} \text{ mg}}{\frac{15}{3} \text{ mg}} \times 1 \text{ mL} = \dfrac{1}{3} \begin{array}{r} .333 \\ 3\overline{)1.000} \end{array}$

$1 \text{ mL} : 15 \text{ mg} :: x : 5 \text{ mg}$

$\dfrac{1 \text{ mL}}{15 \text{ mg}} \times \dfrac{x}{5 \text{ mg}}$

$$\frac{5}{15} = x$$

$$0.33 \text{ mL} = x$$

Give 0.33 mL IV.

Dimensional Analysis Method

$\dfrac{\frac{1}{\cancel{5}} \text{ mg}}{} \left| \dfrac{1 \text{ (mL)}}{\frac{15}{3} \text{ mg}} \right| \dfrac{1}{3} = 0.33 \text{ mL}$

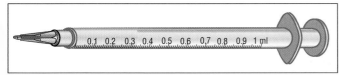

Formula Method	Proportion Expressed as Two Ratios	Proportion Expressed as Two Fractions

3. $\dfrac{\frac{1}{25} \text{ mg}}{\frac{50}{2} \text{ mg}} \times \overset{1}{\cancel{2}} \text{ mL} = 1 \text{ mL}$

$2 \text{ mL} : 50 \text{ mg} :: x : 25 \text{ mg}$

$\dfrac{2 \text{ mL}}{50 \text{ mg}} \times \dfrac{x}{25 \text{ mg}}$

$$2 \times 25 = 50x$$

$$\frac{50}{50} = x$$

$$1 \text{ mL} = x$$

Give 1 mL IM.

Dimensional Analysis Method

$\dfrac{\frac{1}{25} \text{ mg}}{} \left| \dfrac{2 \text{ (mL)}}{\frac{50}{2} \text{ mg}} \right| \dfrac{2}{2} = 1 \text{ mL}$

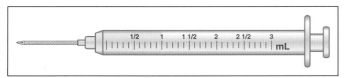

4. 20 units. Remember that Humulin R insulin is a type of regular insulin and so must be drawn up first into the syringe.

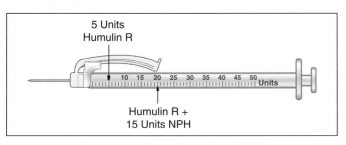

Formula Method	Proportion Expressed as Two Ratios	Proportion Expressed as Two Fractions

5. $\dfrac{\overset{1}{\cancel{20}}\ \cancel{mEq}}{\underset{\underset{1}{2}}{\cancel{40}}\ \cancel{mEq}} \times \overset{10}{\cancel{20}}\ mL = 10\ mL$

20 mL : 40 mEq : : x : 20 mEq

$\dfrac{20\ mL}{40\ mEq} \times \dfrac{x}{20\ mEq}$

$$20 \times 20 = 40x$$

$$\frac{400}{40} = x$$

$$10\ mL = x$$

Add 10 mL to IV.

Dimensional Analysis Method

$$\dfrac{\overset{1}{\cancel{20}}\ \cancel{mEq}}{} \quad \Bigg| \quad \dfrac{20\ \boxed{mL}}{\underset{2}{\cancel{40}}\ \cancel{mEq}} \quad \Bigg| \quad \dfrac{20}{2} = 10\ mL$$

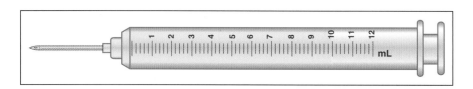

Formula Method	Proportion Expressed as Two Ratios	Proportion Expressed as Two Fractions

6. $\dfrac{\overset{3}{\cancel{0.6}}\ \cancel{mg}}{\underset{2}{\cancel{0.4}}\ \cancel{mg}} \times 1\ mL = \dfrac{3}{2}\ \overset{1.5}{\overline{)3.0}}$

1 mL : 0.4 mg : : x : 0.6 mg

$\dfrac{1\ mL}{0.4\ mg} \times \dfrac{x}{0.6\ mg}$

$$\frac{0.6}{0.4} = x$$

$$1.5\ mL = x$$

Give 1.5 mL subcutaneous.

Dimensional Analysis Method

$$\dfrac{0.6\ \cancel{mg}}{} \quad \Bigg| \quad \dfrac{1\ \boxed{mL}}{0.4\ \cancel{mg}} \quad \Bigg| \quad \dfrac{0.6}{0.4} = 1.5\ mL$$

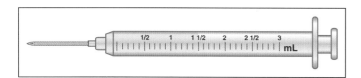

Formula Method	Proportion Expressed as Two Ratios	Proportion Expressed as Two Fractions
7. $\dfrac{\overset{2}{\cancel{0.8}}\ \text{mg}}{\underset{1}{\cancel{0.4}}\ \text{mg}} \times 1\ \text{mL} = 2\ \text{mL}$	$1\ \text{mL} : 0.4\ \text{mg} :: x : 0.8\ \text{mg}$	$\dfrac{1\ \text{mL}}{0.4\ \text{mg}} \times \dfrac{x}{0.8\ \text{mg}}$

$$\frac{0.8}{0.4} = x$$
$$2\ \text{mL} = x$$

Give 2 mL IV.

Dimensional Analysis Method

$$\frac{0.8\ \text{mg}}{} \left| \frac{1\ \cancel{\text{mL}}}{0.4\ \text{mg}} \right| \frac{0.8}{0.4} = 2\ \text{mL}$$

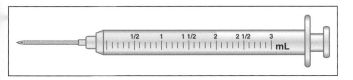

8. Equivalent 0.5 g = 500 mg

Formula Method	Proportion Expressed as Two Ratios	Proportion Expressed as Two Fractions
$\dfrac{\overset{2}{\cancel{500}}\ \text{mg}}{\underset{1}{\cancel{250}}\ \text{mg}} \times 1\ \text{mL} = 2\ \text{mL}$	$1\ \text{mL} : 250\ \text{mg} :: x : 500\ \text{mg}$	$\dfrac{1\ \text{mL}}{250\ \text{mg}} \times \dfrac{x}{500\ \text{mg}}$

$$\frac{500}{250} = x$$
$$2\ \text{mL} = x$$

Dimensional Analysis Method

$$\frac{0.5\ \cancel{\text{g}}}{} \left| \frac{1\ \cancel{\text{mL}}}{250\ \cancel{\text{mg}}} \right| \frac{\overset{4}{\cancel{1000}}\ \cancel{\text{mg}}}{1\ \cancel{\text{g}}} \left| \frac{0.5 \times 4}{} = 2\ \text{mL} \right.$$

Add 2 mL to IV.

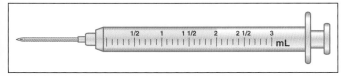

Formula Method	*Proportion Expressed as Two Ratios*	*Proportion Expressed as Two Fractions*
9. $\dfrac{200 \text{ mg}}{500 \text{ mg}} \times 2 \text{ mL} = \dfrac{4}{5}\overline{)\dfrac{.8}{4.0}}$ 0.8 mL	2 mL : 500 mg :: x : 200 mg	$\dfrac{2 \text{ mL}}{500 \text{ mg}} \times \dfrac{x}{200 \text{ mg}}$

$$2 \times 200 = 500x$$
$$\frac{400}{500} = x$$
$$0.8 \text{ mL} = x$$

Dimensional Analysis Method

$$\frac{200 \text{ mg}}{} \left| \frac{2 \text{ mL}}{500 \text{ mg}} \right| \frac{2 \times 2}{5} = 0.8 \text{ mL}$$

Give 0.8 mL IM.

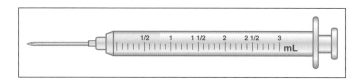

10. Equivalent 1:100 means 1 g in 100 mL

$$1 \text{ g} = 1000 \text{ mg}$$

Hence, the solution is 1000 mg/100 mL.

Formula Method	*Proportion Expressed as Two Ratios*	*Proportion Expressed as Two Fractions*
$\dfrac{7.5 \text{ mg}}{1000 \text{ mg}} \times 100 \text{ mL} = \dfrac{7.5}{10}\overline{)\dfrac{.75}{7.50}}$ $\underline{7\,0}$ 50 $\underline{50}$ $0.75 \text{ or } 0.8 \text{ mL}$	100 mL : 1000 mg :: x : 7.5 mg	$\dfrac{100 \text{ mL}}{1000 \text{ mg}} \times \dfrac{x}{7.5 \text{ mg}}$

$$100 \times 7.5 = 1000x$$
$$\frac{7500}{1000} = x$$
$$0.75 \text{ or } 0.8 \text{ mL} = x$$

Dimensional Analysis Method

$$\frac{7.5 \text{ mg}}{} \left| \frac{\overset{1}{100} \text{ mL}}{1 \text{ g}} \right| \frac{1 \text{ g}}{\underset{10}{1000} \text{ mg}} \left| \frac{7.5}{10} \right. = 0.75 \text{ mL}$$

Give 0.8 mL subcutaneous.

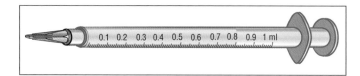

Formula Method	Proportion Expressed as Two Ratios	Proportion Expressed as Two Fractions

11. $\dfrac{\overset{2}{\cancel{10}}\text{ mg}}{\underset{1}{\cancel{5}}\text{ mg}} \times 1\text{ mL} = 2\text{ mL}$

$\overset{\longleftrightarrow}{1\text{ mL} : 5\text{ mg} :: x : 10\text{ mg}}$

$\dfrac{1\text{ mL}}{5\text{ mg}} \times \dfrac{x}{10\text{ mg}}$

$$10 = 5x$$
$$\dfrac{10}{5} = x$$
$$2\text{ mL} = x$$

Dimensional Analysis Method

$\dfrac{10\text{ mg}}{} \;\bigg|\; \dfrac{1\,\cancel{mL}}{5\text{ mg}} \;\bigg|\; \dfrac{10}{5} = 2\text{ mL}$

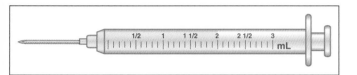

Formula Method	Proportion Expressed as Two Ratios	Proportion Expressed as Two Fractions

12. $\dfrac{\overset{1}{\cancel{25}}\text{ mg}}{\underset{4}{\cancel{100}}\text{ mg}} \times 2\text{ mL} = x$

$\dfrac{2}{4} = x$

$0.5\text{ mL} = x$

$\overset{\longleftrightarrow}{2\text{ mL} : 100\text{ mg} :: x : 25\text{ mg}}$

$\dfrac{2\text{ mL}}{100\text{ mg}} \times \dfrac{x}{25\text{ mg}}$

$$25 \times 2 = 100x$$
$$\dfrac{50}{100} = x$$
$$0.5\text{ mL} = x$$

Dimensional Analysis Method

$\dfrac{\overset{1}{\cancel{25}}\text{ mg}}{} \;\bigg|\; \dfrac{2\,\cancel{mL}}{\underset{4}{\cancel{100}}\text{ mg}} \;\bigg|\; \dfrac{2}{4} = 0.5\text{ mL}$

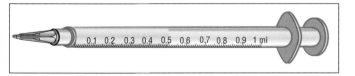

Formula Method	Proportion Expressed as Two Ratios	Proportion Expressed as Two Fractions
13. $\frac{50 \text{ mg}}{25 \text{ mg}} \times 1 \text{ mL} = x$ $2 \text{ mL} = x$	$1 \text{ mL} : 25 \text{ mg} :: x : 50 \text{ mg}$	$\frac{1 \text{ mL}}{25 \text{ mg}} \times \frac{x}{50 \text{ mg}}$

$$\frac{50}{25} = x$$
$$2 \text{ mL} = x$$

Dimensional Analysis Method

$$\frac{50 \text{ mg}}{} \left| \frac{1 \text{ mL}}{25 \text{ mg}} \right| \frac{50}{25} = 2 \text{ mL}$$

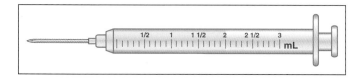

Formula Method	Proportion Expressed as Two Ratios	Proportion Expressed as Two Fractions
14. $\frac{0.5 \text{ mg}}{2 \text{ mg}} \times 1 \text{ mL} = x$ $\frac{0.5}{2} = x$ $0.25 \text{ mL} = x$	$1 \text{ mL} : 2 \text{ mg} :: x : 0.5 \text{ mg}$	$\frac{1 \text{ mL}}{2 \text{ mg}} \times \frac{x}{0.5 \text{ mg}}$

$$\frac{0.5}{2} = x$$
$$0.25 \text{ mL} = x$$

Dimensional Analysis Method

$$\frac{0.5 \text{ mg}}{} \left| \frac{1 \text{ mL}}{2 \text{ mg}} \right| \frac{0.5}{2} = 0.25 \text{ mL}$$

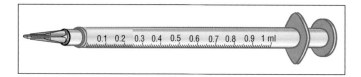

15. Equivalent 0.2 g = 200 mg

Formula Method	Proportion Expressed as Two Ratios	Proportion Expressed as Two Fractions
$\dfrac{\overset{1}{\cancel{200}} \text{ mg}}{\underset{1}{\cancel{200}} \text{ mg}} \times 2 \text{ mL} = x$	2 mL : 200 mg :: x : 200 mg	$\dfrac{2 \text{ mL}}{200 \text{ mg}} \times \dfrac{x}{200 \text{ mg}}$
$2 \text{ mL} = x$		

$$2 \times 200 = 200x$$
$$400 = 200x$$
$$\tfrac{400}{200} = x$$
$$2 \text{ mL} = x$$

Dimensional Analysis Method

$$\dfrac{0.2 \,\cancel{g}}{} \left| \dfrac{2 \,\cancel{mL}}{200 \,\cancel{mg}} \right| \dfrac{\overset{5}{\cancel{1000}} \,\cancel{mg}}{1 \,\cancel{g}} \left| \dfrac{0.2 \times 2 \times 5}{} = 2 \text{ mL} \right.$$

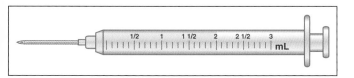

Test 2: Calculations of Liquid Injections

Formula Method	Proportion Expressed as Two Ratios	Proportion Expressed as Two Fractions
1. $\dfrac{\overset{2}{\cancel{10}} \text{ mg}}{\underset{3}{\cancel{15}} \text{ mg}} \times 1 \text{ mL} = \dfrac{2}{3} \overset{0.66}{\overline{)2.00}}$	1 mL : 15 mg :: x : 10 mg	$\dfrac{1 \text{ mL}}{15 \text{ mg}} \times \dfrac{x}{10 \text{ mg}}$
0.66 mL		

$$\tfrac{10}{15} = x$$
$$0.66 \text{ or } 0.7 \text{ mL} = x$$

Dimensional Analysis Method

$$\dfrac{10 \,\cancel{mg}}{} \left| \dfrac{1 \,\cancel{mL}}{15 \,\cancel{mg}} \right| \dfrac{10}{15} = 0.66 \text{ mL}$$

Give 0.7 mL IV.

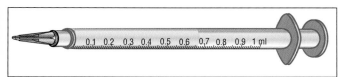

Formula Method	**Proportion Expressed as Two Ratios**	**Proportion Expressed as Two Fractions**

2. $\dfrac{\overset{1}{\cancel{25}}\ \text{mg}}{\underset{4}{\cancel{100}}\ \text{mg}} \times 1\ \text{mL} = \dfrac{1}{4}\,\overline{)\!\begin{array}{r}0.25\\1.00\end{array}}$

$1\ \text{mL} : 100\ \text{mg} :: x : 25\ \text{mg}$

$\dfrac{1\ \text{mL}}{100\ \text{mg}} \times \dfrac{x}{25\ \text{mg}}$

$\dfrac{25}{100} = x$

$0.25\ \text{mL} = x$

Dimensional Analysis Method

$\dfrac{\overset{1}{\cancel{25}}\ \cancel{\text{mg}}}{}\ \bigg|\ \dfrac{1\ \text{(mL)}}{\underset{4}{\cancel{100}}\ \cancel{\text{mg}}}\ \bigg|\ \dfrac{1}{4} = 0.25\ \text{mL}$

Give 0.25 mL. You are using a 1-mL precision syringe; therefore, the answer is solved to the nearest hundredth.

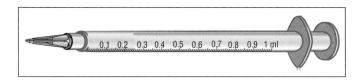

3. Equivalent 0.1 g = 100 mg

Formula Method	**Proportion Expressed as Two Ratios**	**Proportion Expressed as Two Fractions**

$\dfrac{\overset{1}{\cancel{100}}\ \text{mg}}{\underset{2}{\cancel{200}}\ \text{mg}} \times 3\ \text{mL} = \dfrac{3}{2}\,\overline{)\!\begin{array}{r}1.5\\3.0\end{array}}$

$3\ \text{mL} : 200\ \text{mg} :: x : 100\ \text{mg}$

$\dfrac{3\ \text{mL}}{200\ \text{mg}} \times \dfrac{x}{100\ \text{mg}}$

$3 \times 100 = 200x$

$\dfrac{300}{200} = x$

$1.5\ \text{mL} = x$

Dimensional Analysis Method

$\dfrac{0.1\ \cancel{\text{g}}}{}\ \bigg|\ \dfrac{3\ \text{(mL)}}{\underset{1}{\cancel{200}}\ \cancel{\text{mg}}}\ \bigg|\ \dfrac{\overset{5}{\cancel{1000}}\ \cancel{\text{mg}}}{1\ \cancel{\text{g}}}\ \bigg|\ \dfrac{0.1 \times 3 \times 5}{} = 1.5\ \text{mL}$

Give 1.5 mL IM.

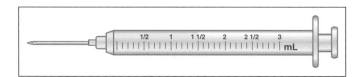

Formula Method	Proportion Expressed as Two Ratios	Proportion Expressed as Two Fractions

4. $\dfrac{\overset{1}{\cancel{1000}}\ \cancel{mcg}}{\underset{5}{\cancel{5000}}\ \cancel{mcg}} \times 1\ mL = \dfrac{1}{5}\overline{\smash{)}\,\begin{matrix}0.2\\1.0\end{matrix}}$

$1\ mL : 5000\ mcg :: x : 1000\ mcg$

$\dfrac{1\ mL}{5000\ mcg} \times \dfrac{x}{1000\ mcg}$

$\dfrac{1000}{5000} = x$

$0.2\ mL = x$

Dimensional Analysis Method

$\dfrac{\overset{1}{\cancel{1000}}\ \cancel{mcg}}{} \left| \dfrac{1\ \cancel{mL}}{\underset{5}{\cancel{5000}}\ \cancel{mcg}} \right| \dfrac{1}{5} = 0.2\ mL$

Give 0.2 mL IM.

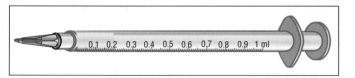

5. Equivalent 1% means 1 g in 100 mL

$$1\ g = 1000\ mg$$

Hence, the solution is 1000 mg in 100 mL.

Formula Method	Proportion Expressed as Two Ratios	Proportion Expressed as Two Fractions

$\dfrac{\overset{5}{\cancel{25}}\ \cancel{mg}}{\underset{\underset{2}{10}}{\cancel{1000}}\ \cancel{mg}} \times \overset{1}{\cancel{100}}\ mL = \dfrac{5}{2}\overline{\smash{)}\,\begin{matrix}2.5\\5.0\end{matrix}}$

$100\ mL : 1000\ mg :: x : 25\ mg$

$\dfrac{100\ mL}{1000\ mg} \times \dfrac{x}{25\ mg}$

$100 \times 25 = 1000x$

$\dfrac{2500}{1000} = x$

$2.5\ mL = x$

Dimensional Analysis Method

$\dfrac{25\ \cancel{mg}}{} \left| \dfrac{\overset{1}{\cancel{100}}\ \text{(mL)}}{\cancel{1}\ \cancel{g}} \right| \dfrac{\cancel{1}\ \cancel{g}}{\underset{10}{\cancel{1000}}\ \cancel{mg}} \left| \dfrac{25}{10} = 2.5\ mL \right.$

Prepare 2.5 mL.

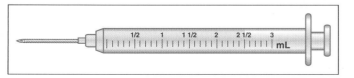

Formula Method	Proportion Expressed as Two Ratios	Proportion Expressed as Two Fractions

6. $\dfrac{0.5\,\text{mg}}{0.4\,\text{mg}} \times 1\ \text{mL} = \dfrac{5}{4}\overline{)\begin{array}{l}1.25\\5.00\end{array}}$

$\qquad\qquad\qquad\quad 1.25 \text{ or } 1.3 \text{ mL}$

$1\ \text{mL} : 0.4\ \text{mg} :: x : 0.5\ \text{mg}$

$\dfrac{1\ \text{mL}}{0.4\ \text{mg}} \times \dfrac{x}{0.5\ \text{mg}}$

$$\dfrac{0.5\ \text{mg}}{0.4\ \text{mg}} = x$$

$$1.25 \text{ or } 1.3 \text{ mL} = x$$

Dimensional Analysis Method

$$\dfrac{0.5\ \cancel{\text{mg}}}{} \left|\ \dfrac{1\ \cancel{\text{mL}}}{0.4\ \cancel{\text{mg}}}\ \right|\ \dfrac{0.5}{0.4} = 1.25 \text{ or } 1.3 \text{ mL}$$

Give 1.3 mL subcutaneous.

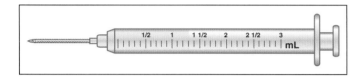

7. 13 units. Humulin R insulin is a type of regular insulin and so must be drawn up first into the syringe.

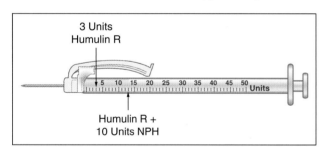

Formula Method	Proportion Expressed as Two Ratios	Proportion Expressed as Two Fractions

8. $\dfrac{1.2\,\text{mEq}}{0.5\,\text{mEq}} \times 1\ \text{mL} = \dfrac{1.2}{0.5}\overline{)\begin{array}{l}2.4\\1.20\end{array}}$

$1\ \text{mL} : 0.5\ \text{mEq} :: x : 1.2\ \text{mEq}$

$\dfrac{1\ \text{mL}}{0.5\ \text{mEq}} \times \dfrac{x}{1.2\ \text{mEq}}$

$$\dfrac{1.2}{0.5} = x$$

$$2.4\ \text{mL} = x$$

Dimensional Analysis Method

$$\dfrac{1.2\ \cancel{\text{mEq}}}{} \left|\ \dfrac{1\ \cancel{\text{mL}}}{0.5\ \cancel{\text{mEq}}}\ \right|\ \dfrac{1.2}{0.5} = 2.4\ \text{mL}$$

Add 2.4 mL to the IV stat.

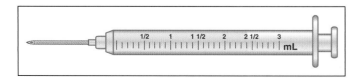

Formula Method	Proportion Expressed as Two Ratios	Proportion Expressed as Two Fractions
9. $\dfrac{\overset{3}{\cancel{75}\text{ mg}}}{\underset{2}{\cancel{50}\text{ mg}}} \times 1\text{ mL} = \dfrac{3}{2}\overline{)3.0}^{1.5}$	1 mL : 50 mg : : x : 75 mg	$\dfrac{1\text{ mL}}{50\text{ mg}} \times \dfrac{\text{x}}{75\text{ mg}}$

$$\frac{75}{50} = \text{x}$$

$$1.5\text{ mL} = \text{x}$$

Dimensional Analysis Method

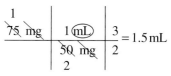

$$\frac{1}{\cancel{75}\text{ mg}} \left| \frac{1\ \cancel{\text{mL}}}{\cancel{50}\text{ mg}} \right| \frac{3}{2} = 1.5\text{ mL}$$

Give 1.5 mL IM.

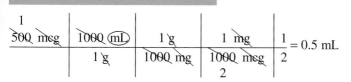

10. Equivalent 1:1000 means 1 g in 1000 mL

$$1\text{ g} = 1000\text{ mg}$$

Hence, the solution is 1000 mg in 1000 mL.

$$500\text{ mcg} = 0.5\text{ mg}$$

Formula Method	Proportion Expressed as Two Ratios	Proportion Expressed as Two Fractions
$\dfrac{0.5\text{ mg}}{\cancel{1000}\text{ mg}} \times \overset{1}{\cancel{1000}}\text{ mL} = 0.5\text{ mL}$	1000 mL : 1000 mg : : x : 0.5 mg	$\dfrac{1000\text{ mL}}{1000\text{ mg}} \times \dfrac{\text{x}}{0.5\text{ mg}}$

$$1000 \times 0.5 = 1000\text{x}$$

$$\frac{500}{1000} = \text{x}$$

$$0.5\text{ mL} = \text{x}$$

Dimensional Analysis Method

$$\frac{1}{\cancel{500}\text{ mcg}} \left| \frac{\cancel{1000}\ \cancel{\text{mL}}}{1\ \cancel{\text{g}}} \right| \frac{1\ \cancel{\text{g}}}{\cancel{1000}\text{ mg}} \left| \frac{1\ \cancel{\text{mg}}}{\cancel{1000}\text{ mcg}} \right| \frac{1}{2} = 0.5\text{ mL}$$

Give 0.5 mL subcutaneous stat.

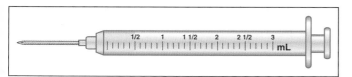

Test 3: Calculations of Liquid Injections

Formula Method	Proportion Expressed as Two Ratios	Proportion Expressed as Two Fractions

1. $\dfrac{\overset{1}{\cancel{0.25 \text{ mg}}}}{\underset{\underset{1}{2}}{\cancel{0.50 \text{ mg}}}} \times \overset{1}{\cancel{2}} \text{ mL} = 1 \text{ mL}$

$2 \text{ mL} : 0.5 \text{ mg} :: x : 0.25 \text{ mg}$

$$\frac{2 \text{ mL}}{0.5 \text{ mg}} \times \frac{x}{0.25 \text{ mg}}$$

$$2 \times 0.25 = 0.5x$$

$$\frac{0.50}{0.50} = x$$

$$1 \text{ mL} = x$$

Dimensional Analysis Method

$$\frac{\overset{1}{\cancel{0.25}} \text{ mg}}{} \left| \frac{2 \text{ } \cancel{\text{mL}}}{\underset{2}{\cancel{0.5}} \text{ mg}} \right| \frac{2}{2} = 1 \text{ mL}$$

Formula Method	Proportion Expressed as Two Ratios	Proportion Expressed as Two Fractions

2. $\dfrac{\cancel{40} \text{ mg}}{\cancel{50} \text{ mg}} \times 2 \text{ mL} = \overset{8}{\underset{5}{}} \, 5\overline{)\overset{1.6}{8.0}} = 1.6 \text{ mL}$

$2 \text{ mL} : 50 \text{ mg} :: x : 40 \text{ mg}$

$$\frac{2 \text{ mL}}{50 \text{ mg}} \times \frac{x}{40 \text{ mg}}$$

$$2 \times 40 = 50x$$

$$\frac{80}{50} = x$$

$$1.6 \text{ mL} = x$$

Dimensional Analysis Method

$$\frac{\cancel{40} \text{ mg}}{} \left| \frac{2 \text{ } \cancel{\text{mL}}}{\cancel{50} \text{ mg}} \right| \frac{4 \times 2}{5} = \frac{8}{5} = 1.6 \text{ mL}$$

Formula Method	Proportion Expressed as Two Ratios	Proportion Expressed as Two Fractions

3. $\dfrac{8 \text{ mg}}{15 \text{ mg}} \times 1 \text{ mL} = \overset{8}{\underset{15}{}} \, 15\overline{)\overset{0.53}{8.00}} = 0.5 \text{ mL}$

$\qquad\qquad\qquad \dfrac{7\ 5}{50}$

$\qquad\qquad\qquad \underline{45}$

$1 \text{ mL} : 15 \text{ mg} :: x : 8 \text{ mg}$

$$\frac{1 \text{ mL}}{15 \text{ mg}} \times \frac{x}{8 \text{ mg}}$$

$$\frac{8}{15} = x$$

$$0.53 \text{ or } 0.5 \text{ mL} = x$$

Dimensional Analysis Method

$$\frac{8 \text{ } \cancel{\text{mg}}}{} \left| \frac{1 \text{ } \cancel{\text{mL}}}{15 \text{ } \cancel{\text{mg}}} \right| \frac{8}{15} = 0.53 \text{ or } 0.5 \text{ mL}$$

Formula Method	Proportion Expressed as Two Ratios	Proportion Expressed as Two Fractions

4.

$$\frac{\overset{1}{\cancel{25 \text{ mg}}}}{\underset{4}{\cancel{100 \text{ mg}}}} \times 1 \text{ mL} = \overset{0.25}{4)\overline{1.00}}$$

$$= 0.25 \text{ or } 0.3 \text{ mL}$$

$$1 \text{ mL} : 100 \text{ mg} :: x : 25 \text{ mg}$$

$$\frac{1 \text{ mL}}{100 \text{ mg}} \times \frac{x}{25 \text{ mg}}$$

$$\frac{25}{100} = x$$

$$0.25 \text{ or } 0.3 \text{ mL} = x$$

Dimensional Analysis Method

$$\frac{\overset{1}{\cancel{25 \text{ mg}}}}{} \; \Bigg| \; \frac{1 \text{ mL}}{\underset{4}{\cancel{100 \text{ mg}}}} \; \Bigg| \; \frac{1}{4} \; = \; 0.25 \text{ or } 0.3 \text{ mL}$$

Formula Method	Proportion Expressed as Two Ratios	Proportion Expressed as Two Fractions

5.

$$\frac{\cancel{200 \text{ mg}}}{\cancel{500 \text{ mg}}} \times 2 \text{ mL} \quad \overset{0.8}{5)\overline{4.0}} = 0.8 \text{ mL}$$

$$2 \text{ mL} : 500 \text{ mg} :: x : 200 \text{ mg}$$

$$\frac{2 \text{ mL}}{500 \text{ mg}} \times \frac{x}{200 \text{ mg}}$$

$$2 \times 200 = 500x$$

$$\frac{400}{500} = x$$

$$0.8 \text{ mL} = x$$

Dimensional Analysis Method

$$\frac{\cancel{200 \text{ mg}}}{} \; \Bigg| \; \frac{2 \text{ mL}}{\cancel{500 \text{ mg}}} \; \Bigg| \; \frac{2 \times 2}{5} \; = \; \frac{4}{5} \; = \; 0.8 \text{ mL}$$

Formula Method	Proportion Expressed as Two Ratios	Proportion Expressed as Two Fractions

6.

$$\frac{\overset{3}{\cancel{1500 \text{ mcg}}}}{\underset{10}{\cancel{5000 \text{ mcg}}}} \times 1 \text{ mL} = \overset{0.3}{10)\overline{3.0}}$$

$$= 0.3 \text{ mL}$$

$$1 \text{ mL} : 5000 \text{ mcg} :: x : 1500 \text{ mcg}$$

$$\frac{1 \text{ mL}}{5000 \text{ mcg}} \times \frac{x}{1500 \text{ mcg}}$$

$$\frac{1500}{5000} = x$$

$$0.3 \text{ mL} = x$$

Dimensional Analysis Method

$$\frac{\overset{3}{\cancel{1500 \text{ mcg}}}}{} \; \Bigg| \; \frac{1 \text{ mL}}{\underset{10}{\cancel{5000 \text{ mcg}}}} \; \Bigg| \; \frac{3}{10} = 0.3 \text{ mL}$$

Formula Method	Proportion Expressed as Two Ratios	Proportion Expressed as Two Fractions

7. $\dfrac{\overset{3}{\cancel{0.6 \text{ mg}}}}{\underset{2}{\cancel{0.4 \text{ mg}}}} \times 1 \text{ mL} = \dfrac{3}{2}\overline{\smash{\big)}3.0}^{\,1.5} = 1.5 \text{ mL}$

$1 \text{ mL} : 0.4 \text{ mg} : : x : 0.6 \text{ mg}$

$\dfrac{1 \text{ mL}}{0.4 \text{ mg}} \times \dfrac{x}{0.6 \text{ mg}}$

$$\frac{0.6}{0.4} = x$$

$$1.5 \text{ mL} = x$$

Dimensional Analysis Method

$$\frac{\overset{3}{\cancel{0.6 \text{ mg}}}}{} \;\middle|\; \frac{1 \text{ mL}}{\underset{2}{\cancel{0.4 \text{ mg}}}} \;\middle|\; \frac{3}{2} = 1.5 \text{ mL}$$

Formula Method	Proportion Expressed as Two Ratios	Proportion Expressed as Two Fractions

8. $0.1 \text{ g} = 100 \text{ mg}$

$\dfrac{\overset{1}{\cancel{100 \text{ mg}}}}{\underset{2}{\cancel{200 \text{ mg}}}} \times 3 \text{ mL} = \dfrac{3}{2}\overline{\smash{\big)}3.0}^{\,1.5} = 1.5 \text{ mL}$

$3 \text{ mL} : 200 \text{ mg} : : x : 100 \text{ mg}$

$\dfrac{3 \text{ mL}}{200 \text{ mg}} \times \dfrac{x}{100 \text{ mg}}$

$$3 \times 100 = 200x$$

$$\frac{300}{200} = x$$

$$1.5 \text{ mL} = x$$

Dimensional Analysis Method

$$\frac{0.1 \text{ g}}{} \;\middle|\; \frac{3 \text{ mL}}{200 \text{ mg}} \;\middle|\; \frac{\overset{5}{\cancel{1000}} \text{ mg}}{1 \text{ g}} \;\middle|\; 0.1 \times 3 \times 5 = 1.5 \text{ mL}$$

Formula Method	Proportion Expressed as Two Ratios	Proportion Expressed as Two Fractions

9. $\dfrac{\overset{3}{\cancel{1.5 \text{ mg}}}}{\underset{4}{\cancel{2.0 \text{ mg}}}} \times 1 \text{ mL} = \dfrac{3}{4}\overline{\smash{\big)}3.00}^{\,0.75}$

$= 0.75 \text{ or } 0.8 \text{ mL}$

$1 \text{ mL} : 2 \text{ mg} : : x : 1.5 \text{ mg}$

$\dfrac{1 \text{ mL}}{2 \text{ mg}} \times \dfrac{x}{1.5 \text{ mg}}$

$$\frac{1.5}{2} = x$$

$$0.75 \text{ or } 0.8 \text{ mL} = x$$

Dimensional Analysis Method

$$\frac{1.5 \text{ mg}}{} \;\middle|\; \frac{1 \text{ mL}}{2 \text{ mg}} \;\middle|\; \frac{1.5}{2} = 0.75 \text{ or } 0.8 \text{ mL}$$

Formula Method	Proportion Expressed as Two Ratios	Proportion Expressed as Two Fractions

10. $\dfrac{600,000 \text{ units}}{500,000 \text{ units}} \times 1 \text{ mL}$

$= \dfrac{6}{5} \overline{)6.0}^{1.2} = 1.2 \text{ mL}$

1 mL : 500,000 units :: x : 600,000 units

$\dfrac{1 \text{ mL}}{500,000 \text{ units}} \times \dfrac{x}{600,000 \text{ units}}$

$\dfrac{600,000}{500,000} = x$

$1.2 \text{ mL} = x$

Dimensional Analysis Method

$\dfrac{600,000 \text{ units}}{1} \left| \dfrac{1 \text{ mL}}{500,000 \text{ units}} \right| \dfrac{6}{5} = 1.2 \text{ mL}$

Formula Method	Proportion Expressed as Two Ratios	Proportion Expressed as Two Fractions

11. 200 mcg = 0.2 mg

$\dfrac{\overset{1}{0.2} \text{ mg}}{\underset{4}{0.8} \text{ mg}} \times 1 \text{ mL} = \dfrac{1}{4} \overline{)1.00}^{0.25}$

$= 0.25 \text{ or } 0.3 \text{ mL}$

1 mL : 0.8 mg :: x : 0.2 mg

$\dfrac{1 \text{ mL}}{0.8 \text{ mg}} \times \dfrac{x}{0.2 \text{ mg}}$

$\dfrac{0.2}{0.8} = x$

0.25 or 0.3 mL = x

Dimensional Analysis Method

$\dfrac{\overset{1}{200 \text{ mcg}}}{1} \left| \dfrac{1 \text{ mL}}{0.8 \text{ mg}} \right| \dfrac{1 \text{ mg}}{\underset{5}{1000 \text{ mcg}}} \left| \dfrac{1}{0.8 \times 5} \right| \dfrac{1}{4} = 0.25 \text{ or } 0.3 \text{ mL}$

12. 1:4000 means   1 g in 4000 mL

1 g = 1000 mg

500 mcg = 0.5 mg

Formula Method	Proportion Expressed as Two Ratios	Proportion Expressed as Two Fractions

$\dfrac{0.5 \text{ mg}}{\underset{1}{1000 \text{ mg}}} \times \overset{4}{4000} \text{ mL} = \dfrac{\overset{}{0.5} \times 4}{2.0 \text{ mL}}$

4000 mL : 1000 mg :: x : 0.5 mg

$\dfrac{4000 \text{ mL}}{1000 \text{ mg}} \times \dfrac{x}{0.5 \text{ mg}}$

$4000 \times 0.5 = 1000x$

$\dfrac{2000}{1000} = 2 \text{ mL}$

Dimensional Analysis Method

$\dfrac{\overset{1}{500 \text{ mcg}}}{1} \left| \dfrac{\overset{4}{4000 \text{ mL}}}{1 \text{ g}} \right| \dfrac{1 \text{ g}}{\underset{2}{1000 \text{ mg}}} \left| \dfrac{1 \text{ mg}}{\underset{1}{1000 \text{ mcg}}} \right| \dfrac{4}{2} = 2 \text{ mL}$

Formula Method	Proportion Expressed as Two Ratios	Proportion Expressed as Two Fractions

13. $\frac{3\,mg}{2\,mg} \times 1\ mL = \frac{3}{2}\overline{)\overset{1.5}{3.0}} = 1.5\ mL$

$\overleftrightarrow{1\ mL : 2\ mg} :: \overleftrightarrow{x : 3\ mg}$

$\dfrac{1\ mL}{2\ mg} \times \dfrac{x}{3\ mg}$

$$\frac{3}{2} = x$$

$$1.5\ mL = x$$

Dimensional Analysis Method

$$\frac{3\ \cancel{mg} \ \left|\ 1\ \text{(mL)}\ \right|\ 3}{2\ \cancel{mg}\ |\ 2} = 1.5\ mL$$

14. 1:1000 means   1 g = 1000 mL
                        1 g = 1000 mg

Formula Method	Proportion Expressed as Two Ratios	Proportion Expressed as Two Fractions

$\dfrac{0.4\ mg}{1000\ mg} \times \overset{1}{1000}\ mL = 0.4\ mL$

$\overleftrightarrow{1000\ mL . 1000\ mg} :: \overleftrightarrow{x . 0.4\ mg}$

$\dfrac{1000\ mL}{1000\ mg} \times \dfrac{x}{0.4\ mg}$

$$1000 \times 0.4 = 1000x$$

$$\frac{400}{1000} = x$$

$$0.4\ mL = x$$

Dimensional Analysis Method

$$\frac{0.4\ \cancel{mg}\ \left|\ \overset{1}{1000}\,\text{(mL)}\ \right|\ 1\ \cancel{g}\ \left|\ 0.4\right.}{1\ \cancel{g}\ |\ 1000\ \cancel{mg}\ |\ 1} = 0.4\ mL$$

15. 50% means   50 g in 100 mL
                     500 mg = 0.5 g

Formula Method	Proportion Expressed as Two Ratios	Proportion Expressed as Two Fractions

$\dfrac{0.5\,g}{\underset{1}{50\,g}} \times \overset{2}{100}\ mL = 1\ mL$

$\overleftrightarrow{100\ mL : 50\ g} :: \overleftrightarrow{x : 0.5\ g}$

$\dfrac{100\ mL}{50\ g} \times \dfrac{x}{0.5\ g}$

$$100 \times 0.5 = 50x$$

$$\frac{\cancel{50}}{\cancel{50}} = x$$

$$1\ mL = x$$

Dimensional Analysis Method

$$\frac{1}{500 \ \text{mg}} \left| \frac{\overset{2}{100} \ \text{mL}}{\underset{1}{50 \ \text{g}}} \right| \frac{1 \ \text{g}}{\underset{2}{1000 \ \text{mg}}} \left| \frac{2}{2} \right. = 1 \ \text{mL}$$

Formula Method

16. $\dfrac{\overset{1}{\cancel{0.75} \ \text{mg}}}{\underset{2}{\cancel{1.50} \ \text{mg}}} \times 1 \ \text{mL} = \frac{1}{2} \ \text{mL}$ or $0.5 \ \text{mL}$

Proportion Expressed as Two Ratios

$1 \ \text{mL} : 1.5 \ \text{mg} :: x : 0.75 \ \text{mg}$

Proportion Expressed as Two Fractions

$$\frac{1 \ \text{mL}}{1.5 \ \text{mg}} \times \frac{x}{0.75 \ \text{mg}}$$

$$\frac{0.75}{1.5} = x$$

$$0.5 \ \text{mL} = x$$

Dimensional Analysis Method

$$\frac{1}{0.75 \ \text{mg}} \left| \frac{1 \ \text{mL}}{\underset{2}{1.5 \ \text{mg}}} \right| \frac{1}{2} = 0.5 \ \text{mL}$$

17. 20% means   20 g in 100 mL

        100 mg = 0.1 g

Formula Method

$\dfrac{0.1 \, \text{g}}{\underset{1}{20 \, \text{g}}} \times \overset{5}{100} \ \text{mL} = 0.5 \ \text{mL}$

Proportion Expressed as Two Ratios

$100 \ \text{mL} : 20 \ \text{g} :: x : 0.1 \ \text{g}$

Proportion Expressed as Two Fractions

$$\frac{100 \ \text{mL}}{20 \ \text{g}} \times \frac{x}{0.1 \ \text{g}}$$

$$100 \times 0.1 = 20x$$

$$\frac{10}{20} = x$$

$$0.5 \ \text{mL} = x$$

Dimensional Analysis Method

$$\frac{1}{100 \ \text{mg}} \left| \frac{\overset{5}{100} \ \text{mL}}{\underset{1}{20 \ \text{g}}} \right| \frac{1 \ \text{g}}{\underset{10}{1000 \ \text{mg}}} \left| \frac{5}{10} \right. = 0.5 \ \text{mL}$$

Formula Method	Proportion Expressed as Two Ratios	Proportion Expressed as Two Fractions

18. $\dfrac{\overset{1}{\cancel{0.125 \text{ mg}}}}{\underset{\underset{1}{2}}{\cancel{0.250 \text{ mg}}}} \times \overset{1}{\cancel{2}} \text{ mL} = 1 \text{ mL}$

2 mL : 0.25 mg : : x : 0.125 mg

$\dfrac{2 \text{ mL}}{0.25 \text{ mg}} \times \dfrac{\text{x}}{0.125 \text{ mg}}$

$$2 \times 0.125 = 0.25\text{x}$$

$$\frac{0.25}{0.25} = \text{x}$$

$$1 \text{ mL} = \text{x}$$

Dimensional Analysis Method

$\dfrac{1}{\cancel{0.125} \text{ mg}} \Bigg| \dfrac{\overset{1}{\cancel{2}} \, \textcircled{mL}}{\underset{\underset{1}{\cancel{2}}}{\cancel{0.25} \text{ mg}}} \Bigg| \dfrac{1}{} = 1 \text{ mL}$

Formula Method	Proportion Expressed as Two Ratios	Proportion Expressed as Two Fractions

19. $\dfrac{\overset{6}{\cancel{12 \text{ mg}}}}{\underset{5}{\cancel{10 \text{ mg}}}} \times 1 \text{ mL} = 5 \overset{1.2}{\overline{\smash{)}6.0}} = 1.2 \text{ mL}$

1 mL : 10 mg : : x : 12 mg

$\dfrac{1 \text{ mL}}{10 \text{ mg}} \times \dfrac{\text{x}}{12 \text{ mg}}$

$$\frac{12}{10} = \text{x}$$

$$1.2 \text{ mL} = \text{x}$$

Dimensional Analysis Method

$\dfrac{6}{\cancel{12} \text{ mg}} \Bigg| \dfrac{1 \, \textcircled{mL}}{\underset{5}{\cancel{10} \text{ mg}}} \Bigg| \dfrac{6}{5} = 1.2 \text{ mL}$

Formula Method	Proportion Expressed as Two Ratios	Proportion Expressed as Two Fractions

20. $\dfrac{\overset{5}{\cancel{10 \text{ mEq}}}}{\underset{\underset{1}{2}}{\cancel{40 \text{ mEq}}}} \times \overset{1}{\cancel{20}} \text{ mL} = 5 \text{ mL}$

20 mL : 40 mEq : : x : 10 mEq

$\dfrac{20 \text{ mL}}{40 \text{ mEq}} \times \dfrac{\text{x}}{10 \text{ mEq}}$

$$20 \times 10 = 40\text{x}$$

$$\frac{200}{40} = \text{x}$$

$$5 \text{ mL} = \text{x}$$

Dimensional Analysis Method

$10 \text{ mEq} \Bigg| \dfrac{\overset{1}{\cancel{20}} \, \textcircled{mL}}{\underset{2}{\cancel{40} \text{ mEq}}} \Bigg| \dfrac{10}{2} = 5 \text{ mL}$

Test 4: Mental Drill in Liquids-for-Injection Problems

1. 2 mL	**7.** 0.75 mL	**13.** 2 mL
2. 5 mL	**8.** 1 mL	**14.** 1.5 mL
3. 2 mL	**9.** 20 mL	**15.** 1.5 mL
4. 1 mL	**10.** 2.5 mL	**16.** 0.35 mL
5. 0.5 mL	**11.** 0.8 mL	**17.** 1.5 mL
6. 1 mL	**12.** 2 mL	**18.** 1.5 mL

Test 5: Injections from Powders

1. a. 2.5 mL, sterile water

   b. 334 mg/mL

   c.

Formula Method	Proportion Expressed as Two Ratios	Proportion Expressed as Two Fractions
$\frac{250 \text{ mg}}{334 \text{ mg}} \times 1 \text{ mL} = x$	$1 \text{ mL} : 334 \text{ mg} :: x : 250 \text{ mg}$	$\frac{1 \text{ mL}}{334 \text{ mg}} \times \frac{x}{250 \text{ mg}}$
$0.75 \times 1 \text{ mL} = x$		
$0.75 \text{ mL} = x$		$\frac{250}{334} = x$
		$0.75 = x$

Dimensional Analysis Method

$$\frac{250 \text{ mg}}{} \left| \frac{1 \text{ mL}}{334 \text{ mg}} \right| \frac{250}{334} = 0.75 \text{ mL}$$

   d. 0.75 mL

   e. 334 mg/mL, date, time, expiration date (7 days after reconstitution), initials

   f. 24 hours at room temperature or 72 hours if refrigerated.

2. a. 2 mL sterile water for injection, sodium chloride injection for 1% lidocaine without preservative

   b. 1 g/2.6 mL (385 mg/mL)

   c.

Formula Method	Proportion Expressed as Two Ratios	Proportion Expressed as Two Fractions
$\frac{1 \text{ g}}{1 \text{ g}} \times 2.6 \text{ mL} = 2.6 \text{ mL}$	$2.6 \text{ mL} : 1 \text{ g} :: x : 1 \text{ g}$	$\frac{2.6 \text{ mL}}{1 \text{ g}} \times \frac{x}{1 \text{ g}}$
		$2.6 \text{ mL} = x$

Dimensional Analysis Method

$$\frac{1 \text{ g}}{} \left| \frac{2.6 \text{ mL}}{1 \text{ g}} \right| \frac{2.6}{} = 2.6 \text{ mL}$$

   d. 2.6 mL

   e. Nothing is left in the vial.

   f. Discard the vial in a proper receptacle.

3. a. 1.8 mL sterile water for injection or bacteriostatic water for injection

   b. 250 mg/mL

   c.

Formula Method	Proportion Expressed as Two Ratios	Proportion Expressed as Two Fractions
$$\dfrac{\overset{6}{\cancel{300}\ \text{mg}}}{\underset{5}{\cancel{250}\ \text{mg}}} \times 1\ \text{mL} = \dfrac{6}{5}\overline{\smash{\big)}6.0}\ \overset{1.2}{}$$ $$1.2\ \text{mL}$$	$$1\ \text{mL} : 250\ \text{mg} :: x : 300\ \text{mg}$$	$$\dfrac{1\ \text{mL}}{250\ \text{mg}} \times \dfrac{x}{300\ \text{mg}}$$ $$\dfrac{300}{250} = x$$ $$1.2\ \text{mL} = x$$

Dimensional Analysis Method
$$\dfrac{\overset{6}{\cancel{300}}\ \text{mg}}{} \ \bigg|\ \dfrac{1\ \widehat{\text{mL}}}{\underset{5}{\cancel{250}}\ \text{mg}} \ \bigg|\ \dfrac{6}{5} = 1.2\ \text{mL}$$

   d. 1.2 mL

   e. Discard the vial. Directions say solution must be used within 1 hour.

   f. No. Discard the vial in an appropriate receptacle.

4. a. 2 mL sterile water for injection

   b. 400 mg/mL

   c.

Formula Method	Proportion Expressed as Two Ratios	Proportion Expressed as Two Fractions
$$\dfrac{\cancel{300}\ \text{mg}}{\cancel{400}\ \text{mg}} \times 1\ \text{mL} = \dfrac{3}{4}\overline{\smash{\big)}3.00}\ \overset{0.75}{}$$ $$0.75\ \text{mL}$$	$$1\ \text{mL} : 400\ \text{mg} :: x : 300\ \text{mg}$$	$$\dfrac{1\ \text{mL}}{400\ \text{mg}} \times \dfrac{x}{300\ \text{mg}}$$ $$\dfrac{\cancel{300}}{\cancel{400}} = x$$ $$0.75\ \text{mL} = x$$

Dimensional Analysis Method
$$\dfrac{\cancel{300}\ \text{mg}}{} \ \bigg|\ \dfrac{1\ \widehat{\text{mL}}}{\cancel{400}\ \text{mg}} \ \bigg|\ \dfrac{3}{4} = 0.75\ \text{mL}$$

   d. 0.75 mL

   e. 400 mg/mL, date, time, expiration date (1 week after reconstitution), initials

   f. Refrigerate; stable for 1 week

5. a. 2.5 mL sterile water for injection

   b. 330 mg/mL

   c.

Formula Method	Proportion Expressed as Two Ratios	Proportion Expressed as Two Fractions
0.33 g is 330 mg.	1 mL : 330 mg : : x : 330 mg	$\dfrac{1\ mL}{330\ mg} \times \dfrac{x}{330\ mg}$

$$\frac{330}{330} = x$$

$$1\ mL = x$$

Dimensional Analysis Method

$$\frac{\overset{1}{0.33}\ \cancel{g}}{} \left| \frac{1\ \cancel{mL}}{\underset{1000}{330}\ mg} \right| \frac{\overset{1000}{1000}\ \cancel{mg}}{1\ \cancel{g}} = 1\ mL$$

   d. 1 mL IM

   e. 330 mg/mL, date, time, expiration date (96 days after reconstitution), initials

   f. Refrigerate; stable for 96 hours

Chapter 8

Test 1: Basic IV Problems

1. a. You have 1000 mL running at 150 mL/hr, therefore

$$\frac{\overset{20}{\cancel{1000}}}{\underset{3}{\cancel{150}}} = \frac{20}{3}\ \overset{6.6}{\overline{)20.0}} = \text{approximately 6.6 hours}$$
$$\phantom{\frac{20}{3}}\underline{18}$$
$$\phantom{\frac{20}{3}}\ \ 2\,0$$
$$\phantom{\frac{20}{3}}\ \ \underline{1\,8}$$

Dimensional Analysis Method

$$\frac{\overset{200}{\cancel{1000}}\ \cancel{mL}}{} \left| \frac{\cancel{hr}}{\underset{30}{\cancel{150}}\ \cancel{mL}} \right| \frac{200}{30} = 6.6\ \text{hours}$$

   b. $\dfrac{\text{number mL} \times \text{TF}}{\text{number min}} = \text{gtt/min}$

      $\dfrac{150 \times 10}{60} = 25\ \text{gtt/min macrodrip tubing}$

      $\dfrac{150 \times 60}{60} = 150\ \text{gtt/min microdrip tubing}$

   Choose macrotubing.

Dimensional Analysis Method

$$\frac{150 \text{ mL}}{\text{hr}} \left| \frac{\overset{1}{10} \text{ gtt}}{\text{mL}} \right| \frac{1 \text{ hr}}{\underset{6}{60} \text{ min}} \right| \frac{150}{6} = 25 \text{ gtt/min macrodrip tubing}$$

$$\frac{150 \text{ mL}}{\text{hr}} \left| \frac{60 \text{ gtt}}{\text{mL}} \right| \frac{1 \text{ hr}}{60 \text{ min}} = 150 \text{ gtt/min microdrip tubing}$$

  c. 25 gtt/min macro

  Note: You could choose microtubing; however, the drip rate is hard to count.

2. a. Because the amount is small and will run over 6 hours, choose *microdrip tubing.*

  b. 6 hours = 360 minutes

$$\frac{100 \times \overset{1}{60}}{\underset{6}{360}} =$$

$$\frac{100}{6} = 16.6 \text{ or } 17 \text{ gtt/min}$$

Dimensional Analysis Method

$$\frac{100 \text{ mL}}{6 \text{ hr}} \left| \frac{\overset{1}{60} \text{ gtt}}{\text{mL}} \right| \frac{1 \text{ hr}}{\underset{1}{60} \text{ min}} \right| \frac{100}{6} = 16.6 \text{ or } 17 \text{ gtt/min}$$

3. a. Because the stock bag is 250 mL NS, you would aseptically withdraw 100 mL. This will leave 150 mL NS. If using an infusion pump, you could set the volume to be infused at 150 mL.

  b. *Microdrip* because

$$3 \text{ hours} = 180 \text{ minutes}$$

$$\text{Macrodrip tubing: } \frac{150 \times \overset{1}{15}}{\underset{12}{180}} =$$

$$\frac{150}{12} = 12.5 \text{ or } 13 \text{ gtt/min}$$

$$\text{Macrodrip tubing: } \frac{150 \times \overset{1}{60}}{\underset{3}{180}} =$$

$$\frac{150}{3} = 50 \text{ gtt/min}$$

c. 50 gtt/min (microdrip)

Note: It would not be incorrect to choose the macrodrip. However, 50 gtt/min provides a better flow.

> ### Dimensional Analysis Method

$$\frac{\overset{50}{\cancel{150}}\ \cancel{mL}}{\underset{1}{\cancel{3}\ \cancel{hr}}}\ \left|\ \frac{1}{\cancel{15}\ \cancel{(gtt)}\ \cancel{mL}}\ \right|\ \frac{1\ \cancel{hr}}{\underset{4}{\cancel{60}\ \cancel{(min)}}}\ \right|\ \frac{50}{4} = 12.5 \text{ or } 13 \text{ gtt/min}$$

$$\frac{\overset{50}{\cancel{150}}\ \cancel{mL}}{\underset{1}{\cancel{3}\ \cancel{hr}}}\ \left|\ \frac{1}{\cancel{60}\ \cancel{(gtt)}\ \cancel{mL}}\ \right|\ \frac{1\ \cancel{hr}}{\underset{1}{\cancel{60}\ \cancel{(min)}}}\ \right|\ \frac{50}{1} = 50 \text{ gtt/min}$$

4. 21 mL/hr

Step 1. $\frac{\text{number mL}}{\text{number hr}} = \text{mL/hr}$

$$\frac{500 \text{ mL}}{24 \text{ hr}}\qquad 24 \overset{\displaystyle 20.8}{\overline{\smash{)}500.0}} = 21 \text{ mL/hr}$$
$$\underline{48}$$
$$20\ 0$$
$$\underline{19\ 2}$$

Step 2 is not necessary because you have an infusion pump that delivers millilitres per hour.

> ### Dimensional Analysis Method

$$\frac{500\ \cancel{(mL)}}{24\ \cancel{(hr)}}\ \left|\ \frac{500}{24}\ \right. = 20.8 \text{ or } 21 \text{ mL/hr}$$

5. Use a reconstitution device to add 100 mg powder to 250 mL D5W and give IVPB over 1 hour (60 min); TF = 10 gtt/mL.

$$\frac{\text{number mL} \times \text{TF}}{\text{number min}} = \text{gtt/min}$$

$$\frac{250 \times 10}{60} = \frac{250}{6} \qquad 6\overset{\displaystyle 41.6}{\overline{\smash{)}250.0}} = 42 \text{ gtt/min}$$

Label the IVPB.

Set the rate at 42 gtt/min.

> ### Dimensional Analysis Method

$$\frac{250\ \cancel{mL}}{1\ \cancel{hr}}\ \left|\ \frac{1}{\cancel{10}\ \cancel{(gtt)}\ \cancel{mL}}\ \right|\ \frac{1\ \cancel{hr}}{\underset{6}{\cancel{60}\ \cancel{(min)}}}\ \right|\ \frac{250}{6} = 41.6 \text{ or } 42 \text{ gtt/min}$$

6 a. Order is 500 mg. Stock is 1 g in 10 mL.

1 g = 1000 mg

Formula Method	Proportion Expressed as Two Ratios	Proportion Expressed as Two Fractions
$\frac{500 \text{ mg}}{1000 \text{ mg}} \times 10 \text{ mL}$ $= 5 \text{ mL}$	10 mL : 1000 mg : : x : 500 mg	$\frac{10 \text{ mL}}{1000 \text{ mg}} \times \frac{x}{500}$ $10 \times 500 = 1000x$ $\frac{5000}{1000} = x$ $5 \text{ mL} = x$

Dimensional Analysis Method

$$\frac{1}{500 \text{ mg}} \left| \frac{1}{10 \text{ mL}} \right| \frac{1 \text{ g}}{1 \text{ g}} \left| \frac{10}{1000 \text{ mg}} \right| \frac{10}{2} = 5 \text{ mL}$$

Add 5 mL aminophylline to make 500 mg in 250 mL D5W.

b. $\frac{\text{number mL}}{\text{number hr}} = \text{mL/hr}$

$\frac{250 \text{ mL}}{8 \text{ hr}} = 31.2 = 31 \text{ mL/hr}$

mL/hr = microgtt/min

No math necessary.

Microdip: 31 mL/hr = 31 gtt/min

Label IV.

Set the rate at 31 gtt/min.

Dimensional Analysis Method

$$\frac{250 \text{ mL}}{8 \text{ hr}} \left| \frac{125}{4} \right. = 31 \text{ mL/hr}$$

7. 2800 mL

Logic: The patient gets 125 mL/hr and there are 24 hours in a day; four times a day the patient receives cefoxitin. That leaves 20 hours (24 − 4) times 125 mL/hr:

```
  125
× 20
2500 mL
```

The patient gets 75 mL q6h and, therefore, is receiving 75 mL four times in 24 hours.

So
```
  75          2500 mL
×  4        + 300 mL
 300         2800 mL
```

8. a. 90 mL/hr—no math necessary—using an infusion pump

b.

$\frac{\text{total number mL}}{\text{mL/hr}} = \text{hr}$

```
         11.1
    90 )1000.0
         90
        100
         90
        100
         10 0
```

Dimensional Analysis Method

$$\frac{1000 \text{ mL}}{\text{hr}} \left| \frac{100}{90 \text{ mL}} \right| \frac{100}{9} = 11.1 \text{ hr}$$

Approximately 11 hours

9. 50 mg

   You have 0.5 g in 500 mL. 0.5 g = 500 mg. The solution is 500 mg in 500 mL. Reducing this amount equals 1 mg in 1 mL. Because the patient is receiving 50 mL/hr, the patient is receiving 50 mg amino-phylline per hour.

10. **a.** You need 75 mL D5W. Take a 100-mL bag of D5W and aseptically remove 25 mL. Add 5 mL Bactrim to the 75 mL. Time is 60 minutes. The order is 75 mL/hr. No math is necessary. You have a pump in millilitres per hour.

    Label the IVPB.

    b. Set the pump:

    For 60 minutes:

    Secondary volume (mL): 75

    Secondary rate (mL/hr): 75

    For 90 minutes: $\dfrac{75 \times 60}{90} = 50$ mL/hr

    Secondary volume (mL): 75

    Secondary rate (mL/hr): 50

11. $\frac{3}{4} \times 150$ mL $= 112.5$ mL Isocal

    150 mL $-$ 112.5 mL $=$ 37.5 mL water

12. $\frac{1}{2} \times 500$ mL $= 250$ mL Vivonex

    500 mL $-$ 250 mL $=$ 250 mL water

13. $25\% = 0.25 = \frac{1}{4}$ (use any of these)

    $\frac{1}{4} \times 400$ mL $= 100$ mL Osmolite

    400 mL $-$ 100 mL $=$ 300 mL water

14. 500 mL Isocal

    0 mL water

Chapter 9

Test 1: Special IV Calculations

1.

Formula Method	Proportion Expressed as Two Ratios	Proportion Expressed as Two Fractions
$\dfrac{15 \text{ units/hr}}{\underset{1}{125 \text{ units}}} \times \overset{2}{250} \text{ mL} = x$	250 mL : 125 units : : x : 15 units	$\dfrac{x \text{ mL}}{15 \text{ units}} \times \dfrac{250 \text{ mL}}{125 \text{ units}}$
$15 \times 2 = 30$ mL/hr on a pump	$15 \times 250 = 125x$	
	$\dfrac{3750}{125} = x$	
Set the pump.	30 mL/hr $= x$	
Total number mL: 250		
mL/hr: 30		

Dimensional Analysis Method

$$\frac{15 \text{ units}}{\text{hr}} \left| \frac{\overset{2}{\cancel{250}} \text{ mL}}{\overset{}{\cancel{125}} \text{ units}} \right| \frac{15 \times 2}{1} = 30 \text{ mL/hr}$$

2.

Formula Method	Proportion Expressed as Two Ratios	Proportion Expressed as Two Fractions
$\dfrac{\overset{3}{\cancel{1500}} \text{ units/hr}}{\underset{\underset{1}{50}}{\cancel{25000}} \text{ units}} \times \overset{10}{\cancel{500}} = 30 \text{ mL/hr}$	$500 \text{ mL} : 25000 \text{ units} :: x : 1500 \text{ units}$	$\dfrac{x \text{ mL}}{1500 \text{ units}} \times \dfrac{500 \text{ mL}}{\underset{50}{25000} \text{ units}}$

$$1500 \times 500 = 25000x$$

$$\frac{750,000}{25,000} = x$$

$$30 \text{ mL/hr} = x$$

Dimensional Analysis Method

$$\frac{\overset{30}{\cancel{1500}} \text{ units}}{\text{hr}} \left| \frac{\overset{1}{\cancel{500}} \text{ mL}}{\underset{\underset{1}{50}}{\cancel{25000}} \text{ units}} \right| 30 = 30 \text{ mL/hr}$$

Set the pump.

Total number mL = 500 mL

mL/hr = 30

3. 2 mg/min × 60 minutes = 120 mg/hr

2 g = 2000 mg

Formula Method	Proportion Expressed as Two Ratios	Proportion Expressed as Two Fractions
$\dfrac{120 \text{ mg/hr}}{\underset{4}{2000} \text{ mg}} \times \overset{1}{\cancel{500}} \text{ mL}$ $= 30 \text{ mL/hr on a pump}$	$500 \text{ mL} : 2000 \text{ mg} :: x : 120 \text{ mg}$	$\dfrac{500 \text{ mL}}{2000 \text{ mg}} \times \dfrac{x}{120 \text{ mg}}$

$$500 \times 120 = 2000x$$

$$\frac{60000}{2000} = x$$

$$\frac{120}{4} = x$$

$$30 \text{ mL} = x$$

Dimensional Analysis Method

$$\frac{2 \text{ mg}}{\text{min}} \left| \frac{\overset{1}{\cancel{500}} \text{ mL}}{\cancel{2} \text{ g}} \right| \frac{1 \text{ g}}{\underset{\underset{1}{2}}{\cancel{1000}} \text{ mg}} \left| \frac{\overset{30}{\cancel{60}} \text{ min}}{1 \text{ hr}} \right| 30 = 30 \text{ mL/hr}$$

Set the pump.

Total number mL: 500

mL/hr: 30

4. a. Add diltiazem to the IV.

Formula Method	Proportion Expressed as Two Ratios	Proportion Expressed as Two Fractions

$$\frac{\overset{1}{\cancel{5}\text{ mg}}}{\underset{\underset{1}{25}}{\cancel{125}\text{ mg}}} \times \overset{4}{\cancel{100}}\text{ mL} = 4\text{ mL/hr}$$

$$100\text{ mL} : 125\text{ mg} :: x : 5\text{ mg}$$

$$\frac{100\text{ mL}}{125\text{ mg}} \times \frac{x}{5\text{ mg}}$$

$$100 \times 5 = 125x$$

$$\frac{500}{125} = x$$

$$4\text{ mL/hr} = x$$

Dimensional Analysis Method

$$\frac{\overset{1}{\cancel{5}\text{ mg}}}{\cancel{hr}} \; \middle| \; \frac{100\;\cancel{mL}}{\underset{25}{\cancel{125}\text{ mg}}} \; \middle| \; \frac{100}{25} = 4\text{ mL/hr}$$

Second way: If you add 25 mL of drug to the 100 mL D5W, you make 125 mL (a 1:1 solution). Because the order is 5 mg/hr, set the pump at 5 mL/hr.

Formula Method	Proportion Expressed as Two Ratios	Proportion Expressed as Two Fractions

$$\frac{\overset{}{\cancel{5}\text{ mg}}}{\underset{\underset{1}{25}}{\cancel{125}\text{ mg}}} \times \overset{5}{\cancel{125}}\text{ mL} = 5\text{ mL/hr}$$

$$125\text{ mL} : 125\text{ mg} :: x : 5\text{ mg}$$

$$\frac{125\text{ mL}}{125\text{ mg}} \times \frac{x}{5\text{ mg}}$$

$$\frac{625}{125} = x$$

$$5\text{ mL/hr} = x$$

Dimensional Analysis Method

$$\frac{5\text{ mg}}{\cancel{hr}} \; \middle| \; \frac{125\;\cancel{mL}}{125\text{ mg}} \; \middle| \; 5 = 5\text{ mL/hr}$$

It is considered better to remove fluid from the IV bag so the volume remains the same.

b.

Formula Method	Proportion Expressed as Two Ratios	Proportion Expressed as Two Fractions

$$\frac{\overset{25}{\cancel{125}\text{ mg}}}{\underset{1}{\cancel{5}\text{ mg}}} \times 1\text{ mL} = 25\text{ mL}$$

$$1\text{ mL} : 5\text{ mg} :: x : 125\text{ mg}$$

$$\frac{1\text{ mL}}{5\text{ mg}} \times \frac{x}{125\text{ mg}}$$

$$\frac{125}{5} = x$$

$$25\text{ mL} = x$$

Dimensional Analysis Method

$$\frac{\overset{25}{\cancel{125}}\;\cancel{mg}}{} \; \middle| \; \frac{1\text{ mL}}{\underset{1}{\cancel{5}\;\cancel{mg}}} \; \middle| \; 25 = 25\text{ mL}$$

Remove 25 mL IV fluid from the IV bag and add 25 mL diltiazem = 100 mL total.

5. 2 g = 2000 mg

Order calls for 4 mg/min. Pumps are set in millilitres per hour. Multiply 4 mg/min × 60 min = 240 mg/hr.

Formula Method	Proportion Expressed as Two Ratios	Proportion Expressed as Two Fractions

$$\frac{\overset{60}{\cancel{240}}\text{ mg/hr}}{\underset{4}{\underset{1}{\cancel{2000}}}\text{ mg}} \times \overset{1}{\cancel{500}}\text{ mL} = 60\text{ mL/hr}$$

$$500\text{ mL} : 2000\text{ mg} :: x : 240\text{ mg}$$

$$\frac{500\text{ mL}}{2000\text{ mg}} \times \frac{x}{240\text{ mg}}$$

$$500 \times 240 = 2000x$$

$$\frac{120,000}{2000} = x$$

$$\frac{240}{4} = x$$

$$60\text{ mL} = x$$

Dimensional Analysis Method

$$\frac{\overset{2}{\cancel{4}}\text{ mg}}{\text{min}} \left| \frac{\overset{1}{\cancel{500}}\;\textcircled{mL}}{\underset{1}{\cancel{2}}\;\cancel{g}} \right| \frac{1\;\cancel{g}}{\underset{\underset{1}{\cancel{2}}}{\cancel{1000}}\;\text{mg}} \left| \frac{\overset{30}{\cancel{60}}\;\text{min}}{1\,\textcircled{hr}} \right| \frac{2 \times 30}{} = 60\text{ mL/hr}$$

Set the pump.
Total number mL: 500
Number mL/hr: 60

6. **a.** Add KCl to the IV.

Formula Method	Proportion Expressed as Two Ratios	Proportion Expressed as Two Fractions

$$\frac{\overset{2}{\cancel{40}}\text{ mEq}}{\underset{1}{\cancel{20}}\text{ mEq}} \times 10\text{ mL} = 20\text{ mL}$$

$$10\text{ mL} : 20\text{ mEq} :: x : 40\text{ mEq}$$

$$\frac{10\text{ mL}}{20\text{ mEq}} \times \frac{x}{40\text{ mEq}}$$

$$10 \times 40 = 20x$$

$$\frac{400}{20} = x$$

$$20\text{ mL} = x$$

Dimensional Analysis Method

$$\frac{\overset{2}{\cancel{40}}\text{ mEq}}{} \left| \frac{\overset{}{\cancel{10}}\;\textcircled{mL}}{\underset{1}{\cancel{20}}\;\text{mEq}} \right| \frac{2 \times 10}{} = 20\text{ mL}$$

b. Remove 20 mL IV fluid and add the 20 mL of KCl to make 1000 mL.

Formula Method	Proportion Expressed as Two Ratios	Proportion Expressed as Two Fractions
1 L = 1000 mL	1000 mL : 40 mEq : : x : 10 mEq	$\dfrac{1000\ mL}{40\ mEq} \times \dfrac{x}{10\ mEq}$

$$\dfrac{\overset{1}{\cancel{10}}\ mEq/hr}{\underset{\underset{1}{4}}{\cancel{40}}\ mEq} \times \overset{250}{\cancel{1000}}\ mL = 250\ mL/hr$$

$$1000 \times 10 = 40x$$

$$\dfrac{10000}{40} = x$$

$$250\ mL = x$$

Dimensional Analysis Method

$$\dfrac{10\ mEq}{\cancel{hr}} \left| \dfrac{\cancel{1\ L}}{40\ mEq}\atop 1 \right| \dfrac{\overset{25}{\cancel{1000}}\ \cancel{mL}}{\cancel{1\ L}} \left| \dfrac{10 \times 25}{} = 250\ mL/hr \right.$$

Set pump at 250 mL/hr. This is a large volume and KCl is a potent electrolyte; therefore, the patient must be on a cardiac monitor for safety. Check the order with the doctor or healthcare provider.

Total number mL: 1000

Number mL/hr: 250

7. 2 g = 2000 mL

Order calls for 1 mg/min. Pumps are set in millilitres per hour. Multiply 1 mg/min × 60 mg = 60 mg/hr.

Formula Method	Proportion Expressed as Two Ratios	Proportion Expressed as Two Fractions
	500 mL : 2000 mg : : x : 60 mg	$\dfrac{500\ mL}{2000\ mg} \times \dfrac{x}{60\ mg/hr}$

$$\dfrac{\overset{15}{\cancel{60}}\ mg/hr}{\underset{\underset{1}{4}}{\cancel{2000}}\ mg} \times \overset{1}{\cancel{500}}\ mL = 15\ mL/hr$$

$$500 \times 60 = 2000x$$

$$\dfrac{30000}{2000} = x$$

$$15\ mL/hr = x$$

Dimensional Analysis Method

$$\dfrac{1\ mg}{min} \left| \dfrac{\overset{1}{\cancel{500}}\ \cancel{mL}}{2\ \cancel{g}} \right| \dfrac{1\ \cancel{g}}{\underset{\underset{1}{2}}{\cancel{1000}}\ mg} \left| \dfrac{\overset{30}{\cancel{60}}\ \cancel{min}}{1\cancel{hr}} \right| \dfrac{30}{2} = 15\ mL/hr$$

Set the pump.

Total number mL: 500

Number mL/hr: 15

8. Use a reconstitution device (see Chapter 8) to add 50 mg of drug to 500 mL D5W.

$$\frac{\text{number mL}}{\text{number hr}} = \text{mL/hr}$$

$$\frac{500 \text{ mL}}{6 \text{ hr}} \quad \frac{83.0}{\overline{)500.0}} = 83 \text{ mL/hr}$$
$$\underline{48}$$
$$20$$
$$\underline{18}$$
$$2\,0$$
$$\underline{1\,8}$$

Dimensional Analysis Method

$$\frac{500 \;\text{(mL)}}{6 \;\text{(hr)}} \Big| \frac{500}{6} = 83.33 \text{ or } 83 \text{ mL/hr}$$

Set the pump.

Total number mL: 500

Number mL/hr: 83

9. Add vasopressin to the IV.

Formula Method	Proportion Expressed as Two Ratios	Proportion Expressed as Two Fractions
$\dfrac{\overset{10}{\cancel{200} \text{ units}}}{\underset{1}{\cancel{20} \text{ units}}} \times 1 \text{ mL} = 10 \text{ mL}$	$1 \text{ mL} : 20 \text{ units} :: x : 200 \text{ units}$	$\dfrac{1 \text{ mL}}{20 \text{ units}} \times \dfrac{x}{200 \text{ units}}$

$$\frac{200}{20} = x$$

$$10 \text{ mL} = x$$

Dimensional Analysis Method

$$\frac{\overset{10}{\cancel{200} \text{ units}}}{} \Bigg| \frac{1 \;\text{(mL)}}{\underset{1}{\cancel{20} \text{ units}}} \Bigg| \frac{10}{} = 10 \text{ mL}$$

Remove 10 mL fluid from the IV and add 10 mL drug = 500 mL.

Formula Method	Proportion Expressed as Two Ratios	Proportion Expressed as Two Fractions
$\dfrac{\overset{9}{\cancel{18} \text{ units/hr}}}{\underset{1}{\cancel{200} \text{ units}}} \times \cancel{500} \text{ mL} = 45 \text{ mL/hr}$	$500 \text{ mL} : 200 \text{ units} :: x : 18 \text{ units}$	$\dfrac{500 \text{ mL}}{200 \text{ units}} \times \dfrac{x}{18 \text{ units}}$

$$500 \times 18 = 200x$$

$$\frac{900}{20} = x$$

$$45 \text{ mL} = x$$

Dimensional Analysis Method

$$\frac{18 \ \cancel{units}}{\cancel{hr}} \left| \frac{500 \ mL}{200 \ \cancel{units}} \right| \frac{18 \times 5}{2} = 45 \ mL/hr$$

Set the pump.

Total number mL: 500

Number mL/hr: 45

10. Order: 250 mcg/min

Solution: 500 mg in 500 mL D5W

Step 1. $\dfrac{500 \ mg}{500 \ mL} = 1 \ mg/mL$

Step 2. $1 \ mg = 1000 \ mcg/mL$

Step 3. Divide by 60 to get mcg/min. $\frac{1000}{60} = 16.67 \ mcg/min.$

Step 4.

Formula Method	Proportion Expressed as Two Ratios	Proportion Expressed as Two Fractions
$\dfrac{250 \ mcg/min}{16.67 \ mcg/min} \times 1 \ mL = x$ 14.99 or $15 \ mL = x$	$1 \ mL : 16.67 \ mcg/min :: x : 250 \ mcg/min$	$\dfrac{1 \ mL}{16.67 \ mcg/min} \times \dfrac{x}{250 \ mcg/min}$ $250 = 16.67x$ $\dfrac{250}{16.67} = x$ 14.99 or $15 \ mL = x$

Dimensional Analysis Method

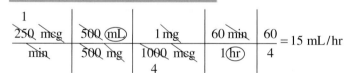

$$\frac{250 \ \cancel{mcg}}{\cancel{min}} \left| \frac{500 \ \cancel{mL}}{500 \ \cancel{mg}} \right| \frac{1 \ \cancel{mg}}{1000 \ \cancel{mcg}} \left| \frac{60 \ \cancel{min}}{1 \ \cancel{hr}} \right| \frac{60}{4} = 15 \ mL/hr$$

Set the pump.

Total mL: 500

mL/hr: 15

11. Order: 2.5 mcg/kg/min
Solution: 400 mg in 250 mL
Weight: 60 kg
Multiply 60 kg × 2.5 mcg = 150 mcg.

Step 1. $\dfrac{400 \text{ mg}}{250 \text{ mL}} = 1.6 \text{ mg/mL}$

Step 2. $1.6 \times 1000 = 1600 \text{ mcg/mL}$

Step 3. Divide by 60 $\dfrac{1600}{60} = 26.67 \text{ mcg/min}$

Step 4.

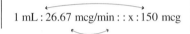

Formula Method	Proportion Expressed as Two Ratios	Proportion Expressed as Two Fractions
$\frac{150 \text{ mcg/min}}{26.67 \text{ mcg/min}} \times 1 \text{ mL} = 5.6 \text{ or } 6 \text{ mL/hr}$	1 mL : 26.67 mcg/min : : x : 150 mcg	$\dfrac{1 \text{ mL}}{26.67 \text{ mcg/min}} \times \dfrac{x}{150 \text{ mcg/min}}$

$$\frac{150}{26.67} = 5.6 \text{ or } 6 \text{ mL/hr} = x$$

Dimensional Analysis Method

$$\frac{2.5 \text{ mcg}}{\text{kg / min}} \left| \frac{250 \text{ mL}}{400 \text{ mg}} \right| \frac{1 \text{ mg}}{1000 \text{ mcg}} \left| \frac{60 \text{ min}}{1 \text{ hr}} \right| 60 \text{ kg} \left| \frac{2.5 \times 6 \times 6}{4 \times 4} = 5.625 \text{ or } 6 \text{ mL / hr} \right.$$

6 gtt/min = 6 mL/hr

Set the pump.
Total number mL: 250
Number mL/hr: 6

12. Order: 2 milliunits/min
Solution: 5 units in 500 mL NS

Step 1. $\dfrac{5 \text{ units}}{500 \text{ mL}} = 0.01 \text{ units/mL}$

Step 2. $0.01 \text{ units} \times 1000 = 10 \text{ milliunits/mL}$

Step 3. Divide by 60 $\dfrac{10}{60} = 0.167 \text{ milliunits/min}$

Step 4.

Formula Method	*Proportion Expressed as Two Ratios*	*Proportion Expressed as Two Fractions*
$\dfrac{2 \text{ milliunits}}{0.167 \text{ milliunit}} \times 1 \text{ mL} = x$	1 mL : 0.167 milliunit :: x : 2 milliunits	$\dfrac{1 \text{ mL}}{0.167 \text{ milliunit}} \times \dfrac{x}{2 \text{ milliunits}}$
11.76 or 12 mL = x		

11.76 or 12 mL = x

2 gtt/min = 12 mL/hr

Set the pump.

Total number mL: 500 mL

Number mL/hr: 12

Dimensional Analysis Method

$$\dfrac{2 \text{ milliunits}}{\text{minute}} \left| \dfrac{\overset{100}{\cancel{500}} \text{ mL}}{\underset{1}{\cancel{5} \text{ units}}} \right| \dfrac{1 \text{ unit}}{1000 \text{ milliunits}} \left| \dfrac{60 \text{ minutes}}{1 \text{ hr}} \right| \dfrac{2 \times 60 \times 2}{5} = \dfrac{120}{10}$$

13. **a.** Correct; $100 \text{ mg/m}^2 \times 1.7 = 170 \text{ mg}$

   b. 1 L = 1000 mL

$$\dfrac{\text{number mL}}{\text{number hr}} = \text{mL/hr}$$

$$\begin{array}{r} 41.6 \\ 24 \overline{)1000.0} = 42 \text{ mL/hr} \\ \underline{96} \\ 40 \\ \underline{24} \\ 160 \\ \underline{144} \end{array}$$

Dimensional Analysis Method

$$\dfrac{\cancel{1 \text{ L}}}{24 \text{ hr}} \left| \dfrac{1000 \text{ mL}}{\cancel{1 \text{ L}}} \right| \dfrac{1000}{24} = 41.66 \text{ or } 42 \text{ mL/hr}$$

Set the pump.

Total number mL: 1000

Number mL/hr: 42

14. Order: 5 mcg/kg/min

   Solution: 50 mg in 250 mL

   Weight: 90 kg

   Multiply: 5 mcg × 90 kg = 450 mcg/min

Step 1. $\dfrac{50 \text{ mg}}{250 \text{ mL}} = 0.2 \text{ mg/mL}$

Step 2. $0.2 \times 1000 = 200 \text{ mcg/mL}$

Step 3. Divide by 60 $\dfrac{200}{60} = 3.33$ mcg/min

Step 4.

Formula Method	Proportion Expressed as Two Ratios	Proportion Expressed as Two Fractions
$\dfrac{450 \text{ mcg/min}}{3.33 \text{ mcg/min}} \times 1 \text{ mL} = 135 \text{ mL}$	1 mL : 3.33 mcg/min : : x : 450 mcg/min	$\dfrac{1 \text{ mL}}{3.33 \text{ mcg}} \times \dfrac{x}{450 \text{ mcg}}$

$$\dfrac{450}{3.33} = x$$

$$135 \text{ mL} = x$$

Dimensional Analysis Method

$$\dfrac{1}{\cancel{5} \text{ mcg}}{\Big/} \dfrac{\overset{1}{\cancel{250}} \text{ mL}}{\underset{10}{\cancel{50} \text{ mg}}} \Big| \dfrac{1 \text{ mg}}{\underset{4}{\cancel{1000} \text{ mcg}}} \Big| \dfrac{60 \text{ min}}{1 \text{ hr}} \Big| 90 \text{ kg} \Big| \dfrac{60 \times 90}{10 \times 4} = 135 \text{ mL/hr}$$

Set the pump.

Total number mL: 250 mL

Number mL/hr: 135 mL/hr

15. Order: 2 mcg/min

Solution: 4 mg in 250 mL

Step 1. $\dfrac{4 \text{ mg}}{250 \text{ mL}} = 0.016$ mg/mL

Step 2. $0.016 \text{ mg} \times 1000 = 16$ mcg

Step 3. Divide by 60 $\dfrac{16}{60} = 0.267$ mcg/min

Step 4.

Formula Method	Proportion Expressed as Two Ratios	Proportion Expressed as Two Fractions
$\dfrac{2 \text{ mcg/min}}{0.267 \text{ mcg/min}} \times 1 \text{ mL}$ $= 7.5 \text{ or } 8 \text{ mL}$	1 mL : 0.267 mcg/min : : x : 2 mcg/min	$\dfrac{1 \text{ mL}}{0.267 \text{ mcg/min}} \times \dfrac{x}{2 \text{ mcg/min}}$

$$\dfrac{2}{0.267} = x$$

$$7.49 \text{ or } 7 \text{ mL} = x$$

Set the pump.

Total number mL: 250 mL

Number mL/hr: 8 mL/hr

Dimensional Analysis Method

$$\dfrac{1}{\cancel{2} \text{ mcg}}{\Big/} \dfrac{\overset{1}{\cancel{250}} \text{ mL}}{\underset{2}{\cancel{4} \text{ mg}}} \Big| \dfrac{1 \text{ mg}}{\underset{4}{\underset{1}{\cancel{1000} \text{ mcg}}}} \Big| \dfrac{\overset{15}{\cancel{60} \text{ minute}}}{1 \text{ hr}} \Big| \dfrac{15}{2} = 7.5 \text{ or } 8 \text{ mL/hr}$$

16. a. Yes. 40 units $\times$ 90 kg = 3600 units

   b. Yes. Increase rate by 2 units/kg/hr

   2 units $\times$ 90 kg = 180 units

Formula Method	*Proportion Expressed as Two Ratios*	*Proportion Expressed as Two Fractions*
$\dfrac{\cancel{180} \text{ units}}{\underset{50}{\cancel{25000}} \text{ units}} \times \overset{1}{\cancel{500}} \text{ mL} = 3.6 \text{ mL}$	500 mL : 25000 units : : x : 180 units	$\dfrac{500 \text{ mL}}{25000 \text{ units}} \times \dfrac{x}{180 \text{ units}}$

$$500 \times 180 = 25000x$$

$$3.6 \text{ mL} = x$$

Dimensional Analysis Method

$$\dfrac{180 \text{ units}}{\cancel{hr}} \left|\; \dfrac{\overset{1}{\cancel{500}} \;\cancel{mL}}{\underset{50}{\cancel{25000}} \;\cancel{units}} \;\right| \dfrac{180}{50} = 3.6 \text{ mL}$$

New infusion rate: 32 + 3.6 = 35.6 or 36 mL/hr

17. a. Yes. 40 units $\times$ 90 kg = 3600 units

   b. Yes. Increase rate by 3 units/kg/hr

   3 units $\times$ 90 kg = 270 units

Formula Method	*Proportion Expressed as Two Ratios*	*Proportion Expressed as Two Fractions*
$\dfrac{\cancel{270} \text{ units}}{\underset{50}{\cancel{25000}} \text{ units}} \times \overset{1}{\cancel{500}} \text{ mL} =$ $\dfrac{270}{50} = x$ $5.4 \text{ mL} = x$	500 mL : 25000 units : : x : 270 units	$\dfrac{500 \text{ mL}}{2500 \text{ units}} \times \dfrac{x}{270 \text{ units}}$

$$500 \times 270 = 25000x$$

$$5.4 \text{ mL} = x$$

Dimensional Analysis Method

$$\dfrac{270 \text{ units}}{} \left|\; \dfrac{\overset{1}{\cancel{500}} \;\cancel{mL}}{\underset{50}{\cancel{25000}} \;\cancel{units}} \;\right| \dfrac{270}{50} = 5.4 \text{ mL}$$

New infusion rate: 32 + 5.4 = 37.4 or 37 mL/hr

18. a. No. Bolus.

   b. Yes. Decrease by 1 unit/kg/hr

   1 unit × 90 kg = 90 units

Formula Method	Proportion Expressed as Two Ratios	Proportion Expressed as Two Fractions
$\dfrac{\overset{}{90 \text{ units}}}{\underset{50}{25000 \text{ units}}} \times \overset{1}{500} \text{ mL} = x$ $1.8 \text{ mL} = x$	500 mL : 25000 units : : x : 90 units	$\dfrac{500 \text{ mL}}{25000 \text{ units}} \times \dfrac{x}{90 \text{ units}}$ $500 \times 90 = 25000x$ $1.8 \text{ mL} = x$

Dimensional Analysis Method

$$\frac{90 \text{ units}}{\text{hr}} \left| \frac{\overset{1}{500} \text{ mL}}{\underset{50}{25000} \text{ units}} \right| \frac{90}{50} = 1.8 \text{ mL}$$

New infusion rate: 32 − 1.8 = 30.2 or 30 mL/hr

19. a. Infusion rate is increased by 1 unit/hr

   3 units/h + 1 unit/h = 4 units/hr

Formula Method	Proportion Expressed as Two Ratios	Proportion Expressed as Two Fractions
$\dfrac{4 \text{ units/hr}}{0.5 \text{ units}} \times 1 \text{ mL} = 8 \text{ mL/hr}$	1 mL : 0.5 units :: x : 4 units/hr	$\dfrac{1 \text{ mL}}{0.5 \text{ units}} \times \dfrac{x}{4 \text{ units/hr}}$ $1 \times 4 = 0.5x$ $4/0.5 = x$ $8 \text{ mL/hr} = x$

Dimensional Analysis Method

$$\frac{4 \text{ units/hr}}{} \left| \frac{1 \text{ mL}}{0.5 \text{ units}} \right| \frac{4}{0.5} \left| 8 \text{ mL/hr} \right.$$

Set IV pump at 8 mL/hr.

   b. Infusion rate is increased by 1 unit/hr

   4 units/hr + 1 unit/hr = 5 units/hr

Formula Method	Proportion Expressed as Two Ratios	Proportion Expressed as Two Fractions
$\dfrac{5 \text{ units/hr}}{0.5 \text{ units}} \times 1 \text{ mL} = 10 \text{ mL/hr}$	1 mL: 0.5 units :: x: 5 units/hr	$\dfrac{1 \text{ mL}}{0.5 \text{ units}} \times \dfrac{x}{5 \text{ units/hr}}$ $1 \times 5 = 0.5x$ $5/0.5 = x$ $10 \text{ mL/hr} = x$

Dimensional Analysis Method

$$\frac{5 \text{ units/hr}}{} \left| \frac{1 \text{ mL}}{0.5 \text{ units}} \right| \frac{5}{0.5} = 10 \text{ mL/hr}$$

Set IV pump at 10 mL/hr.

Chapter 10

Test 1: Infants and Children Dosage Problems

1. Safe dose 0.5 mg to 1 mg/dose IM. The order is safe.

Formula Method	**Proportion Expressed as Two Ratios**	**Proportion Expressed as Two Fractions**
$\frac{1 \text{ mg}}{10 \text{ mg}} \times 1 \text{ mL}$ $= 0.1 \text{ mL IM}$	$1 \text{ mL} : 10 \text{ mg} :: x : 1 \text{ mg}$	$\frac{1 \text{ mL}}{10 \text{ mg}} \times \frac{x}{1 \text{ mg}}$

$$\frac{1}{10} = x$$
$$0.1 \text{ mL} = x$$

Dimensional Analysis Method

$$\frac{1 \text{ mg}}{} \left| \frac{1 \text{ mL}}{10 \text{ mg}} \right| \frac{1}{10} = 0.1 \text{ mL}$$

Use a precision syringe.

2. Safe dose: 20 to 40 mg/kg/24 hr given q8h.

Low Dose	*High Dose*
20 mg	40 mg
× 10 kg	× 10 kg
200 mg/24 hr	400 mg/24 hr

Order is 125 mg q8h (3 doses).

125 mg × 3 doses = 375. Dose is safe.

No math necessary. Supply is 125 mg/5 mL.

Give 5 mL.

3. Safe dose: 50,000 units/kg × 1 dose

50,000 units
× 10 kg
500,000 units

The order is safe.

Formula Method	Proportion Expressed as Two Ratios	Proportion Expressed as Two Fractions
$\dfrac{500,000 \text{ units}}{600,000 \text{ units}} \times 1 \text{ mL} = \dfrac{5}{6} = 0.83 \text{ mL}$	$1 \text{ mL} : 600,000 \text{ units} :: x : 500,000 \text{ units}$	$\dfrac{1 \text{ mL}}{600,000 \text{ units}} \times \dfrac{x}{500,000 \text{ units}}$

$$\frac{500,000}{600,000} = x$$

$$0.83 \text{ mL} = x$$

Dimensional Analysis Method

$$\frac{500,000 \text{ units}}{} \left| \frac{1 \text{ mL}}{600,000 \text{ units}} \right| \frac{5}{6} = 0.83 \text{ mL}$$

Use a precision syringe. Give 0.83 mL IM.

4. Step 1. Safe dose: 2.5 mg/kg/dose q8h

$$\begin{array}{r} 2.5 \text{ mg} \\ \times\ 3.6 \text{ kg} \\ \hline 9 \text{ mg} \end{array}$$

Order is safe.

Step 2. Minimum safe dilution: 2 mg/mL

$$2 \text{ mg} \overline{)\ 9 \text{ mg}}^{\ 4.5 \text{ mL}} \text{ is the minimum safe dilution. 10 mL is safe.}$$

Formula Method	Proportion Expressed as Two Ratios	Proportion Expressed as Two Fractions
Step 3. $\dfrac{9 \text{ mg}}{40 \text{ mg}} \times 1 \text{ mL} = \dfrac{9}{40}\overline{)9.000}^{.225}$ $= 0.23 \text{ mL}$	$1 \text{ mL} : 40 \text{ mg} :: x : 9 \text{ mg}$	$\dfrac{1 \text{ mL}}{40 \text{ mg}} \times \dfrac{x}{9 \text{ mg}}$

$$\frac{9}{40} = x$$

$$0.23 \text{ mL} = x$$

Dimensional Analysis Method

$$\frac{9 \text{ mg}}{} \left| \frac{1 \text{ mL}}{40 \text{ mg}} \right| \frac{9}{40} = 0.23 \text{ mL}$$

Use a precision syringe to draw up 0.23 mL.

Step 4. Add about 5 mL D5½NS to the Buretrol. Add the 0.23 mL drug. Add more D5½NS to make 10 mL.

Step 5. Set the pump at 20 because 20 mL in 1 hour will deliver the 10 mL in 30 min.

Step 6. When the IV is completed, add a flush of 20 mL D5½NS to the Buretrol to clear the tubing of medication.

5. Safe dose: infants and children younger than 3 years: 10 to 40 mg. The dose is safe.

Formula Method	Proportion Expressed as Two Ratios	Proportion Expressed as Two Fractions
$\dfrac{10\ \cancel{mg}}{20\ \cancel{mg}} \times 5\ mL = \dfrac{5}{2} = 2.5\ mL\ po$	$5\ mL : 20\ mg :: x : 10\ mg$	$\dfrac{5\ mL}{20\ mg} \times \dfrac{x}{10\ mg}$

$$5 \times 10 = 20x$$
$$50 = 20x$$
$$\frac{50}{20} = x$$
$$\frac{10}{4} = x$$
$$2.5\ mL = x$$

Dimensional Analysis Method

$$\dfrac{1}{\cancel{10}\ \cancel{mg}} \left| \dfrac{5\ \cancel{mL}}{\underset{2}{\cancel{20}\ \cancel{mg}}} \right| \dfrac{5}{2} = 2.5\ mL$$

6. Step 1. Safe dose: 10 mg/kg q8h IV

$$\begin{array}{r} 10\ mg \\ \times\ 5.5\ kg \\ \hline 55\ mg\ q8h \end{array}$$

Dose is safe.

Step 2. Minimum safe dilution: 5 mg/mL; infuse over 1 hour.

$$5\ mg\overline{)\,54\ mg\,}^{\,10.8\ mL} = 11\ mL;\ \text{infuse over 1 hour}$$

Step 3. To the 500-mg powder add 10 mL sterile water for injection to make 50 mg/mL.

Formula Method	Proportion Expressed as Two Ratios	Proportion Expressed as Two Fractions
$\dfrac{54\ \cancel{mg}}{50\ \cancel{mg}} \times 1\ mL = \dfrac{54}{50} = 50\overline{)54.00}^{\,1.08}$ $\underline{4\ 00}$ $= 1.1\ mL$	$1\ mL : 50\ mg :: x : 54\ mg$	$\dfrac{1\ mL}{50\ mg} \times \dfrac{x}{54\ mg}$ $\dfrac{54}{50} = x$

$$1.08\ \text{or}\ 1.1\ mL = x$$

Dimensional Analysis Method

$$\dfrac{54\ \cancel{mg}}{\,}\left| \dfrac{1\ \cancel{mL}}{50\ \cancel{mg}} \right| \dfrac{54}{50} = 1.08\ \text{or}\ 1.1\ mL$$

Withdraw 1.1 mL of the drug, label the vial, refrigerate.

Step 4. Add about 5 mL D5½NS to the Buretrol. Add 1.1 mL drug. Add more D5½NS to make 12 mL.

Step 5. Set the pump for 12 (12 mL over 1 hour).

Step 6. When the IV is completed, add 20 mL D5½NS as a flush to the Buretrol to clear the tubing of medication.

7. Safe dose: 25 to 50 mg/kg/dose

Low Dose	High Dose
25 mg	50 mg
× 6.7 kg	× 6.7 kg
167.5 mg/dose	335 mg/dose

Order of 350 mg is not safe. Consult the physician or healthcare provider.

8. Step 1. BSA is 1.32

Step 2. Safe dose: 7.5 to 30 mg/m^2

Low Dose	High Dose
1.32 BSA	1.32 BSA
× 7.5 mg	× 30 mg
9.9 mg/dose	39.6 mg/dose

Step 3. Order is 10 mg. Dose is safe.

Step 4.

Formula Method	*Proportion Expressed as Two Ratios*	*Proportion Expressed as Two Fractions*
$\dfrac{10\ \text{mg}}{2.5\ \text{mg}} \times 1\ \text{tablet} = 4\ \text{tablets}$	1 tablet : 2.5 mg :: x : 10 mg	$\dfrac{1\ \text{tablet}}{2.5\ \text{mg}} \times \dfrac{x}{10\ \text{mg}}$

$$\frac{10}{2.5} = x$$

$$4\ \text{tablets} = x$$

Dimensional Analysis Method

$$\frac{10\ \text{mg}}{} \left| \frac{1\ \text{tablet}}{2.5\ \text{mg}} \right| \frac{10}{2.5} = 4\ \text{tablets}$$

9. Step 1: Safe dose is 2 to 6 g in a 24-hour period divided into either q8h or q12h.

The order is 2 g q8h (3 doses).

2 g × 3 doses = 6 g. The order is safe.

Step 2. Minimum safe dilution is 50 mg/mL over 15 to 30 min. 2 g = 2000 mg

$$50\ \text{mg}\,)\overline{2000\ \text{mg}}\quad \frac{40\ \text{mL}}{}$$

is the minimum safe dilution: 50 mL is safe.

Step 3. Order is 2 g. Stock is a 2-g powder.

Directions say to dilute initially with 10 mL sterile water for injection. Draw the total amount into a syringe.

Step 4. Add about 20 mL D5⅓NS to the Buretrol. Add the medication from the syringe. Then add more D5½NS to make 50 mL.

Step 5. Set the pump for 100. It will deliver 50 mL in 30 min.

Step 6. When the IV is completed, add 20 mL D5½NS as a flush to the Buretrol to clear the tubing of medication.

10. Usual dose is 1 to 1.5 mg/kg/dose.

Low Dose	*High Dose*
1 mg	1.5 mg
×15.9 kg	×15.9 kg
15.9 mg/dose	23.85 mg/dose

20 mg is a safe dose.

Formula Method

$$\frac{20 \text{ mg}}{50 \text{ mg}} \times 1 \text{ mL} = \frac{2}{5} = 0.4 \text{ mL IV}$$

Proportion Expressed as Two Ratios

$$1 \text{ mL} : 50 \text{ mg} :: x : 20 \text{ mg}$$

Proportion Expressed as Two Fractions

$$\frac{1 \text{ mL}}{50 \text{ mg}} \times \frac{x}{20 \text{ mg}}$$

$$\frac{20}{50} = x$$

$$0.4 \text{ mL} = x$$

Dimensional Analysis Method

$$\frac{20 \text{ mg}}{} \left| \frac{1 \text{ mL}}{50 \text{ mg}} \right| \frac{2}{5} = 0.4 \text{ mL}$$

Use a precision syringe to draw up 0.4 mL. Follow hospital policy to give Demerol IV stat.

Chapter 11

Test 1: Dimensional Analysis

1.
$$\frac{500 \text{ mg}}{} \left| \frac{5 \text{ mL}}{125 \text{ mg}} \right.$$

$$\frac{\overset{4}{500 \text{ mg}}}{} \left| \frac{5 \text{ mL}}{\underset{1}{125 \text{ mg}}} \right| 4 \times 5 = 20 \text{ mL}$$

2.
$$\frac{5000 \text{ units}}{} \left| \frac{1 \text{ mL}}{10000 \text{ units}} \right.$$

$$\frac{\overset{1}{5000 \text{ units}}}{} \left| \frac{1 \text{ mL}}{\underset{2}{10000 \text{ units}}} \right| \frac{1}{2} = \frac{1}{2} \text{ or } 0.5 \text{ mL}$$

3. $\dfrac{20 \text{ mg}}{} \bigg| \dfrac{4 \text{ mL}}{40 \text{ mg}}$

$$\dfrac{\overset{1}{\cancel{20} \text{ mg}}}{} \bigg| \dfrac{4 \,\cancel{(\text{mL})}}{\underset{2}{\cancel{40} \text{ mg}}} \bigg| \dfrac{4}{2} = 2 \text{ mL}$$

4. $\dfrac{0.25 \text{ mg}}{} \bigg| \dfrac{1 \text{ tablet}}{0.125 \text{ mg}}$

$$\dfrac{\overset{2}{\cancel{0.25} \text{ mg}}}{} \bigg| \dfrac{1 \,\cancel{(\text{tablet})}}{\underset{1}{\cancel{0.125} \text{ mg}}} \bigg| \dfrac{2 \times 1}{} = 2 \text{ tablets}$$

5. $\dfrac{650 \text{ mg}}{} \bigg| \dfrac{5 \text{ mL}}{325 \text{ mg}}$

$$\dfrac{\overset{2}{\cancel{650} \text{ mg}}}{} \bigg| \dfrac{5 \,\cancel{(\text{mL})}}{\underset{1}{\cancel{325} \text{ mg}}} \bigg| \dfrac{2 \times 5}{} = 10 \text{ mL}$$

6. 10% = 10 g in 100 mL

$\dfrac{0.5 \text{ g}}{} \bigg| \dfrac{100 \text{ mL}}{10 \text{ g}}$

$$\dfrac{\overset{1}{\cancel{0.5} \text{ g}}}{} \bigg| \dfrac{100 \,\cancel{(\text{mL})}}{\underset{20}{\cancel{10} \text{ g}}} \bigg| \dfrac{100}{20} = 5 \text{ mL}$$

7. $\dfrac{125 \text{ mcg}}{} \bigg| \dfrac{1 \text{ mL}}{0.25 \text{ mg}} \bigg| \dfrac{1 \text{ mg}}{1000 \text{ mcg}}$

$$\dfrac{\overset{1}{\cancel{125} \text{ mcg}}}{} \bigg| \dfrac{1 \,\cancel{(\text{mL})}}{0.25 \text{ mg}} \bigg| \dfrac{1 \,\cancel{\text{mg}}}{\underset{8}{\cancel{1000} \,\cancel{\text{mcg}}}} \bigg| \dfrac{1 \times 1 \times 1}{0.25 \times 8} = \dfrac{1}{2} \text{ or } 0.5 \text{ mL}$$

8. $\dfrac{\overset{3}{\cancel{375} \text{ mg}}}{} \bigg| \dfrac{5 \text{ mL}}{\underset{1}{\cancel{125} \text{ mg}}} \bigg| \dfrac{3 \times 5}{1} = 15 \text{ mL}$

$$\dfrac{\overset{15}{\cancel{375} \text{ mg}}}{} \bigg| \dfrac{5 \,\cancel{\text{mL}}}{\underset{5}{\cancel{125} \text{ mg}}} \bigg| \dfrac{1 \,\cancel{(\text{tsp})}}{5 \,\cancel{\text{mL}}} \bigg| \dfrac{15 \times 5 \times 1}{5 \times 5} = \dfrac{75}{25}$$

9. $\dfrac{40 \text{ mg}}{\text{m}^2} \left| \begin{array}{c} 0.44 \text{ m}^2 \\ \\ \end{array} \right.$

$\dfrac{40 \text{ mg}}{\cancel{\text{m}^2}} \left| \dfrac{0.44 \ \cancel{\text{m}^2}}{} \right| \dfrac{40 \times 0.44}{} = 17.6 \text{ mg}$

10. $\dfrac{0.1 \text{ mg}}{\text{kg}} \left| \dfrac{1 \text{ mL}}{10 \text{ mg}} \right| \dfrac{15 \text{ kg}}{}$ $\dfrac{0.2 \text{ mg}}{\text{kg}} \left| \dfrac{1 \text{ mL}}{10 \text{ mL}} \right| \dfrac{15 \text{ kg}}{}$

$\dfrac{0.1 \ \cancel{\text{mg}}}{\cancel{\text{kg}}} \left| \dfrac{1 \text{ mL}}{10 \ \cancel{\text{mg}}} \right| \dfrac{15 \ \cancel{\text{kg}}}{}$ $\dfrac{0.2 \ \cancel{\text{mg}}}{\cancel{\text{kg}}} \left| \dfrac{1 \text{ mL}}{10 \ \cancel{\text{mg}}} \right| \dfrac{15 \ \cancel{\text{kg}}}{}$

$\dfrac{0.1 \times 1 \times 15}{10} = \dfrac{1.5}{10} = 0.15 \text{ mL}$ $\dfrac{0.2 \times 1 \times 15}{10} = \dfrac{3}{10} = 0.3 \text{ mL}$

11. $\dfrac{0.44 \text{ g}}{} \left| \dfrac{1 \text{ mL}}{330 \text{ mg}} \right| \dfrac{1000 \text{ mg}}{1 \text{ g}}$

$\dfrac{0.44 \ \cancel{\text{g}}}{} \left| \dfrac{1 \ \cancel{\text{mL}}}{330 \ \cancel{\text{mg}}} \right| \dfrac{1000 \ \cancel{\text{mg}}}{1 \ \cancel{\text{g}}} \left| \dfrac{0.44 \times 100}{33} \right. = \dfrac{44}{33} = 1.33 \text{ or } 1.3 \text{ mL}$

12. $\dfrac{1{,}000{,}000 \text{ units}}{} \left| \dfrac{1 \text{ mL}}{500{,}000 \text{ units}} \right.$

$\dfrac{\overset{2}{\cancel{1{,}000{,}000 \text{ units}}}}{} \left| \dfrac{1 \ \cancel{\text{mL}}}{\underset{1}{\cancel{500{,}000 \text{ units}}}} \right| \dfrac{2 \times 1}{1} = 2 \text{ mL}$

13. $\dfrac{500 \text{ mL}}{6 \text{ hr}}$

$\dfrac{500 \ \cancel{\text{mL}}}{6 \ \cancel{\text{hr}}} \left| \dfrac{500}{6} \right. = 83.3 \text{ or } 83 \text{ mL/hr}$

14. $\dfrac{1000 \text{ mL}}{16 \text{ hr}}$

$\dfrac{1000 \ \cancel{\text{mL}}}{16 \ \cancel{\text{hr}}} \left| \dfrac{1000}{16} \right. = 62.5 \text{ or } 63 \text{ mL/hr}$

15. $\dfrac{1000 \text{ mL}}{10 \text{ hr}} \left| \dfrac{60 \text{ gtt}}{1 \text{ mL}} \right| \dfrac{1 \text{ hr}}{60 \text{ min}}$

$\dfrac{\overset{100}{\cancel{1000 \ \text{mL}}}}{\underset{}{\cancel{10 \ \text{hr}}}} \left| \dfrac{\overset{1}{\cancel{60 \ \text{gtt}}}}{1 \ \cancel{\text{mL}}} \right| \dfrac{1 \ \cancel{\text{hr}}}{\underset{1}{\cancel{60 \ \text{min}}}} \left| \dfrac{100 \times 1 \times 1}{1 \times 1 \times 1} \right. = 100 \text{ gtt/min}$

16. $\dfrac{250 \text{ mL}}{2 \text{ hr}} \Big| \dfrac{15 \text{ gtt}}{1 \text{ mL}} \Big| \dfrac{1 \text{ hr}}{60 \text{ min}}$

$$\dfrac{250 \text{ mL}}{2 \text{ hr}} \Bigg| \dfrac{15 \overset{1}{\cancel{\text{gtt}}}}{1 \cancel{\text{mL}}} \Bigg| \dfrac{1 \cancel{\text{hr}}}{\underset{4}{60} \cancel{\text{min}}} \Bigg| \dfrac{250 \times 1 \times 1}{2 \times 1 \times 4} = \dfrac{250}{8} = 31.25 \text{ or } 31 \text{ gtt/min}$$

17.

$$\dfrac{5 \cancel{\text{units}}}{\cancel{\text{hr}}} \Bigg| \dfrac{\overset{1}{125} \cancel{\text{mL}}}{\underset{1}{125} \cancel{\text{units}}} \Bigg| \dfrac{5}{} = 5 \text{ mL/hr}$$

18. $\dfrac{1500 \text{ units}}{\text{hr}} \Big| \dfrac{500 \text{ mL}}{25,000 \text{ units}}$

$$\dfrac{1500 \cancel{\text{units}}}{\cancel{\text{hr}}} \Bigg| \dfrac{\overset{1}{500} \cancel{\text{mL}}}{\underset{50}{25,000} \cancel{\text{units}}} \Bigg| \dfrac{1500}{50} = 30 \text{ mL/hr}$$

19. $\dfrac{30 \text{ mL}}{\text{hr}} \Big| \dfrac{25,000 \text{ units}}{250 \text{ mL}}$

$$\dfrac{30 \cancel{\text{mL}}}{\cancel{\text{hr}}} \Bigg| \dfrac{\overset{100}{25,000} \cancel{\text{units}}}{\underset{1}{250} \cancel{\text{mL}}} \Bigg| \dfrac{30 \times 100}{} = 3000 \text{ units/hr}$$

20. $\dfrac{15 \text{ mcg}}{\text{min}} \Big| \dfrac{250 \text{ mL}}{50 \text{ mg}} \Big| \dfrac{1 \text{ mg}}{1000 \text{ mcg}} \Big| \dfrac{60 \text{ min}}{1 \text{ hr}}$

$$\dfrac{15 \cancel{\text{mcg}}}{\cancel{\text{min}}} \Bigg| \dfrac{\overset{5}{250} \cancel{\text{mL}}}{\underset{1}{50} \cancel{\text{mg}}} \Bigg| \dfrac{1 \cancel{\text{mg}}}{1000 \cancel{\text{mcg}}} \Bigg| \dfrac{60 \cancel{\text{min}}}{1 \cancel{\text{hr}}} \Bigg| \dfrac{15 \times 5 \times 60}{1000} = \dfrac{4500}{1000} = 4.5 \text{ or } 5 \text{ mL}$$

21. $\dfrac{2 \text{ mg}}{\text{min}} \Big| \dfrac{500 \text{ mL}}{2 \text{ g}} \Big| \dfrac{1 \text{ g}}{1000 \text{ mg}} \Big| \dfrac{60 \text{ min}}{1 \text{ hr}}$

$$\dfrac{\overset{1}{\cancel{2}} \text{ mg}}{\cancel{\text{min}}} \Bigg| \dfrac{\overset{1}{500} \cancel{\text{mL}}}{\underset{1}{\cancel{2}} \cancel{\text{g}}} \Bigg| \dfrac{1 \cancel{\text{g}}}{\underset{2}{1000} \cancel{\text{mg}}} \Bigg| \dfrac{60 \cancel{\text{min}}}{1 \cancel{\text{hr}}} \Bigg| \dfrac{60}{2} = 30 \text{ mL/hr}$$

22.

$$\frac{10 \text{ mcg}}{\text{kg/min}} \left| \frac{500 \text{ mL}}{500 \text{ mg}} \right| \frac{1 \text{ mg}}{1000 \text{ mcg}} \left| \frac{100 \text{ kg}}{} \right| \frac{60 \text{ min}}{1 \text{ hr}}$$

$$\frac{10 \text{ mcg}}{\text{kg / min}} \left| \frac{\overset{1}{\cancel{500}} \cancel{\text{mL}}}{\underset{1}{\cancel{500}} \cancel{\text{mg}}} \right| \frac{1 \text{ mg}}{\underset{10}{\cancel{1000}} \cancel{\text{mcg}}} \left| \frac{\overset{1}{\cancel{100}} \cancel{\text{kg}}}{} \right| \frac{60 \cancel{\text{min}}}{1 \cancel{\text{hr}}} \left| \frac{10 \times 1 \times 1 \times 1 \times 60}{1 \times 10 \times 1} \right. = \frac{600}{10} = 60 \text{ mL/hr}$$

23.

$$\frac{5 \text{ mcg}}{\text{kg/min}} \left| \frac{250 \text{ mL}}{50 \text{ mg}} \right| \frac{1 \text{ mg}}{1000 \text{ mcg}} \left| \frac{60 \text{ min}}{1 \text{ hr}} \right| \frac{100 \text{ kg}}{}$$

$$\frac{\cancel{5} \text{ mcg}}{\text{kg / min}} \left| \frac{\overset{1}{\cancel{250}} \cancel{\text{mL}}}{\cancel{50} \cancel{\text{mg}}} \right| \frac{1 \text{ mg}}{\underset{-4 \quad 1}{\cancel{1000}} \cancel{\text{mcg}}} \left| \frac{\overset{15}{\cancel{60}} \cancel{\text{min}}}{1 \cancel{\text{hr}}} \right| \overset{2}{\cancel{100}} \cancel{\text{kg}}$$

24.

$$\frac{4.8 \cancel{\text{units}}}{\cancel{\text{hr}}} \left| \frac{\overset{1}{\cancel{100}} \cancel{\text{mL}}}{\underset{1}{\cancel{100}} \cancel{\text{units}}} \right. = 4.8 \text{ mL/hr}$$

25.

$$\frac{6.8 \cancel{\text{units}}}{\cancel{\text{hr}}} \left| \frac{\overset{1}{\cancel{100}} \cancel{\text{mL}}}{\underset{1}{\cancel{100}} \cancel{\text{units}}} \right. = 6.8 \text{ mL/hr}$$

26.

$$\frac{16 \cancel{\text{units}}}{\cancel{\text{kg}} / \cancel{\text{hr}}} \left| \frac{50 \cancel{\text{kg}}}{} \right| \frac{\overset{1}{\cancel{500}} \cancel{\text{mL}}}{\underset{50}{\cancel{25000}} \cancel{\text{units}}} \left| \frac{16 \times 50}{50} \right. = 16 \text{ mL/hr}$$

27.

$$\frac{60 \cancel{\text{units}}}{\cancel{\text{kg}}} \left| \frac{50 \cancel{\text{kg}}}{} \right| \frac{60 \times 50}{} = 3000 \text{ units}$$

28.

$$\frac{2 \cancel{\text{units}}}{\cancel{\text{kg}} / \cancel{\text{hr}}} \left| \frac{55 \cancel{\text{kg}}}{} \right| \frac{\overset{1}{\cancel{500}} \cancel{\text{mL}}}{\underset{50}{\cancel{2500}} \cancel{\text{units}}} \left| \frac{2 \times 55}{50} \right. = 2.2 \text{ mL/hr}$$

21.5 mL/hr + 2.2 mL/hr = 23.7 mL

Chapter 12

Test 1: Basic Drug Information

1. a	**5.** b	**9.** a	**13.** a	**17.** d
2. c	**6.** a	**10.** b	**14.** a	**18.** d
3. d	**7.** a	**11.** d	**15.** a	**19.** a
4. b	**8.** d	**12.** c	**16.** b	

Chapter 13

Test 1: Administration Procedures

Part A

1. c	**5.** c	**9.** d	**13.** b	**17.** d
2. d	**6.** b	**10.** a	**14.** a	**18.** c
3. b	**7.** a	**11.** c	**15.** d	**19.** c
4. d	**8.** d	**12.** a	**16.** b	

Part B

1. Correct. As the needle or catheter is removed, there is a possibility of bleeding at the site.
2. Incorrect. The nurse must wash his or her hands before leaving the room.
3. Incorrect. It is not necessary to wear gloves to prepare an IV because there is no contact at this time with the patient's blood or body fluids.
4. Correct. Standard precautions state that a mask must be worn when the patient is on strict or respiratory isolation precautions.
5. Correct. There is a potential risk of exposure to hepatitis B virus and HIV. Laboratory testing may not show the presence of the virus or antibodies to the virus.
6. Correct. Although transdermal pads are applied to intact skin, standard precautions require gloves.
7. Correct. In carrying out the vaginal douche, there is a possibility of exposure to vaginal secretions.

8. Incorrect. All needle-stick injuries should be reported to the proper authority and the protocol for exposure to blood, including postexposure prophylaxis, if deemed necessary, should be carried out. Standard precautions apply to all patients regardless of the diagnosis.
9. Incorrect. There is always a possibility or risk when doing an invasive procedure such as an injection.
10. Incorrect. Because the patient is alert and can take the medicine cup from the nurse, hand washing is adequate.
11. Incorrect. The CDC guidelines advise the nurse not to recap a needle, but to place it immediately in a puncture-proof container.
12. Incorrect. The nurse's fingers may come in contact with mucous membranes in administering eye drops.

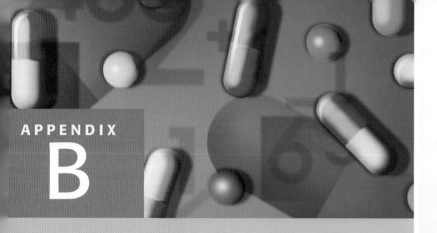

Chapter 6

Calculations

Formula Method	Proportion Expressed as Two Ratios	Proportion Expressed as Two Fractions
1. $\dfrac{7.5 \text{ mg}}{5 \text{ mg}} \times 1 \text{ tab} = x$ $1\frac{1}{2} \text{ tablets} = x$	$1 \text{ tablet} : 5 \text{ mg} :: x : 7.5 \text{ tablets}$	$\dfrac{1 \text{ tablet}}{5 \text{ mg}} \times \dfrac{x}{7.5 \text{ tablets}}$

$$\frac{7.5}{5} = x \qquad 7.5 = 5x$$

$$1\frac{1}{2} \text{ tablets} = x$$

Dimensional Analysis Method

$$\frac{7.5 \text{ mg}}{} \bigg| \frac{1 \text{ tablet}}{5 \text{ mg}} \bigg| \frac{7.5}{5} = 1.5 \text{ or } 1\frac{1}{2} \text{ tablets}$$

Formula Method	Proportion Expressed as Two Ratios	Proportion Expressed as Two Fractions
2. $\dfrac{20 \text{ mg}}{10 \text{ mg}} \times 1 \text{ tablet} = x$ $2 \text{ tablets} = x$	$1 \text{ tablet} : 10 \text{ mg} :: x : 20 \text{ mg}$	$\dfrac{1 \text{ tablet}}{10 \text{ mg}} \times \dfrac{x}{20 \text{ mg}}$

$$\frac{20}{10} = x \qquad 20 = 10$$

$$2 \text{ tablets} = x$$

Dimensional Analysis Method

$$\frac{20 \text{ mg}}{} \bigg| \frac{1 \text{ tablet}}{10 \text{ mg}} \bigg| \frac{20}{10} = 2 \text{ tablets}$$

3. 500 mcg = 0.5 mg
250 mcg = 0.25 mg

Formula Method	**Proportion Expressed as Two Ratios**	**Proportion Expressed as Two Fractions**

$\dfrac{0.75 \text{ mg}}{0.5 \text{ mg}} \times 1 \text{ tablet} = x$

1½ tablets

1 tablet : 0.5 mg : : x : 0.75 mg

$\dfrac{1 \text{ tablet}}{0.5 \text{ mg}} \times \dfrac{x}{0.75 \text{ mg}}$

$\dfrac{0.75}{0.5} = x$

1½ tablets = x

0.75 mg = 0.5x

OR

$\dfrac{0.75 \text{ mg}}{0.25 \text{ mg}} \times 1 \text{ tablet} = x$

3 tablets

1 tablet : 1.25 mg : : x : 0.75 mg

$\dfrac{1 \text{ tablet}}{0.25 \text{ mg}} \times \dfrac{x}{0.75 \text{ mg}}$

$\dfrac{0.75}{0.25} = x$

3 tablets = x

0.75 mg = 0.25x

Dimensional Analysis Method

$$\dfrac{0.75 \text{ mg}}{} \left| \dfrac{1 \text{ tablet}}{500 \text{ mcg}} \right| \dfrac{1000 \text{ mcg}}{1 \text{ mg}} \quad \dfrac{0.75 \times 2}{} = 1.5$$

OR

$$\dfrac{0.75 \text{ mg}}{} \left| \dfrac{1 \text{ tablet}}{250 \text{ mcg}} \right| \dfrac{1000 \text{ mcg}}{1 \text{ mg}} \quad \dfrac{0.75 \times 4}{} = 3 \text{ tablets}$$

4. 500 mg = 0.5 mg
250 mcg = 0.25 mg

Formula Method	**Proportion Expressed as Two Ratios**	**Proportion Expressed as Two Fractions**

$\dfrac{0.25 \text{ mg}}{0.5 \text{ mg}} \times 1 \text{ tablet} = x$

½ tablet

1 tablet : 0.5 mg : : x : 0.25 mg

$\dfrac{1 \text{ tablet}}{0.5 \text{ mg}} \times \dfrac{x}{0.25 \text{ mg}}$

$\dfrac{0.5}{0.25} = x$

½ tablet = x

0.25 mg = 0.5x

OR

$\dfrac{0.25 \text{ mg}}{0.25 \text{ mg}} \times 1 \text{ tablet} = x$

1 tablet

OR

1 tablet : 0.25 mg : : x : 0.25 mg

$\dfrac{1 \text{ tablet}}{0.25 \text{ mg}} \times \dfrac{x}{0.25 \text{ mg}}$

$\dfrac{0.25}{0.25} = 1 \text{ tablet} = x$

Dimensional Analysis Method

$$\frac{0.25 \text{ mg}}{} \left| \frac{1 \text{ tablet}}{500 \text{ mg}} \right| \frac{1000 \text{ mcg}}{1 \text{ mg}} \right| \frac{0\ 25 \times 2}{} = 0.5 \text{ or } \frac{1}{2} \text{ tablet}$$

OR

$$\frac{0.25 \text{ mg}}{} \left| \frac{1 \text{ tablet}}{250 \text{ mcg}} \right| \frac{1000 \text{ mcg}}{1 \text{ mg}} \right| \frac{0.25 \times 4}{} = 1 \text{ tablet}$$

5. 500 mcg = 0.5 mg
250 mcg = 0.25 mg

Formula Method	Proportion Expressed as Two Ratios	Proportion Expressed as Two Fractions

$$\frac{0.125 \text{ mg}}{0.5 \text{ mg}} \times 1 \text{ tablet} = x$$

0.25 or ¼ tablet = x

(may be unable to quarter the tablet)

1 tablet : 0.5 mg : : x : 0.125 mg

$$\frac{1 \text{ tablet}}{0.5 \text{ mg}} \times \frac{x}{0.125 \text{ mg}}$$

$$\frac{0.125 \text{ mg}}{0.5 \text{ mg}} = x \qquad 0.125 \text{ mg} = 0.5x$$

0.25 or ¼ tablet = x

OR   OR

$$\frac{0.125 \text{ mg}}{0.25 \text{ mg}} \times 1 \text{ tablet} = x$$

½ tablet

1 tablet : 0.25 mg : : x : 0.125 mg

$$\frac{1 \text{ tablet}}{0.25 \text{ mg}} \times \frac{x}{0.125 \text{ mg}}$$

$$\frac{0.125}{0.25} = x \qquad 0.125 = 0.25x$$

½ tablet = x

Dimensional Analysis Method

$$\frac{0.125 \text{ mg}}{} \left| \frac{1 \text{ tablet}}{500 \text{ mg}} \right| \frac{1000 \text{ mg}}{1 \text{ mg}} \right| \frac{0\ 125 \times 2}{} = 0.25 \text{ or } \frac{1}{4} \text{ tablet}$$

OR

$$\frac{0.125 \text{ mg}}{} \left| \frac{1 \text{ tablet}}{250 \text{ mg}} \right| \frac{1000 \text{ mg}}{1 \text{ mg}} \right| \frac{0\ 125 \times 4}{} = \frac{1}{2} \text{ tablet}$$

Formula Method	Proportion Expressed as Two Ratios	Proportion Expressed as Two Fractions
6. $\dfrac{15 \text{ mEq}}{10 \text{ mEq}} \times 750 \text{ mg} = x$	$750 \text{ mg} : 10 \text{ mEq} :: x : 15 \text{ mEq}$	$\dfrac{750 \text{ mg}}{10 \text{ mEq}} \times \dfrac{x}{15 \text{ mEq}}$
$1{,}125 \text{ mg}$		

$$750 \times 15 = 10x$$

$$\frac{11{,}250}{10} = x$$

$$1{,}125 \text{ mg} = x$$

Dimensional Analysis Method

$$\frac{\cancel{15}^{3} \text{ mEq}}{} \left| \frac{750 \text{ mg}}{\cancel{10}_{2} \text{ mEq}} \right| \frac{750 \times 3}{2} = 1{,}125 \text{ mg}$$

Formula Method	Proportion Expressed as Two Ratios	Proportion Expressed as Two Fractions
7. $0.25 \text{ mg} = 250 \text{ mcg}$ $0.5 \text{ mg} = 500 \text{ mcg}$ $\dfrac{250 \text{ mcg}}{125 \text{ mcg}} \times 1 \text{ tablet} = x$ 2 tablets $\dfrac{500 \text{ mcg}}{125 \text{ mcg}} \times 1 \text{ tablet} = x$ 4 tablets	$1 \text{ tablet} : 125 \text{ mg} :: x : 250 \text{ mcg}$	$\dfrac{1 \text{ tablet}}{125 \text{ mcg}} \times \dfrac{x}{250 \text{ mg}}$

$$250 = 125$$

$$\frac{250}{125} = x$$

$$2 \text{ tablets} = x$$

$$1 \text{ tablet} : 125 \text{ mg} :: x : 500 \text{ mg}$$

$$\frac{1 \text{ tablet}}{125 \text{ mg}} \times \frac{x}{500 \text{ mg}}$$

$$500 = 125x$$

$$\frac{500}{125} = x$$

$$4 \text{ tablets} = x$$

Dimensional Analysis Method

$$\frac{0.25 \text{ mg}}{} \left| \frac{1 \text{ tablet}}{125 \text{ mcg}} \right| \frac{1000 \text{ mcg}}{1 \text{ mg}} \right| 0.25 \times 8 = 2 \text{ tablets}$$

$$\frac{0.5 \text{ mg}}{} \left| \frac{1 \text{ tablet}}{125 \text{ mcg}} \right| \frac{1000 \text{ mcg}}{1 \text{ mg}} \right| 0.5 \times 8 = 4 \text{ tablets}$$

Formula Method

8. $\dfrac{20 \text{ mg}}{40 \text{ mg}} \times 5 \text{ mL} = x$

$2.5 \text{ mL} = \tfrac{1}{2} \text{ tsp} = x$

Proportion Expressed as Two Ratios

$5 \text{ mL} : 40 \text{ mg} :: x : 20 \text{ mg}$

Proportion Expressed as Two Fractions

$\dfrac{5 \text{ mL}}{40 \text{ mg}} \times \dfrac{x}{20 \text{ mg}}$

$5 \times 20 = 40x$

$\dfrac{100}{40} = x$

$2.5 \text{ mL or } \tfrac{1}{2} \text{ tsp} = x$

Dimensional Analysis Method

$\dfrac{\overset{1}{20} \text{ mg}}{\underset{2}{40} \text{ mg}} \left| 5 \text{ (mL)} \right. = 5 \text{ mL} = 2.5 \text{ mL}$

Formula Method

9. $\dfrac{650 \text{ mg}}{325 \text{ mg}} \times 1 \text{ tablet} = x$

2 tablets

Proportion Expressed as Two Ratios

$1 \text{ tablet} : 325 \text{ mg} :: x : 650 \text{ mg}$

Proportion Expressed as Two Fractions

$\dfrac{1 \text{ tablet}}{325 \text{ mg}} \times \dfrac{x}{650 \text{ mg}}$

$\dfrac{650}{325} = x \qquad 650 = 325x$

$2 \text{ tablets} = x$

Dimensional Analysis Method

$\dfrac{1 \text{ (tablet)}}{\underset{1}{325} \text{ mg}} \left| \overset{2}{650} \text{ mg} \right| \dfrac{2}{1} = 2 \text{ tablets}$

Formula Method

10. $1 \text{ g} = 1000 \text{ mg}$

$\dfrac{1000 \text{ mg}}{200 \text{ mg}} \times 1 \text{ tablet} = x$

4 tablets

Proportion Expressed as Two Ratios

$1 \text{ tablet} : 200 \text{ mg} :: x : 1000 \text{ mg}$

Proportion Expressed as Two Fractions

$\dfrac{1 \text{ tablet}}{200 \text{ mg}} \times \dfrac{x}{1000 \text{ mg}}$

$\dfrac{1000}{200} = x \qquad 1000 = 200x$

$4 \text{ tablets} = x$

Dimensional Analysis Method

$1 \text{ g} \left| \dfrac{1 \text{ (tablet)}}{\underset{1}{200} \text{ mg}} \right| \dfrac{\overset{4}{1000} \text{ mg}}{1 \text{ g}} \left| \dfrac{4}{} \right. = 4 \text{ tablets}$

Critical Thinking Questions

The "answers" are suggested and there may be other correct comments, suggestions, and answers.

1. Any of the medications that need conversion to another measurement system increase the potential for error, since it takes knowledge of the correct conversion and calculation of that conversion. Xanax in mcg, K-Dur in mEq, and digoxin in mcg would have a higher potential for error.

2. Digoxin has the parameter: hold if HR < 60. The heart rate in the scenario is above 60 so it is safe to give. Xanax is given for anxiety, and Tylenol for mild pain. There are no contraindications for these medications but you would assess if the patient is having these symptoms. Since Prinivil is an antihypertensive, you would hold the medication if the blood pressure was too low—without a specific parameter, it would be best to check with the healthcare provider how "low" is "too low."

3. Does the medication come in liquid form? If so, use that instead of the tablets. Does the drug come in a tablet with a higher dosage?

4. Xanax does not have a route. Pepcid does not have a schedule. Tylenol does not have a route.

5. Could any of the pills be safely crushed and mixed with a food or drink? Is there a liquid form of the medication available? Is there another route available to administer the medications? (For example, Pepcid also can be given intravenously.)

Chapter 7

Calculations

Formula Method	Proportion Expressed as Two Ratios	Proportion Expressed as Two Fractions
1. $\dfrac{40 \text{ mg}}{10 \text{ mg}} \times 1 \text{ mL} = 4 \text{ mL}$	1 mL : 10 mg : : x : 40 mg	$\dfrac{1 \text{ mL}}{10 \text{ mg}} \diagup\!\!\!\!\diagdown \dfrac{x}{40 \text{ mg}}$

$$40 = 10x$$

$$\frac{40}{10} = x$$

$$4 \text{ mL} = x$$

Dimensional Analysis Method

$$\frac{40 \text{ mg}}{} \bigg| \frac{1 \text{ mL}}{10 \text{ mg}} \bigg| \frac{40}{10} = 4 \text{ mL}$$

Formula Method	Proportion Expressed as Two Ratios	Proportion Expressed as Two Fractions
2. $\dfrac{2500 \text{ units}}{5000 \text{ units}} \times 1 \text{ mL} = x$ 0.5 mL	1 mL : 5000 units : : x : 2500 units	$\dfrac{1 \text{ mL}}{5000 \text{ units}} \diagup\!\!\!\!\diagdown \dfrac{x}{2500 \text{ units}}$

$$2500 = 5000x$$

$$\frac{2500}{5000} = x$$

$$0.5 \text{ mL} = x$$

Dimensional Analysis Method

$$\frac{\overset{0.5}{2500 \text{ units}}}{} \bigg| \frac{1 \text{ mL}}{\underset{2}{50000 \text{ units}}} \bigg| = 0.5 \text{ mL}$$

Formula Method

3. $\dfrac{8000 \text{ units}}{20000 \text{ units}} \times 1 \text{ mL} = x$

$0.4 \text{ mL} = x$

Proportion Expressed as Two Ratios

1 mL : 20000 units :: x : 8000 units

Proportion Expressed as Two Fractions

$\dfrac{1 \text{ mL}}{20000 \text{ units}} \times \dfrac{x}{8000 \text{ units}}$

$8000 = 20000x$

$\dfrac{8000}{20000} = x$

$0.4 \text{ mL} = x$

Dimensional Analysis Method

$\dfrac{8000 \text{ units}}{} \left| \dfrac{1 \text{ mL}}{20000 \text{ units}} \right| \dfrac{8}{20} = 0.4 \text{ mL}$

4. Yes, give insulin if BG = 12.1 mmol/L.
Give 7.5 units Humulin R subcutaneous
No calculation needed.

Formula Method

5. $\dfrac{100 \text{ mg}}{125 \text{ mg}} \times 2 \text{ mL} = x$

$\dfrac{200}{12} = x$

$1.6 = x$

Proportion Expressed as Two Ratios

2 mL : 125 mg :: x : 100 mg

Proportion Expressed as Two Fractions

$\dfrac{2 \text{ mL}}{125 \text{ mg}} \times \dfrac{x \text{ mL}}{100 \text{ mg}}$

$200 = 125x$

$\dfrac{200}{125} = x$

$1.6 = x$

Dimensional Analysis Method

$\dfrac{100 \text{ mg}}{} \left| \dfrac{2 \text{ mL}}{125 \text{ mg}} \right| \dfrac{200}{125} = 1.6 \text{ mL}$

Formula Method

6. $\dfrac{12.5 \text{ mg}}{25 \text{ mg}} \times 1 \text{ mL} = x$

$0.5 \text{ mL} = x$

Proportion Expressed as Two Ratios

1 mL : 25 mg :: x : 12.5 mg

Proportion Expressed as Two Fractions

$\dfrac{1 \text{ mL}}{25 \text{ mg}} \times \dfrac{x \text{ mL}}{12.5 \text{ mg}}$

$12.5 = 25x$

$\dfrac{12.5}{25} = x$

$0.5 \text{ mL} = x$

Dimensional Analysis Method

$\dfrac{12.5 \text{ mg}}{} \left| \dfrac{1 \text{ mL}}{25 \text{ mg}} \right| \dfrac{12.5}{25} = 0.5 \text{ mL}$

7. Vasotec should be administered.

Formula Method	Proportion Expressed as Two Ratios	Proportion Expressed as Two Fractions

$$\frac{0.625 \text{ mg}}{1.25 \text{ mg}} \times 1 \text{ mL} = x$$

$$0.5 \text{ mL}$$

$$1 \text{ mL} : 1.25 \text{ mg} :: x : 0.625 \text{ mg}$$

$$\frac{1 \text{ mL}}{1.25 \text{ mg}} \times \frac{x}{0.625 \text{ mg}}$$

$$0.625 \text{ mg} = 1.25x$$

$$\frac{0.625}{1.25} = x$$

$$0.5 \text{ mL} = x$$

Dimensional Analysis Method

$$\frac{0.625 \text{ mg}}{} \left| \frac{1 \text{ mL}}{1.25 \text{ mg}} \right| \frac{0.625}{1.25} = 0.5 \text{ mL}$$

8. 1 g = 1000 mg

Formula Method	Proportion Expressed as Two Ratios	Proportion Expressed as Two Fractions

$$\frac{\overset{2}{1000} \text{ mg}}{\underset{1}{500} \text{ mg}} \times 1 \text{ mL} = x$$

$$2 \text{ mL}$$

$$1 \text{ mL} : 500 \text{ mg} :: x : 1000 \text{ mg}$$

$$\frac{1 \text{ mL}}{500 \text{ mg}} \times \frac{x}{1000 \text{ mg}}$$

$$1000 = 500x$$

$$\frac{1000}{500} = x$$

$$2 \text{ mL} = x$$

Dimensional Analysis Method

$$\frac{1 \text{ g}}{} \left| \frac{1 \text{ mL}}{500 \text{ mg}} \right| \frac{\overset{2}{1000} \text{ mg}}{\underset{1}{1 \text{ g}}} = 2 \text{ mL}$$

Critical Thinking Questions

The "answers" are suggested and there may be other correct comments, suggestions, and answers.

1. IV push drugs must be reconstituted and/or diluted according to manufacturer directions and institutional guidelines. IV push drugs must be administered over a certain amount of time as specified in manufacturer directions and/or institutional guidelines. IV push drugs are given through a patent and intact IV site. During administration, if the IV site appears infiltrated, the administration is stopped and further assessment completed.

2. Insulin must be checked with another licensed personnel (in most institutions). This is to ensure accuracy in calculation and preparation.

    Administration precautions include making sure the correct route is used (only regular insulin can be given IV) and choosing a site according to insulin administration guidelines. (See Chapter 13 or any nursing pharmacology textbook.)

3. Insulin dosages can be miscalculated as with any drug. "U" must be written as units per ISMP-Canada recommendations "u" can be mistaken for a number.
4. Heparin doses can be miscalculated as with any drug. "U" must be written as units per ISMP-Canada recommendations "u" can be mistaken for a number. Heparin comes in two different strengths, 10,000 units in 1 mL and 1,000 units in 1 mL and these are often mistaken as the vials are very similar. Many institutions require two licensed personnel to double-check the heparin dose.
5. Type 2 diabetics often experience higher glucose levels and more variance of their glucose level in the hospital because it is a more stressful situation physically and emotionally, increasing the glucocorticoids in their body and therefore raising their blood glucose. This patient is also on Solu-Medrol and any exogenous steroid will raise blood glucose.
6. Phenergan should be held as it is listed under the patient's drug allergies. The patient has a history of renal cell carcinoma a nephrectomy—an assessment of renal function needs to be done. Medications that may need to be given in a lower dose would include Lasix and Vancomycin. These two drugs may also need to be given at separate times because of the renal involvement. The aPTT needs to be checked to determine the safe dose of heparin.

Chapter 8

Calculations

1. $$\frac{100 \text{ mL} \times 60 \text{ gtt}}{60 \text{ min}} = 100 \text{ gtt/min}$$

$$\frac{100 \text{ mL} \times \overset{1}{20}}{\underset{3}{60} \text{ min}} = \frac{100}{3} = 33.33 \text{ or } 33 \text{ gtt/min}$$

2. $$\frac{100 \text{ mL} \times \overset{2}{60} \text{ gtt}}{\underset{1}{30} \text{ min}} = 200 \text{ gtt/min}$$

$$\frac{100 \text{ mL} \times 20 \text{ gtt}}{30 \text{ min}} = \frac{200}{3} = 66.66 \text{ or } 67 \text{ gtt/min}$$

3. $$\frac{50 \text{ mL} \times \overset{2}{60} \text{ gtt}}{\underset{1}{30} \text{ minutes}} = 100 \text{ gtt/min}$$

(guidelines: infuse 50 mL over 30 minutes if no direction is given)

$$\frac{50 \text{ mL} \times 15 \text{ gtt}}{\underset{2}{30} \text{ minutes}} = \frac{50}{2} = 25 \text{ gtt/min}$$

4. $$\frac{1000 \text{ mL}}{40 \text{ mL}} = 25 \text{ hours}$$

5. Gentamicin   100 mL (daily)   NS   40 mL/hr × 20.5 hours
  Cubicin   100 mL (daily)   (24 hours − 3.5 hours that
  Tazocin   50 mL   antibiotics are running)

$$\frac{\times\ \ 4\ \ \ }{200\ mL} \text{(6 hours = 4 doses)}$$

$$\frac{40\ mL/hr}{\times\ 20.5\ hr}$$
$$\overline{820\ mL}$$

  Total intake: 1020 mL

Critical Thinking Questions

The "answers" are suggested and there may be other correct comments, suggestions, and answers.

1. The patient complains of nausea and vomiting. The PO medications may be held and/or another route substituted (check with physician or healthcare provider for an order). Prinivil and Procardia should be held because of the low blood pressure and physician or healthcare provider notified.

2. Each antibiotic works against different organisms (note the suffixes in the names -cillin, -mycin, -micin—they are each a different category of antiinfective). The cause of the infection may not be known yet (usually dependent on the results of cultures) and so the three antibiotics together would kill most bacteria. After the cause of the infection is known, then perhaps only one antibiotic would be used.

3. 40 mL × 6 hours = 240 mL. The IV solution may not be infusing at the correct rate due to miscalculation of rate (if using gtt/min) or setting the wrong rate on the infusion pump. If the infusion is running by gravity, then the patient's position can affect the flow rate. If the patient only has one IV infusion site, then the primary fluid (NS) will be stopped when the antibiotics are infusing.

4. Yes, the dose is 20 mg. The order reads "if over 10 mg must be IVPB." Mix in 50 mL and give over 30 minutes. (If direction is not given as to amount and rate, use 50 mL as a minimum amount over 30 minutes.)

Chapter 9

Calculations

1. 30 mg in 500 mL D5W

$$\frac{30\ mg}{500\ mL} = 0.06\ mg/mL$$

$$0.06\ mg \times 1000\ mcg = 60\ mcg/mL$$

2. Dose 100 mcg/min

$$100\ mcg \times 60\ min = 6000\ mcg/hr$$

Formula Method	Proportion Expressed as Two Ratios	Proportion Expressed as Two Fractions
$\dfrac{\overset{100}{\cancel{6000}\ \cancel{mcg}}}{\underset{1}{\cancel{60}\ \cancel{mcg}}} \times 1\ mL = 100\ mL/hr$	1 mL : 60 mcg : : x : 6000 mcg	$\dfrac{1\ mL}{60\ mcg} \times \dfrac{x}{6000\ mcg}$ $6000 = 60x$ $\dfrac{6000}{60} = x$ $100\ mL = x$

Dimensional Analysis Method

(combines # 1 and # 2)

$$\frac{\overset{1}{100\ \cancel{mcg}}}{\cancel{min}} \left| \frac{500\ \cancel{mL}}{\underset{1}{30\ \cancel{mg}}} \right| \frac{1\ \cancel{mg}}{\underset{10}{1000\ \cancel{mcg}}} \left| \frac{\overset{2}{60\ \cancel{min}}}{1\ \cancel{hr}} \right| \frac{500 \times 2}{10} = 100\ \text{mL/hr}$$

3. $\dfrac{4\ \text{mg}}{500\ \text{mL}} = 0.008\ \text{mg/mL}$

$0.008\ \text{mg} \times 1000\ \text{mcg} = 8\ \text{mcg/mL}$

4. Dose: $0.5\ \text{mcg/min}$

$0.5\ \text{mg} \times 60\ \text{min} = 30\ \text{mcg/hr}$

Formula Method	Proportion Expressed as Two Ratios	Proportion Expressed as Two Fractions
$\dfrac{30\ \text{mcg}}{8\ \text{mcg}} \times 1\ \text{mL} = 3.75\ \text{mL}$	$1\ \text{mL} : 8\ \text{mcg} :: x : 30\ \text{mcg}$	$\dfrac{1\ \text{mL}}{8\ \text{mcg}} \times \dfrac{x}{30\ \text{mcg}}$

$$30 = 8x$$
$$\frac{30}{8} = x$$
$$3.75\ \text{mL} = x$$

Dimensional Analysis Method

(combines # 1 and # 2)

$$\frac{0.5\ \cancel{mcg}}{\cancel{min}} \left| \frac{500\ \cancel{mL}}{\underset{1}{4\ \cancel{mg}}} \right| \frac{1\ \cancel{mg}}{\underset{2}{1000\ \cancel{mcg}}} \left| \frac{\overset{15}{60\ \cancel{min}}}{1\ \cancel{hr}} \right| \frac{0.5 \times 15}{2} = 3.75\ \text{mL} \quad \text{Set the pump at 3.8 or 4 mL/hr}$$

5. $12\ \text{units/kg/hr}$

$12\ \text{units} \times 90\ \text{kg} = 1080\ \text{units/hr}$

6.

Formula Method	Proportion Expressed as Two Ratios	Proportion Expressed as Two Fractions

$$\frac{1080\ \cancel{\text{units}}}{\cancel{25000}\ \cancel{\text{units}}_{50}} \times 500\ \text{mL} = 21.6\ \text{mL/hr}$$

or 22 mL/hr

$$500\ \text{mL} : 25000\ \text{units} :: x : 1080\ \text{units}$$

$$\frac{500\ \text{mL}}{25000\ \text{units}} \times \frac{1\ \text{mL}}{1080\ \text{units}}$$

$$500 \times 1080 = 25000x$$

$$21.6\ \text{mL/hr} = x$$

Dimensional Analysis Method

(combines # 5 and # 6)

$$\frac{12\ \cancel{\text{units}}}{\cancel{\text{kg}}\ \cancel{\text{hr}}} \left|\ \frac{\overset{1}{\cancel{500}}\ \cancel{\text{mL}}}{\cancel{25000}\ \cancel{\text{units}}_{50}}\ \right|\ 90\ \cancel{\text{kg}}\ \left|\ \frac{12 \times 90}{50}\right. = 21.6\ \text{mL/hr}$$ Set the pump at 21.6 or 22 mL/hr

next aPTT due in 6 hours

7.

Formula Method	Proportion Expressed as Two Ratios	Proportion Expressed as Two Fractions

$$\frac{x}{100\ \text{mL}} \times 1\ \text{mL} = 10\ \text{mg/mL}$$

$$\frac{x}{\cancel{100}} \times \cancel{100} = 10 \times 100$$

$$x = 1000\ \text{mg}$$

$$x : 100\ \text{mL} :: 10\ \text{mg} : 1\ \text{mL}$$

$$\frac{x\ \text{mg}}{100\ \text{mL}} \times \frac{10\ \text{mg}}{1\ \text{mL}}$$

$$100 \times 10 = x$$

$$1000\ \text{mg} = x$$

Dimensional Analysis Method

$$\frac{10\ \cancel{\text{mg}}}{1\ \cancel{\text{mL}}}\ \left|\ 100\ \cancel{\text{mL}}\ \right|\ \frac{10 \times 100}{1} = 1000\ \text{mg}$$

8a. Order: 5 mcg/kg/min

5 mcg × 90 kg = 450 mcg/min

Step 1: $\dfrac{1000\ \text{mg}}{100\ \text{mL}} = 10$ mg in 1 mL

Step 2: 10 mg × 1000 = 10000 mcg in 1 mL

Step 3: Divide by 60 to get mcg per min

$$\frac{10000}{60} = 166.67\ \text{mcg/min}$$

Step 4: Solve. Round to the nearest whole number.

Formula Method	Proportion Expressed as Two Ratios	Proportion Expressed as Two Fractions
$\dfrac{450 \text{ mcg/min}}{166.67 \text{ mcg/min}} \times 1 \text{ mL} = 2.69$ or 3 mL	1 mL : 166.67 mcg/min : : x : 450 mcg/min	$\dfrac{1 \text{ mL}}{166.67 \text{ mcg/min}} \times \dfrac{x}{450 \text{ mcg/min}}$

$$450 = 166.67x$$

$$\frac{450}{166.67} = x$$

$$2.69 \text{ or } 3 \text{ mL} = x$$

Dimensional Analysis Method

(combines all steps)

$$\frac{1 \,\cancel{mL}}{\cancel{10}_{2}\,\cancel{mg}} \; \bigg| \; \frac{1\,\cancel{mg}}{1000\,\cancel{mcg}} \; \bigg| \; \frac{\cancel{5}^{1}\,\cancel{mcg}}{\cancel{kg}/\cancel{min}} \; \bigg| \; \frac{90\,\cancel{kg}}{} \; \bigg| \; \frac{60\,\cancel{min}}{1\,\cancel{hr}} \; \bigg| \; \frac{90 \times 60}{2 \times 1000} = \frac{5400}{2000} = 2.7 \text{ or } 3 \text{ mL/hr}$$ Set the pump at 2.7 or 3 mL/hr.

8b. Order: 50 mcg/kg/min

50 mcg × 90 kg = 4500 mcg/min

(Steps 1–4 unchanged)

Formula Method	Proportion Expressed as Two Ratios	Proportion Expressed as Two Fractions
$\dfrac{4500 \text{ mcg/min}}{166.67 \text{ mcg/min}} \times 1 \text{ mL} = 26.99$ or 27 mL/hr	1 mL : 166.67 mcg/min : : x : 4500 mcg/min	$\dfrac{1 \text{ mL}}{166.67 \text{ mcg/min}} \times \dfrac{x}{4500 \text{ mcg/min}}$

$$4500 = 166.67x$$

$$\frac{4500}{166.67} = x$$

$$26.99 \text{ or } 27 \text{ mL} = x$$

Dimensional Analysis Method

(combines all steps)

$$\frac{1 \,\cancel{mL}}{\cancel{10}_{1}\,\cancel{mg}} \; \bigg| \; \frac{1\,\cancel{mg}}{1000\,\cancel{mcg}} \; \bigg| \; \frac{\cancel{50}^{5}\,\cancel{mcg}}{\cancel{kg}/\cancel{min}} \; \bigg| \; \frac{90\,\cancel{kg}}{} \; \bigg| \; \frac{60\,\cancel{min}}{1\,\cancel{hr}} \; \bigg| \; \frac{5 \times 90 \times 60}{1000} = \frac{27000}{1000} = 27 \text{ mL/hr}$$

Set the pump at 26.99 or 27 mL/hr.

Critical Thinking Questions

The "answers" are suggested answers and there may be other correct comments, suggestions, and answers.

1. The medication dosages may need to be adjusted based on the patient's renal failure. Also the dosages and/or administration times may be adjusted based on when the patient receives dialysis.

2. The two vasopressors are different medications and have different actions (Neo-Synephrine—alpha adrenergic agonist; Levophed—alpha adrenergic agonist and beta 1 adrenergic agonist), but the end result is to raise the blood pressure. Different doses of different medications may work better, and different patients react differently.

3. The patient is intubated and there are no immediate plans to extubate her, because of her serious medical condition. Diprivan will sedate and allow the patient to rest on the ventilator. The sedation will also help to decrease oxygen demand on the heart, thereby helping the cardiomyopathy and overall improve the medical condition.

4. A calcium channel blocker such as nifedipine may help atrial fibrillation but the patient is allergic to calcium channel blockers.

5. The two vasopressors may be causing the increased heart rate because of their effect on the alpha and beta receptors.

6. IV push drugs are given slowly to infuse the amount of drug concentration given over a longer time. This may be to prevent side effects, in this case, to prevent nausea.

Chapter 10

Calculations

1a. Dose: 20 mg

Formula Method	Proportion Expressed as Two Ratios	Proportion Expressed as Two Fractions
$$\frac{\overset{1}{\cancel{20\ mg}}}{\underset{1}{\cancel{20\ mg}}} \times 1\ mL = x$$ $$1\ mL = x$$	$1\ mL : 20\ mg :: x : 20\ mg$	$$\frac{1\ mL}{20\ mg} \diagup\frac{x}{20\ mg}$$ $$20 = 20x$$ $$1\ mL = x$$

Dimensional Analysis Method
$$\frac{\overset{1}{\cancel{20\ mg}} \quad 1\ \boxed{mL}}{\underset{1}{\cancel{20\ mg}}} = 1\ mL = x$$

1b. Dose: 10 mg

Formula Method	Proportion Expressed as Two Ratios	Proportion Expressed as Two Fractions
$$\frac{\overset{1}{\cancel{10\ mg}}}{\underset{2}{\cancel{20\ mg}}} \times 1\ mL = x$$ $$\tfrac{1}{2} \text{ or } 0.5\ mL$$	$1\ mL : 20\ mg :: x : 10\ mg$	$$\frac{1\ mL}{20\ mg} \diagup\frac{x}{10\ mg}$$ $$10 = 20x$$ $$\frac{10}{20} = x$$ $$\tfrac{1}{2} \text{ or } 0.5\ mL = x$$

Dimensional Analysis Method

$$\frac{\overset{1}{\cancel{10}\ \text{mg}} \quad \Big|\ 1\,\boxed{\text{mL}}\ \Big|\ 1}{\qquad\ \Big|\ \underset{2}{\cancel{20}\ \text{mg}}\ \Big|\ 2} = 0.5\ \text{mL}$$

2. Dose: 400 mg

Formula Method	Proportion Expressed as Two Ratios	Proportion Expressed as Two Fractions
$\dfrac{400\ \text{mg}}{\underset{32}{\cancel{160}\ \text{mg}}} \times \overset{1}{\cancel{5}}\ \text{mL} = \dfrac{400}{32} = 12.5\ \text{mL}$	$5\ \text{mL} : 160\ \text{mg} :: x : 400\ \text{mg}$	$\dfrac{5\ \text{mL}}{160\ \text{mg}} \diagdown\!\!\!\!\diagup \dfrac{x}{400\ \text{mL}}$

$$5 \times 400 = 160x$$

$$\frac{2000}{160} = x$$

$$12.5\ \text{mL} = x$$

Dimensional Analysis Method

$$\frac{400\ \text{mg}\ \Big|\ 5\ \boxed{\text{mL}}\ \Big|\ 400}{\qquad\ \Big|\ \cancel{160}\ \text{mg}\ \Big|\ 32} = 12.5\ \text{mL}$$
$$\qquad\qquad\ \ 32$$

3. 5 mg/kg
$5 \times 30 = 150$ mg

Formula Method	Proportion Expressed as Two Ratios	Proportion Expressed as Two Fractions
$\dfrac{150\ \text{mg}}{\underset{20}{\cancel{100}\ \text{mg}}} \times \overset{1}{\cancel{5}}\ \text{mL} = x$	$5\ \text{mL} : 100\ \text{mg} :: x : 150\ \text{mg}$	$\dfrac{5\ \text{mL}}{100\ \text{mg}} \diagdown\!\!\!\!\diagup \dfrac{x}{150\ \text{mg}}$
$\dfrac{150}{20} = x$		
$7.5\ \text{mL} = x$		

$$5 \times 150 = 100x$$

$$\frac{750}{100} = x$$

$$7.5\ \text{mL} = x$$

Dimensional Analysis Method

(combines all steps)

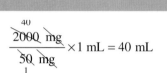

$$\frac{5\ \cancel{mg}}{\cancel{kg}} \left| \frac{30\ \cancel{kg}}{} \right| \frac{\overset{1}{\cancel{5}}\ \cancel{mL}}{\underset{20}{\cancel{100}}\ \cancel{mg}} \left| \frac{5 \times 30}{20} \right. = \frac{150}{20} = 7.5\ \text{mL}$$

4. Dose: 2 g = 2000 mg

Formula Method	Proportion Expressed as Two Ratios	Proportion Expressed as Two Fractions
$\dfrac{\overset{40}{\cancel{2000}}\ \cancel{mg}}{\underset{1}{\cancel{50}}\ \cancel{mg}} \times 1\ \text{mL} = 40\ \text{mL}$	1 mL : 50 mg : : x : 2000 mg	$\dfrac{1\ \text{mL}}{50\ \text{mg}} \times \dfrac{x}{2000\ \text{mg}}$

$$2000 = 50x$$

$$\frac{2000}{50} = x$$

$$40\ \text{mL} = x$$

Dimensional Analysis Method

$$\frac{2\ \text{g}}{} \left| \frac{1\ \cancel{mL}}{\underset{1}{\cancel{50}}\ \cancel{mg}} \right| \frac{\overset{20}{\cancel{1000}}\ \cancel{mg}}{\cancel{1g}} \left| \frac{20 \times 2}{} \right. = 40\ \text{mL}$$

Infuse over 30 min. Set the pump at 80 mL/hr. The pump will deliver 40 mL in 30 minutes. Follow directions to infuse via Buretrol (see Chapter 8).

5. 0.9 BSA

0.72 mg × BSA =

0.72 × 0.9 = 0.648 mg

6. Dose = 150 mg

Formula Method	Proportion Expressed as Two Ratios	Proportion Expressed as Two Fractions
$\dfrac{150\ \cancel{mg}}{125\ \cancel{mg}} \times 1\ \text{mL} = \dfrac{150}{125} = 1.2\ \text{mL}$	1 mL : 125 mg : : x : 150 mg	$\dfrac{1\ \text{mL}}{125\ \text{mg}} \times \dfrac{x}{150\ \text{mg}}$

$$150 = 125x$$

$$\frac{150}{125} = x$$

$$1.2\ \text{mL} = x$$

Dimensional Analysis Method

$$\frac{\overset{30}{\cancel{150}} \text{ mg} \mid 1 \text{ mL} \mid 30}{\underset{25}{\cancel{125}} \text{ mg} \mid 25} = 1.2 \text{ mL}$$

7. 1 mg/kg
 $1 \times 30 = 30$ kg.

The dose is higher than the safe dose (10–25 mg). Check with the physician or healthcare provider, although the ordered dose is a correct prescribing dose.

8. 10 mL/kg/hr
 $10 \times 30 = 300$ mL for 1 hour

Critical Thinking Questions

The "answers" are suggested answers and there may be other correct comments, suggestions, and answers.

1. Hold (and discontinue) the Augmentin—it contains amoxicillin and the patient is allergic to penicillin. Check with the physician or healthcare provider about giving cefazolin—sometimes the patient will have a cross-sensitivity to other antibiotics if allergic to penicillin, especially cephalosporins, which cefazolin is classified as.
2. Digoxin is ordered and there does not seem to be a medical condition that warrants the order. There may be a medical history of a cardiac condition that the nurse is unaware of. Check with the physician or healthcare provider.
3. The PO route may be difficult given the history of "flu-like" symptoms and no food and minimal drink for 28 hours. Check if any of the medications can be given via another route (need to have the physician or healthcare provider order a different route). If the patient has decreased nausea, check to see if the medications can be given in a liquid form.
4. The amount to be infused is 300 mL for 1 hour. Although this is a large dose of fluid for a child, the child's condition (no food and minimal drink for 48 hours) may warrant the fluid in order to prevent further dehydration. 100 mL/hr is also a higher dose, but again may be needed for the child's condition. Close monitoring of the infusion is needed.

Glossary

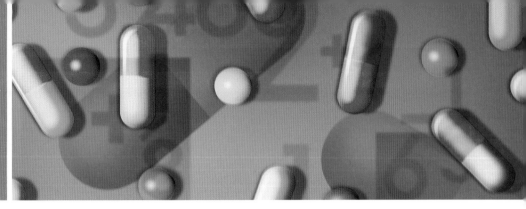

Absorption   the passing of a drug in the body across tissue into the general circulation and becomes active in the body

ac   before meals

ad lib   as desired

Adverse effects   nontherapeutic effects that may be harmful

Aerosol   method of drug administration in which the solid drug is delivered in a liquid spray

Agonist   drug that binds with cell receptors to invoke a cellular response, usually similar to the cell's action

Allergic reaction   reaction to a drug involving the body's antibody response to a perceived antigen (in this case, the medication)

Ampoule   a sealed glass container for powdered or liquid drugs

Amt   amount

Analgesic   drug to relieve or minimize pain

Anaphylactic shock   severe allergic reaction that results in a shock state

Anaphylaxis   severe allergic reaction

Antagonism   the interaction between two drugs in which the combined effect is less than the sum of the effects of the drugs acting separately

Antagonist   drug that binds with cell receptors to block the cellular response

Antibiotic   drug that inhibits or kills bacteria, fungus, or protozoans

Anticoagulant   drug that inhibits formation of blood clots

Antiemetic   drug that prevents vomiting and reduces nausea

Antihypertensive   drug that lowers blood pressure

Antitussive   drug to use to suppress coughing

Anxiolytic   drugs that relieves/anxiety

Apothecary system   a measurement system using grains and minims, considered obselete

ASA   acetylsalicylic acid; medication used in the treatment of mild to moderate pain, inflammation, and fever and in the prevention of heart attacks and strokes

Bactericidal   a drug action that kills an organism

Bacteriostatic   a drug action that inhibits an organism's ability to grow and reproduce

bid   twice a day

Bioavailability   the availability of a drug once it is absorbed and transported in the body to the site of its action

Biotransformation   the conversion of an active drug to an inactive compound

Body surface area (BSA)   calculation of metres squared based on height and weight, as shown in a nomogram

BP   blood pressure

Bronchodilator   drug that dilates the bronchioles of the lungs

Buccal   the route of administration in which a drug is placed in the pouch between the teeth and the cheek

Cap or Capsule   a gelatin container that holds a drug in a solid or liquid form

Cardiac glycoside   a drug that increases cardiac contractility and increases cardiac output. Lanoxin (digoxin) is the most common cardiac glycoside used

CDC   Centers for Disease Control and Prevention

Celsius (C)   a temperature scale (0°C = freezing; 100°C = boiling); human body temperature is approximately 37°C

Centimetre   unit of length in the metric system; equal to 0.01 metre

Chemical name   the drug name derived from its chemical structure

Chemotherapy   drug treatment of cancer

Civil law statutes concerned with the rights and duties of individuals

Combination drugs drugs that contain more than one active medication

Common factor a number that is a factor of two different numbers (that is, 3 is a factor of 6 and 9)

Common fraction a fraction with a whole number in the numerator and denominator (i.e., ⅚)

Compliance taking a medication as prescribed or following label instructions

Concentration the amount of drug in a solution; in fraction, decimal, or percentage form

Contraindication a situation in which a drug should be avoided

Controlled drug a drug controlled by federal law; a drug that may be lead to drug abuse or dependence

Corticosteroid hormones that help the body respond to stress; also used in immune response, anti-inflammatory. In the body, produced by the adrenal cortex

CR controlled release

Cream a semisolid drug preparation applied externally to the skin or mucous membrane

Criminal law statutes that protect the public again actions harmful to society

Cross tolerance becoming tolerant to one drug and then acquiring tolerance to another drug; this could be with a similar drug or a drug from a similar category or a drug with a similar classification

CSF cerebrospinal fluid

Cumulation or Accumulation the inability of the body to metabolize one dose of a drug before another dose is administered; cumulation leads to increased concentration of the drug in the body and possible toxicity

d day

D/C discharge or discontinue; Do not use, write out "discharge" or "discontinue" as appropriate

Denominator the bottom number in a fraction

Dermal route the topical application of a drug to the skin

Diluent a liquid used to dissolve a solid, usually a powder, into a solution

Displacement the increase in the volume of fluid added to a powder when the powder dissolves and goes into solution

Distribution the movement of a drug through body fluids, chiefly blood, to cells

Dividend the number to be divided (e.g., 40 divided by 5, 40 is the dividend)

Divisor the number by which the dividend is divided; in the previous example, 5 is the divisor

Dose the amount of drug to be administered at one time or the total amount to be given

DR delayed release

Drip or Drop factor the number of drops of an IV fluid in 1 mL; listed on the IV tubing set or package

Drip rate the number of drops of an IV solution to be infused per minute

Drop (gtt) an acceptable unit of measurement for medication dispensed by a dropper

Drug a chemical agent used in the treatment, diagnosis, or prevention of disease

Dry powder inhaler (DPI) inhaler that converts a solid drug into a fine powder

Elixir a clear, aromatic, sweetened alcoholic preparation

Emulsion suspension of a fat or oil in water with the aid of an agent to reduce surface tension

Enteral refers to the small intestine

Enteral feedings delivery of liquid feedings through a tube

Enteral route drugs given orally or through nasogastric (N/G) or percutaneous endoscopic gastrostomy (PEG) tubes

Enteric coating a layer placed over a tablet or capsule to prevent dissolution in the stomach; used to protect the drug from gastric acid or to protect the stomach from drug irritation

Epidural route medication is administered into the space around the dura mater of the spinal column

ER extended release

Ethics a system of values and morals

Excretion the physiologic elimination of substances from the body

Expectorant drug to increase bronchial secretions

Expiration date a drug cannot be administered after the last day of the month stamped on the label

Film-coated tablets compressed, powdered drugs that are smooth and easy to swallow because of their outer shell covering

First-pass effect drugs that are administered orally that pass from the intestine to the liver and are partially metabolized before entering the circulation

Flow rate number of millilitres per hour of IV fluid to be infused

Fluid extract or fluidextract potent alcoholic liquid concentration of a drug

Food and Drugs Act the Statute within the Department of Justice Canada that prescribes the standards of composition, strength, potency, purity, quality, or other property of the article of food or drug to which they refer

Formulary reference for pharmacists and other healthcare providers with lists of drugs, drug combinations, etc.

Fraction division of one number by another

G-tube gastrostomy tube; inserted into the stomach. Can be used for drug administration and enteral feedings

Gauge the diameter or width of a needle; the higher the gauge number, the finer the needle

Gel an aqueous suspension of small particles of an insoluble drug in a hydrated form

Generic name the official name of a drug as listed in the United States or other pharmacopoeia

Glucocorticoid hormones that help the body to respond to stress. In the body, manufactured by the adrenal cortex

Gram (g) basic unit of weight in the metric system

gtt drop or drops

h hour

Half-life the time that a drug is metabolized by 50% in the body

Health Canada the federal department responsible for helping Canadians maintain and improve their health, while respecting individual choices and circumstances

Hepatotoxic a drug or side effects of a drug that may affect the liver

Household system a measurement system based on household items of measurement; uses teaspoon, tablespoon, cup; should not be used in medication orders in Canada

I & O intake and output

Idiosyncratic an unexplained or unusual reaction to a drug

Improper fraction a fraction with the numerator larger or equal to the denominator

Incompatibility a mixture of two or more drugs that results in a harmful chemical or physical interaction

Inhalant vapor that is inhaled via the nose, lungs, or trachea

Inhaler a device used to spray liquid or powder in a fine mist into the lungs during inspiration

inj injection

Institute for Safe Medication Practices (ISMP) Canada an independent national non-profit agency committed to the advancement of medication safety in all healthcare settings.

Interaction either desirable or undesirable effects produced by giving two or more drugs together

Intra-articular medication injected into the joints

Intradermal (ID) an injection given into the upper layers of the skin

Intramuscular (IM) an injection given into the muscle

Intrathecal administration into the cerebrospinal fluid via the subarachnoid space

Intravenous (IV) medication given by injection or infusion into a vein

Intravenous piggyback (IVPB) used to administer medication via the IV route using a secondary infusion set attached to the primary IV

Isotonic solutions that have the same osmotic pressure as physiologic body fluids

IU international unit; do not use, write out "international units"

J-tube a tube placed in the jejunum, can be used for drug administration and enteral feedings

Kilogram (kg) basic unit of mass in the metric system; equal to 1000 grams

Litre (L) 1 unit of fluid volume in the metric system; equal to one tenth of a cubic metre

Loading dose higher dose given at the initiation of drug therapy in order to build up the therapeutic effect

Lotion liquid suspension intended for external use

Lowest common denominator the smallest number that is a multiple of the denominators

Lowest terms the smallest numbers possible in the numerator and denominator of a fraction; reducing a fraction to lowest terms means the numerator and denominator cannot be reduced further

Lozenge a flat, round, or rectangular preparation held in the mouth until it dissolves

Magma a bulky suspension of an insoluble preparation in water that must be shaken before pouring

MAO inhibitor monoamine oxidase (MAO) inhibitor; a type of medication used in the treatment of depression and Parkinson's disease

MDI metered-dose inhaler; an aerosol device that consists of two parts: a canister under pressure and a mouthpiece; finger pressure on the mouthpiece opens a valve that discharges one dose

Medication another word for drug. Sometimes used to refer a drug that has been administered

Medication Administration Record (MAR) documentation of drugs received by the patient or schedule of drugs to be received

Medication error a preventable error in medication administration, usually related to one of the six rights

Meniscus the curved surface of a liquid in a container

Metabolism the chemical biotransformation of a drug to a form that can be excreted

Metre (m) unit of length in the metric system; equal to 1/1000 of a kilometre

Metric system a measurement system that uses meters, litres, grams; common system used worldwide except in the United States; widely used system in dosages of drugs; based on units of 10

mg milligram

MgSO$_4$ magnesium sulfate; JCAHO states do not use; write out "magnesium sulfate" because this abbreviation can be confused with MSO$_4$

Microgram (mcg) smallest unit of mass in the metric system; equal to 1/1000 of a milligram

Military time time based on a 24-hour clock rather than the traditional 12-hour clock

Milliequivalent (mEq) the number of grams of solute in a 1-mL solution; used to measure electrolytes and some medications

Milligram (mg) unit of mass in the metric system; equal to 1/1000 of a gram

Millilitre (mL) unit of volume in the metric system; equal to 1/1000 of a litre

Millimetre (mm) unit of length in the metric system; equal to 1/1000 of a metre

min minute

Mixed number a whole number and a fraction (e.g., 1 $^{11}/_{42}$)

Multidose large stock containers of medication

Narcotic natural or synthetic drug related to morphine; a large classification of drugs that include hallucinogens, CNS stimulants, and illegal drugs

Nebulizer device to convert liquid drugs into a fine mist to use as an inhaled route

Nephrotoxic a drug or side effects of a drug that may affect the renal system

N/G tube nasogastric tube inserted through the nasal opening into the stomach. Can be used for drug administration and enteral feedings.

Nomogram a tabular illustration of body surface area based on height and weight

Nonmaleficence ethical principle to not harm the patient. "Do no harm"

Nonparenteral drugs drugs administered by topical, rectal, or oral route

Nonprescription drug a drug obtained without a prescription; also called over the counter or OTC

NPO nothing by mouth

NSAIDs nonsteroidal anti-inflammatory drugs; used in the treatment of mild to moderate pain and inflammation

Numerator the top number in a fraction

O/G tube orogastric tube inserted through the oral cavity into the stomach. Can be used for drug administration and enteral feedings

Ointment a semisolid preparation in a petroleum or lanolin base for external use

Ophthalmic pertaining to the eye

Oral route abbreviated po; drugs given through the mouth

OTC over the counter

Otic pertaining to the ear

Ototoxic a drug or side effects of the drug that may affect the ear

Parenteral a general term that means administration by injection (IV, IM, or subcutaneous)

Paste a thick ointment used to protect the skin

Pastille a disklike solid that slowly dissolves in the mouth

Patch a small adhesive that releases medication over an extended period of time; applied topically

pc after meals

PEG tube a special type of gastrostomy tube, percutaneous endoscopic gastrotomy. Is designed to be more permanent. Can be used for drug administration and enteral feedings

Percentage parts per hundred, designated by a percent sign (%)

Percentage solution the solid that is dissolved in a liquid represents a percentage of the total weight of the solution; measured in grams per 100 mL solution

Pharmacodynamics the study of the chemical and physical effects of drugs in the body

Pharmacogenetics chemical and physical effects in the body to a drug related to a person's genetics

Pharmacokinetics the science of the factors that determine how much drug reaches the site of action in the body and is excreted

Pharmacology the study of the origin, nature, chemistry effects, and uses of drugs

Pharmacopoeia medical reference containing information about drugs

Pharmacotherapeutics the study of the use of drugs to treat, prevent, and diagnose diseases

Piggyback medication placed in an IV infusion set attached to the mainline IV for delivery to the patient

Placebo an inert substance used in place of a drug to determine its psychological effect and the physiologic changes caused by the psychological response

PO by mouth, oral

Potency strength of a drug at a specific concentration or dose

Powder a finely ground solid drug or mixture of drugs for internal or external use

PR per rectum

Prefilled cartridge a small vial with a needle attached that fits into a metal or plastic holder for injection

Prefilled syringe a liquid, sterile medication that is ready to administer without further preparation

Prescription an order for medication written by an authorized prescriber

Prescription drug a drug that requires a prescription; regulated usually by state laws

Prime number a whole number divisible only by one and itself; a whole number that cannot be reduced any further (i.e., 3, 5, 7)

PRN when required

Protocol a specific set of drug orders referring to certain physical conditions, or lab values that must be met before drug administration. Also used when titrating certain drugs, that is, insulin and heparin

Product the answer in multiplication

Prolonged-release or slow-release tablet a powdered, compressed drug that disintegrates more slowly and has a longer duration of action

Proper fraction a fraction with a numerator smaller than the denominator

Proportion a set of ratios or fractions

pt patient

q each, every

q4h every 4 hours

q6h every 6 hours

q8h every 8 hours

q12h every 12 hours

qid four times a day

Quotient the answer in division

Ratio a way to compare numbers; numbers are separated by a colon, such as 1:5, which reads one is to five

Reconstitution dissolving a powder to a liquid form

Rectal route (PR, per rectum) medication administered through the rectum

Reduce to simplify

Rounding reducing decimal places in a number; a number may be rounded off to the nearest tenth, hundredth, thousandth, etc.; a number may also be reduced to the nearest whole number

Routine order order written for a drug that will be administered on a certain schedule or regular basis

Rx a prescription

Scheduled drug a drug in one of five categories (in the United States) that are based on their potential for misuse, abuse, or addiction

Scored tablet a compressed, powdered drug with a line down the centre so that the tablet can be broken in half

Single order medication that is to be given once

SI units Système International d'Unités; a measurement adapted from the metric system, used in most developed countries to provide a standard language

Solution a clear liquid that contains a drug dissolved in water

Spansule a long-acting capsule that contains drug particles coated to dissolve at different times

Spirits concentrated alcoholic solutions of volatile substances

SR sustained release

Standard precautions procedures to protect against infection that are used when caring for all patients and when handling contaminated equipment

Standing order drug order written to cover certain situations; the drug is administered only when those conditions are met

Stat immediately and once only

Subcutaneous the tissue between the skin and muscle

Subcutaneous (Sub Q/Sub-Q) parenteral route of administration for medications required to be given into subcutaneous tissue

Sublingual tablet a powdered drug that is compressed or molded into a solid shape that dissolves quickly under the tongue

Suppository a mixture of a drug with a firm base molded into a shape to be inserted into a body cavity

Suspension solid particles of a drug dispersed in a liquid that must be shaken to obtain an accurate dose

Syrup a solution of sugar in water to disguise the unpleasant taste of a medication

Tablet or Tab a powdered drug that is compressed or molded into a solid shape; may contain additives that bind the powder or aid in its absorption

Teratogen drug that can cause birth defects

tid three times a day

Timed release small beads of drug in a capsule coated to delay absorption

Tincture alcoholic or hydroalcoholic solution of a drug

Tolerance a decreased responsiveness to a drug after repeated exposure

Topical route of administration in which a drug is applied to the skin or mucous membrane

Toxicity a nontherapeutic effect that may result in damage to tissues or organs

TPN total parenteral nutrition

Trade name a brand or proprietary name identified by the symbol ® that follows the name

Transcribe rewriting; in nursing and hospitals, a drug order is transcribed usually to another form that is used to record and document administration of medications

Transdermal medicated drug molecules contained in a unique polymer patch applied to the skin for slow absorption

Troche a flat, round, or rectangular preparation held in the mouth (or placed in the vagina) until it dissolves

Tube feeding method of providing nutrition for a patient through a feeding tube. Can also refer to the high-calorie, high-protein nutritional solution that is used

Unit dose an individually wrapped and labelled dose of a drug

Unit system a measurement system using units to measure amounts of drugs; drugs that use this system include heparin, penicillin, and insulin

Vaginal route medication inserted or injected into the vagina

Vasopressor drug that constricts blood vessels, thereby raising blood pressure

Vial a glass container with a rubber stopper containing one or more doses of a drug

Young's rule a rule used to calculate drug dosages for children ages 1 to 12 years; based on the age of the child

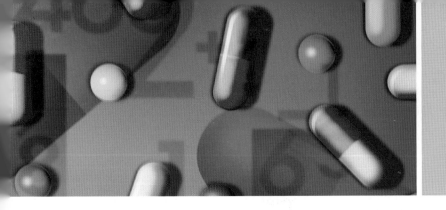

Index

Page numbers followed by *f* indicate figures; those followed by *t* indicate tables.